Thrombolysis and Thrombectomy in Acute Ischemic Stroke

Thrombolysis and Thrombectomy in Acute Ischemic Stroke

Editors

Hyo Suk Nam
Byung Moon Kim

MDPI • Basel • Beijing • Wuhan • Barcelona • Belgrade • Manchester • Tokyo • Cluj • Tianjin

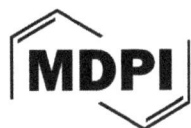

Editors
Hyo Suk Nam
Yonsei University College of
Medicine
Korea

Byung Moon Kim
Yonsei University College of
Medicine
Korea

Editorial Office
MDPI
St. Alban-Anlage 66
4052 Basel, Switzerland

This is a reprint of articles from the Special Issue published online in the open access journal *Journal of Clinical Medicine* (ISSN 2077-0383) (available at: https://www.mdpi.com/journal/jcm/special_issues/acute_stroke).

For citation purposes, cite each article independently as indicated on the article page online and as indicated below:

LastName, A.A.; LastName, B.B.; LastName, C.C. Article Title. *Journal Name* **Year**, *Volume Number*, Page Range.

ISBN 978-3-0365-7598-8 (Hbk)
ISBN 978-3-0365-7599-5 (PDF)

© 2023 by the authors. Articles in this book are Open Access and distributed under the Creative Commons Attribution (CC BY) license, which allows users to download, copy and build upon published articles, as long as the author and publisher are properly credited, which ensures maximum dissemination and a wider impact of our publications.

The book as a whole is distributed by MDPI under the terms and conditions of the Creative Commons license CC BY-NC-ND.

Contents

About the Editors ix

Preface to "Thrombolysis and Thrombectomy in Acute Ischemic Stroke" xi

Hyo Suk Nam and Byung Moon Kim
Advance of Thrombolysis and Thrombectomy in Acute Ischemic Stroke
Reprinted from: *J. Clin. Med.* 2023, 12, 720, doi:10.3390/jcm12020720 1

Hyung Jun Kim, Moo-Seok Park, Joonsang Yoo, Young Dae Kim, Hyungjong Park, Byung Moon Kim, Oh Young Bang, et al.
Association between $CHADS_2$, CHA_2DS_2-VASc, ATRIA, and Essen Stroke Risk Scores and Unsuccessful Recanalization after Endovascular Thrombectomy in Acute Ischemic Stroke Patients
Reprinted from: *J. Clin. Med.* 2022, 11, 274, doi:10.3390/jcm11010274 5

Klearchos Psychogios, Apostolos Safouris, Odysseas Kargiotis, Georgios Magoufis, Athina Andrikopoulou, Ermioni Papageorgiou, Maria Chondrogianni, et al.
Advanced Neuroimaging Preceding Intravenous Thrombolysis in Acute Ischemic Stroke Patients Is Safe and Effective
Reprinted from: *J. Clin. Med.* 2021, 10, 2819, doi:10.3390/jcm10132819 19

Jang-Hyun Baek, Young Dae Kim, Ki Jeong Lee, Jin Kyo Choi, Minyoul Baik, Byung Moon Kim, Dong Joon Kim, Ji Hoe Heo and Hyo Suk Nam
Low Hypoperfusion Intensity Ratio Is Associated with a Favorable Outcome Even in Large Ischemic Core and Delayed Recanalization Time
Reprinted from: *J. Clin. Med.* 2021, 10, 1869, doi:10.3390/jcm10091869 31

Chun-Min Wang, Yu-Ming Chang, Pi-Shan Sung and Chih-Hung Chen
Hypoperfusion Index Ratio as a Surrogate of Collateral Scoring on CT Angiogram in Large Vessel Stroke
Reprinted from: *J. Clin. Med.* 2021, 10, 1296, doi:10.3390/jcm10061296 43

Yoon-Chul Kim, Hyung Jun Kim, Jong-Won Chung, In Gyeong Kim, Min Jung Seong, Keon Ha Kim, Pyoung Jeon, et al.
Novel Estimation of Penumbra Zone Based on Infarct Growth Using Machine Learning Techniques in Acute Ischemic Stroke
Reprinted from: *J. Clin. Med.* 2020, 9, 1977, doi:10.3390/jcm9061977 53

Mustafa Kilic, Christina Wendl, Sibylle Wilfling, David Olmes, Ralf Andreas Linker and Felix Schlachetzki
Acute Middle Cerebral Artery Occlusion Detection Using Mobile Non-Imaging Brain Perfusion Ultrasound—First Case
Reprinted from: *J. Clin. Med.* 2022, 11, 3384, doi:10.3390/jcm11123384 67

Simona Halúsková, Roman Herzig, Dagmar Krajíčková, Abduljabar Hamza, Antonín Krajina, Vendelín Chovanec, Miroslav Lojík, et al.
Acute Management Should Be Optimized in Patients with Less Specific Stroke Symptoms: Findings from a Retrospective Observational Study
Reprinted from: *J. Clin. Med.* 2021, 10, 1143, doi:10.3390/jcm10051143 77

Seungyon Koh, Ji Hyun Park, Bumhee Park, Mun Hee Choi, Sung Eun Lee, Jin Soo Lee, Ji Man Hong, et al.
Prediction of Infarct Growth and Neurological Deterioration in Patients with Vertebrobasilar Artery Occlusions
Reprinted from: *J. Clin. Med.* **2020**, *9*, 3759, doi:10.3390/jcm9113759 . . . . **91**

Moritz Kielkopf, Thomas Meinel, Johannes Kaesmacher, Urs Fischer, Marcel Arnold, Mirjam Heldner, David Seiffge, et al.
Temporal Trends and Risk Factors for Delayed Hospital Admission in Suspected Stroke Patients
Reprinted from: *J. Clin. Med.* **2020**, *9*, 2376, doi:10.3390/jcm9082376 . . . . **105**

Giovanni Merlino, Carmelo Smeralda, Massimo Sponza, Gian Luigi Gigli, Simone Lorenzut, Alessandro Marini, Andrea Surcinelli, et al.
Dynamic Hyperglycemic Patterns Predict Adverse Outcomes in Patients with Acute Ischemic Stroke Undergoing Mechanical Thrombectomy
Reprinted from: *J. Clin. Med.* **2020**, *9*, 1932, doi:10.3390/jcm9061932 . . . . **113**

Marcin Wnuk, Justyna Derbisz, Leszek Drabik, Maciej Malecki and Agnieszka Slowik
Fasting Normoglycemia after Intravenous Thrombolysis Predicts Favorable Long-Term Outcome in Non-Diabetic Patients with Acute Ischemic Stroke
Reprinted from: *J. Clin. Med.* **2021**, *10*, 3005, doi:10.3390/jcm10143005 . . . . **127**

Elena Muiño, Jara Cárcel-Márquez, Caty Carrera, Laia Llucià-Carol, Cristina Gallego-Fabrega, Natalia Cullell, Miquel Lledós, et al.
RP11-362K2.2:RP11-767I20.1 Genetic Variation Is Associated with Post-Reperfusion Therapy Parenchymal Hematoma. A GWAS Meta-Analysis
Reprinted from: *J. Clin. Med.* **2021**, *10*, 3137, doi:10.3390/jcm10143137 . . . . **141**

Justina Jurkevičienė, Mantas Vaišvilas, Rytis Masiliūnas, Vaidas Matijošaitis, Antanas Vaitkus, Dovilė Geštautaitė, Saulius Taroza, et al.
Reperfusion Therapies for Acute Ischemic Stroke in COVID-19 Patients: A Nationwide Multi-Center Study
Reprinted from: *J. Clin. Med.* **2022**, *11*, 3004, doi:10.3390/jcm11113004 . . . . **161**

Marlena Schnieder, Mathias Bähr, Mareike Kirsch, Ilko Maier, Daniel Behme, Christian Heiner Riedel, Marios-Nikos Psychogios, et al.
Analysis of Frailty in Geriatric Patients as a Prognostic Factor in Endovascular Treated Patients with Large Vessel Occlusion Strokes
Reprinted from: *J. Clin. Med.* **2021**, *10*, 2171, doi:10.3390/jcm10102171 . . . . **173**

Dagmar Krajíčková, Antonín Krajina, Roman Herzig, Oldřich Vyšata, Libor Šimůnek and Martin Vališ
Acute Recanalization of Large Vessel Occlusion in the Anterior Circulation Stroke: Is Mechanical Thrombectomy Alone Better in Patients over 80 Years of Age? Findings from a Retrospective Observational Study
Reprinted from: *J. Clin. Med.* **2021**, *10*, 4266, doi:10.3390/jcm10184266 . . . . **185**

Marcin Wnuk, Justyna Derbisz, Leszek Drabik and Agnieszka Slowik
C-Reactive Protein and White Blood Cell Count in Non-Infective Acute Ischemic Stroke Patients Treated with Intravenous Thrombolysis
Reprinted from: *J. Clin. Med.* **2021**, *10*, 1610, doi:10.3390/jcm10081610 . . . . **197**

**PauloÁvila-Gómez, Pablo Hervella, Andrés Da Silva-Candal, María Pérez-Mato,
Manuel Rodríguez-Yáñez, Iria López-Dequidt, José M. Pumar, et al.**
Temperature-Induced Changes in Reperfused Stroke: Inflammatory and
Thrombolytic Biomarkers
Reprinted from: *J. Clin. Med.* **2020**, *9*, 2108, doi:10.3390/jcm9072108 . . . . **209**

**Joonsang Yoo, Jeong-Ho Hong, Seong-Joon Lee, Yong-Won Kim, Ji Man Hong,
Chang-Hyun Kim, Jin Wook Choi, et al.**
Acute Kidney Injury after Endovascular Treatment in Patients with Acute Ischemic Stroke
Reprinted from: *J. Clin. Med.* **2020**, *9*, 1471, doi:10.3390/jcm9051471 . . . . **221**

About the Editors

Hyo Suk Nam

Hyo Suk Nam is currently employed at the Department of Neurology at Yonsei University College of Medicine in Seoul, South Korea. He completed a fellowship in clinical and research neurology at the same institution and earned a Ph.D. in neurology from Yonsei in 2010. His areas of research include clinical stroke, acute patient management, care pathway improvement, mobile health, and basic stroke research. He has published over 50 papers as a corresponding or first author and over 160 papers as a co-author in peer-reviewed journals. He conducted the SECRET (SElection CRiteria in Endovascular thrombectomy and Thrombolytic therapy) study, which was a nationwide, multicenter study that aimed to examine the impact of comorbidities in thrombolysis and thrombectomy. This study has been extensively analyzed, and many articles on the SECRET registry have been published in peer-reviewed journals. Additionally, he is a primary investigator for a randomized controlled trial entitled "Outcome in Patients Treated with Intraarterial thrombectomy - optiMAL Blood Pressure control (OPTIMAL-BP) trial." The trial aims to determine the effectiveness of intensive blood pressure lowering compared to conventional treatment after endovascular treatment.

Byung Moon Kim

Byung Moon Kim is a Professor of Interventional Neuroradiology at the Department of Radiology, Severance Stroke Center, Severance Hospital, Yonsei University College of Medicine, Seoul, Republic of Korea. His research interests include the endovascular treatment of acute stroke, cerebral atherosclerotic stenosis, cerebral aneurysms, CNS shunt disease, and vascular malformations. With more than 25 years of experience in the fields of interventional neuroradiology, he has published around 100 papers as the first/corresponding author in peer-reviewed journals and has presented more than 50 proceedings at international conferences. In his scientific and professional career, he has been the president of the Korean Society of Interventional Neuroradiology (2018–2019), the Chairman of Organizing Committee of Asian-Australasian Federation of Interventional and Therapeutic Neuroradiology (AAFITN) 3030, and the Vice President of Korean Interventional Medical Society (2022–2023).

Preface to "Thrombolysis and Thrombectomy in Acute Ischemic Stroke"

Stroke is a major health concern worldwide, being the second-leading cause of death and the third-leading cause of death and disability. The burden of stroke has been increasing significantly. Until the early 1990s, the management of patients with stroke was primarily conservative in nature. However, with the approval of intravenous recombinant tissue plasminogen activator (IVT) by the US FDA in 1995, significant improvements were made in the management of stroke. Currently, endovascular treatment (EVT) has become a standard of care for patients with acute large vessel occlusion. Advancements in treatment methods and post-reperfusion care have led to better patient outcomes. While the future looks promising, ongoing research and development will continue to improve reperfusion therapy and care for stroke patients.

The primary objective of this Special Issue is to address the current knowledge gaps and promote advancements in the use of IVT and EVT for the treatment of acute ischemic stroke. The eighteen articles submitted to the *Journal of Clinical Medicine* were carefully selected and are presented in this book. The published articles explore a diverse range of topics and applications of reperfusion therapy in acute ischemic stroke. Although submissions for this Special Issue have been closed, the need for continued research and development in this field remains vital.

Finally, we would like to extend our deepest gratitude to the staff of MDPI Books, the editorial team of *JCM*—particularly Ms. Niya Wu, the assistant editor of this Special Issue—the accomplished authors, and the dedicated and professional reviewers for their contributions.

Hyo Suk Nam and Byung Moon Kim
Editors

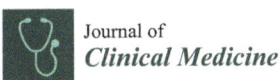

Editorial

Advance of Thrombolysis and Thrombectomy in Acute Ischemic Stroke

Hyo Suk Nam [1,*] and Byung Moon Kim [2]

1 Department of Neurology, Yonsei University College of Medicine, Seoul 03722, Republic of Korea
2 Department of Radiology, Yonsei University College of Medicine, Seoul 03722, Republic of Korea
* Correspondence: hsnam@yuhs.ac; Tel.: +82-2-2228-1617; Fax: +82-2-393-0705

Globally, stroke remains the second leading cause of death, and the third-leading cause of death and disability, in the world. Stroke burden increased substantially [1]. The use of intravenous recombinant tissue plasminogen activator (IVT) has been the standard of care for treating acute ischemic stroke for over two decades; however, its low efficacy and potential harmfulness limit its effectiveness. After successful randomized clinical trials, endovascular thrombectomy (EVT) has become the mainstay treatment of large vessel occlusion in patients with acute ischemic stroke. However, the guidelines still recommend that patients eligible for IVT should receive it. Two randomized clinical trials showed that EVT was effective even in the late time window of up to 16 or 24 h [2,3]. Many researchers have conducted research into more effective treatments, evaluation tools, and efficient care pathways in thrombolysis and thrombectomy in patients with acute ischemic stroke.

The recanalization rate of EVT is about 70–80% and the number needed to treat is 2.6 with a low complication rate. However, more than half of patients remain functionally dependent 3 months after the initial stroke. It remains unclear whether EVT will be beneficial in all stroke patients. Recanalization is one of the critical factors affecting early and late outcomes following acute ischemic stroke. Kim et al., investigated whether stroke risk scores are associated with unsuccessful recanalization in patients who received EVT [4]. They tested the $CHADS_2$, CHA_2DS_2-VASc, ATRIA, and Essen stroke risk scores, and found that all stroke risk scores were associated with recanalization failure after EVT. This study showed the association between stroke risk scores and the clinical outcomes of patients who received EVT.

Successful recanalization does not always translate into good clinical outcomes. When successful recanalization fails to bring a favorable prognosis, it is called futile recanalization (FR). FR is usually defined as the modified Rankin scale ≥ 3 at 3 months despite successful recanalization (Thrombolysis in Cerebral Infarction grade $\geq$ 2b). The prevalence of FR has been reported to range from 29 to 67%. Causes of FR can be divided into baseline patient characteristics, imaging findings, and postprocedural factors. The baseline characteristics of old age, female gender, higher initial National Institutes of Health Stroke Scale score, comorbidities, systolic blood pressure, glucose and biomarkers, and late treatment are reported. Imaging factors included large infarction, poor collaterals, proximal occlusion, and white matter hyperintensity. Procedural factors included no IVT use, symptomatic intracranial hemorrhage, blood pressure variability, and blood pressure controls after recanalization.

EVT in older people can be challenging, as older people often live with frailty, which may be associated with FR and poor outcomes. Schnieder et al., investigated whether frail patients also face adverse outcomes after EVT [5]. They found that frailty led to poor functional outcomes and higher mortality in patients undergoing EVT. Krajíčková et al., studied real-world data of elderly patients who were treated with EVT [6]. They found that patients $\geq$ 80 years old and undergoing IVT were less likely to achieve a 3-month good clinical outcome. Women were highly associated with 3-month good clinical outcomes and lower 3-month mortality.

Citation: Nam, H.S.; Kim, B.M. Advance of Thrombolysis and Thrombectomy in Acute Ischemic Stroke. *J. Clin. Med.* **2023**, *12*, 720. https://doi.org/10.3390/jcm12020720

Received: 5 January 2023
Accepted: 11 January 2023
Published: 16 January 2023

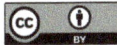

Copyright: © 2023 by the authors. Licensee MDPI, Basel, Switzerland. This article is an open access article distributed under the terms and conditions of the Creative Commons Attribution (CC BY) license (https://creativecommons.org/licenses/by/4.0/).

The prediction of prognosis based on advanced imaging techniques before IVT or EVT is promising. Incorporating advanced neuroimaging in patients with acute ischemic stroke may increase the yield of IVT administration without affecting the treatment's effectiveness and safety [7]. Among various tools, hypoperfusion severity can be estimated using the hypoperfusion intensity ratio (HIR). Baek et al., studied the association between HIR and clinical outcomes [8]. They found that the low-HIR group had a more favorable outcome, even with an unfavorable Alberta Stroke Program Early CT score and onset-to-recanalization time. Using pre-treatment CT angiography, HIR provides an objective numerical value compared to classic tools that provide a qualitative or merely categorical value. Kim et al., demonstrated the feasibility of a machine-learning-based tissue outcome prediction technique using features derived from pre-treatment, perfusion-weighted, and diffusion-weighted imaging [9].

During and after thrombolysis and thrombectomy, contrast-associated acute kidney injury can deteriorate patients. Yoo et al., studied the retrospective cohort of three stroke centers in Korea, finding that AKI occurred in 9.8% of EVT patients [10]. The occurrence of AKI was associated with a poor functional outcome and mortality at 3 months. Accompanying coronavirus disease 2019 (COVID-19) in patients with acute ischemic stroke is problematic. However, safety and efficacy data of IVT and EVT in patients with COVID-19 are scarce. Jurkevičienė et al., found that reperfusion therapies in COVID-19 patients are safe. Functional outcomes at 3 months were significantly worse and 3-month mortality was higher than the control group [11].

Until the early 1990s, managing patients with stroke had long remained a conservative treatment. After the US FDA approved recombinant tissue plasminogen activator in 1995, stroke management was never the same. Likewise, the current method of EVT is a mainstay in patients with acute large vessel occlusion. The development of treatment tools and sophisticated care after reperfusion therapy improves outcomes. As promising as the future looks, we will meet the next generation of reperfusion therapy and care.

Author Contributions: Conceptualization, H.S.N. and B.M.K.; methodology, H.S.N. and B.M.K.; data acquisition, H.S.N. and B.M.K.; writing—original draft preparation, H.S.N. and B.M.K.; writing—review and editing, H.S.N. and B.M.K.; project administration, H.S.N.; funding acquisition, H.S.N. All authors have read and agreed to the published version of the manuscript.

Funding: This work was supported by the National Research Foundation of Korea (NRF) grant funded by the Korea government (MSIT). (No. 2022R1A2C1007948).

Conflicts of Interest: The authors declare no conflict of interest.

References

1. Feigin, V.L.; Stark, B.A.; Johnson, C.O.; Roth, G.A.; Bisignano, C.; Abady, G.G.; Abbasifard, M.; Abbasi-Kangevari, M.; Abd-Allah, F.; Abedi, V.; et al. Global, regional, and national burden of stroke and its risk factors, 1990–2019: A systematic analysis for the global burden of disease study 2019. *Lancet Neurol.* **2021**, *20*, 795–820. [CrossRef] [PubMed]
2. Albers, G.W.; Marks, M.P.; Kemp, S.; Christensen, S.; Tsai, J.P.; Ortega-Gutierrez, S.; McTaggart, R.A.; Torbey, M.T.; Kim-Tenser, M.; Leslie-Mazwi, T.; et al. Thrombectomy for stroke at 6 to 16 hours with selection by perfusion imaging. *N. Engl. J. Med.* **2018**, *378*, 708–718. [CrossRef] [PubMed]
3. Nogueira, R.G.; Jadhav, A.P.; Haussen, D.C.; Bonafe, A.; Budzik, R.F.; Bhuva, P.; Yavagal, D.R.; Ribo, M.; Cognard, C.; Hanel, R.A.; et al. Thrombectomy 6 to 24 hours after stroke with a mismatch between deficit and infarct. *N. Engl. J. Med.* **2018**, *378*, 11–21. [CrossRef] [PubMed]
4. Kim, H.J.; Park, M.S.; Yoo, J.; Kim, Y.D.; Park, H.; Kim, B.M.; Bang, O.Y.; Kim, H.C.; Han, E.; Kim, D.J.; et al. Association between $CHADS_2$, CHA_2DS_2-VASc, ATRIA, and Essen stroke risk scores and unsuccessful recanalization after endovascular thrombectomy in acute ischemic stroke patients. *J. Clin. Med.* **2022**, *11*, 274. [CrossRef] [PubMed]
5. Schnieder, M.; Bahr, M.; Kirsch, M.; Maier, I.; Behme, D.; Riedel, C.H.; Psychogios, M.N.; Brehm, A.; Liman, J.; von Arnim, C.A.F. Analysis of frailty in geriatric patients as a prognostic factor in endovascular treated patients with large vessel occlusion strokes. *J. Clin. Med.* **2021**, *10*, 2171. [CrossRef] [PubMed]
6. Krajickova, D.; Krajina, A.; Herzig, R.; Vysata, O.; Simunek, L.; Valis, M. Acute recanalization of large vessel occlusion in the anterior circulation stroke: Is mechanical thrombectomy alone better in patients over 80 years of age? Findings from a retrospective observational study. *J. Clin. Med.* **2021**, *10*, 4266. [CrossRef] [PubMed]

7. Psychogios, K.; Safouris, A.; Kargiotis, O.; Magoufis, G.; Andrikopoulou, A.; Papageorgiou, E.; Chondrogianni, M.; Papadimitropoulos, G.; Polyzogopoulou, E.; Spiliopoulos, S.; et al. Advanced neuroimaging preceding intravenous thrombolysis in acute ischemic stroke patients is safe and effective. *J. Clin. Med.* **2021**, *10*, 2819. [CrossRef] [PubMed]
8. Baek, J.H.; Kim, Y.D.; Lee, K.J.; Choi, J.K.; Baik, M.; Kim, B.M.; Kim, D.J.; Heo, J.H.; Nam, H.S. Low hypoperfusion intensity ratio is associated with a favorable outcome even in large ischemic core and delayed recanalization time. *J. Clin. Med.* **2021**, *10*, 1869. [CrossRef] [PubMed]
9. Kim, Y.-C.; Kim, H.J.; Chung, J.-W.; Kim, I.G.; Seong, M.J.; Kim, K.H.; Jeon, P.; Nam, H.S.; Seo, W.-K.; Kim, G.-M.; et al. Novel estimation of penumbra zone based on infarct growth using machine learning techniques in acute ischemic stroke. *J. Clin. Med.* **2020**, *9*, 1977. [CrossRef] [PubMed]
10. Yoo, J.; Hong, J.H.; Lee, S.J.; Kim, Y.W.; Hong, J.M.; Kim, C.H.; Choi, J.W.; Kang, D.H.; Kim, Y.S.; Hwang, Y.H.; et al. Acute kidney injury after endovascular treatment in patients with acute ischemic stroke. *J. Clin. Med.* **2020**, *9*, 1471. [CrossRef] [PubMed]
11. Jurkeviciene, J.; Vaisvilas, M.; Masiliunas, R.; Matijosaitis, V.; Vaitkus, A.; Gestautaite, D.; Taroza, S.; Puzinas, P.; Galvanauskaite, E.; Jatuzis, D.; et al. Reperfusion therapies for acute ischemic stroke in COVID-19 patients: A nationwide multi-center study. *J. Clin. Med.* **2022**, *11*, 3004. [CrossRef] [PubMed]

Disclaimer/Publisher's Note: The statements, opinions and data contained in all publications are solely those of the individual author(s) and contributor(s) and not of MDPI and/or the editor(s). MDPI and/or the editor(s) disclaim responsibility for any injury to people or property resulting from any ideas, methods, instructions or products referred to in the content.

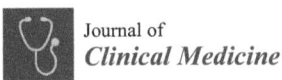

Article

Association between CHADS$_2$, CHA$_2$DS$_2$-VASc, ATRIA, and Essen Stroke Risk Scores and Unsuccessful Recanalization after Endovascular Thrombectomy in Acute Ischemic Stroke Patients

Hyung Jun Kim [1], Moo-Seok Park [1], Joonsang Yoo [2], Young Dae Kim [3], Hyungjong Park [4], Byung Moon Kim [5], Oh Young Bang [6], Hyeon Chang Kim [7], Euna Han [8], Dong Joon Kim [5], JoonNyung Heo [3], Jin Kyo Choi [9], Kyung-Yul Lee [10], Hye Sun Lee [11], Dong Hoon Shin [12], Hye-Yeon Choi [13], Sung-Il Sohn [4], Jeong-Ho Hong [4], Jong Yun Lee [14], Jang-Hyun Baek [15], Gyu Sik Kim [16], Woo-Keun Seo [6], Jong-Won Chung [6], Seo Hyun Kim [17], Sang Won Han [18], Joong Hyun Park [18], Jinkwon Kim [3], Yo Han Jung [10], Han-Jin Cho [19], Seong Hwan Ahn [20], Sung Ik Lee [21], Kwon-Duk Seo [16], Yoonkyung Chang [22], Tae-Jin Song [1,*], Hyo Suk Nam [3,*] and on behalf of the SECRET Study Investigators [†]

Citation: Kim, H.J.; Park, M.-S.; Yoo, J.; Kim, Y.D.; Park, H.; Kim, B.M.; Bang, O.Y.; Kim, H.C.; Han, E.; Kim, D.J.; et al. Association between CHADS$_2$, CHA$_2$DS$_2$-VASc, ATRIA, and Essen Stroke Risk Scores and Unsuccessful Recanalization after Endovascular Thrombectomy in Acute Ischemic Stroke Patients. *J. Clin. Med.* **2022**, *11*, 274. https://doi.org/10.3390/jcm11010274

Academic Editor: Aristeidis H. Katsanos

Received: 8 December 2021
Accepted: 31 December 2021
Published: 5 January 2022

Publisher's Note: MDPI stays neutral with regard to jurisdictional claims in published maps and institutional affiliations.

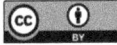

Copyright: © 2022 by the authors. Licensee MDPI, Basel, Switzerland. This article is an open access article distributed under the terms and conditions of the Creative Commons Attribution (CC BY) license (https://creativecommons.org/licenses/by/4.0/).

1. Department of Neurology, Seoul Hospital, College of Medicine, Ewha Woman's University, Seoul 07804, Korea; khhhj7@naver.com (H.J.K.); pierceu@hanmail.net (M.-S.P.)
2. Department of Neurology, Yongin Severance Hospital, Yonsei University College of Medicine, Yongin 16995, Korea; quarksea@gmail.com
3. Department of Neurology, Yonsei University College of Medicine, Seoul 03722, Korea; neuro05@yuhs.ac (Y.D.K.); jnheo@yuhs.ac (J.H.); antithrombus@gmail.com (J.K.)
4. Department of Neurology, Keimyung University School of Medicine, Daegu 42601, Korea; hjpark209042@gmail.com (H.P.); sungil.sohn@gmail.com (S.-I.S.); neurohong79@gmail.com (J.-H.H.)
5. Department of Radiology, Yonsei University College of Medicine, Seoul 03722, Korea; bmoon21@yuhs.ac (B.M.K.); djkimmd@yuhs.ac (D.J.K.)
6. Department of Neurology, Samsung Medical Center, Sungkyunkwan University School of Medicine, Seoul 06351, Korea; ohyoung.bang@samsung.com (O.Y.B.); mcastenosis@gmail.com (W.-K.S.); neurocjw@gmail.com (J.-W.C.)
7. Department of Preventive Medicine, Yonsei University College of Medicine, Seoul 03722, Korea; hckim@yuhs.ac
8. College of Pharmacy, Yonsei Institute for Pharmaceutical Research, Yonsei University, Incheon 21983, Korea; eunahan@yonsei.ac.kr
9. Department of Neurology, Seoul Medical Center, Seoul 02053, Korea; gumicjg@naver.com
10. Department of Neurology, Gangnam Severance Hospital, Yonsei University College of Medicine, Seoul 06273, Korea; kylee@yuhs.ac (K.-Y.L.); yhjung@yuhs.ac (Y.H.J.)
11. Biostatistics Collaboration Unit, Department of Research Affairs, Yonsei University College of Medicine, Seoul 03722, Korea; HSLEE1@yuhs.ac
12. Department of Neurology, Gachon University Gil Medical Center, Incheon 21565, Korea; dr.donghoon.shin@gmail.com
13. Department of Neurology, Kyung Hee University Hospital at Gangdong, Kyung Hee University School of Medicine, Seoul 05278, Korea; hyechoi@gmail.com
14. Department of Neurology, National Medical Center, Seoul 04564, Korea; jjongyl@gmail.com
15. Department of Neurology, Kangbuk Samsung Hospital, Sungkyunkwan University School of Medicine, Seoul 03181, Korea; janghyun.baek@gmail.com
16. Department of Neurology, National Health Insurance Service Ilsan Hospital, Goyang 10444, Korea; myoungsim@naver.com (G.S.K.); seobin7@naver.com (K.-D.S.)
17. Department of Neurology, Yonsei University Wonju College of Medicine, Wonju 26426, Korea; s-hkim@yonsei.ac.kr
18. Department of Neurology, Sanggye Paik Hospital, Inje University College of Medicine, Seoul 01757, Korea; sah1puyo@gmail.com (S.W.H.); truelove1@hanmail.net (J.H.P.)
19. Department of Neurology, Pusan National University School of Medicine, Busan 49241, Korea; chohj75@pusan.ac.kr
20. Department of Neurology, Chosun University School of Medicine, Gwangju 61453, Korea; shahn@Chosun.ac.kr
21. Department of Neurology, Sanbon Hospital, Wonkwang University School of Medicine, Gunpo 15865, Korea; neurologist@hanmail.net
22. Department of Neurology, Mokdong Hospital, College of Medicine, Ewha Woman's University, Seoul 07985, Korea; tin1207@nate.com

* Correspondence: knstar@ewha.ac.kr (T.-J.S.); hsnam@yuhs.ac (H.S.N.); Tel.: +82-2-6986-1672 (T.-J.S.); +82-2-2228-1617 (H.S.N.); Fax: +82-2-6986-7000 (T.-J.S.); +82-2-393-0705 (H.S.N.)
† SECRET Study Investigators are listed in the data Supplementary Materials.

Abstract: Background: The $CHADS_2$, CHA_2DS_2-VASc, ATRIA, and Essen scores have been developed for predicting vascular outcomes in stroke patients. We investigated the association between these stroke risk scores and unsuccessful recanalization after endovascular thrombectomy (EVT). Methods: From the nationwide multicenter registry (Selection Criteria in Endovascular Thrombectomy and Thrombolytic therapy (SECRET)) (Clinicaltrials.gov NCT02964052), we consecutively included 501 patients who underwent EVT. We identified pre-admission stroke risk scores in each included patient. Results: Among 501 patients who underwent EVT, 410 (81.8%) patients achieved successful recanalization (mTICI $\geq$ 2b). Adjusting for body mass index and $p < 0.1$ in univariable analysis revealed the association between all stroke risk scores and unsuccessful recanalization ($CHADS_2$ score: odds ratio (OR) 1.551, 95% confidence interval (CI) 1.198–2.009, $p = 0.001$; CHA_2DS_2VASc score: OR 1.269, 95% CI 1.080–1.492, $p = 0.004$; ATRIA score: OR 1.089, 95% CI 1.011–1.174, $p = 0.024$; and Essen score: OR 1.469, 95% CI 1.167–1.849, $p = 0.001$). The $CHADS_2$ score had the highest AUC value and differed significantly only from the Essen score (AUC of $CHADS_2$ score; 0.618, 95% CI 0.554–0.681). Conclusion: All stroke risk scores were associated with unsuccessful recanalization after EVT. Our study suggests that these stroke risk scores could be used to predict recanalization in stroke patients undergoing EVT.

Keywords: ischemic stroke; stroke risk score; recanalization; thrombectomy

1. Introduction

Endovascular thrombectomy (EVT) plays a pivotal role in improving the prognosis by recanalizing occluded blood vessels in stroke patients [1]. With the recent success of trials on EVT, the number of patients receiving EVT continues to increase [1–5]. Moreover, the time window for EVT has also expanded [4,5]. Nevertheless, a significant number of patients who underwent EVT did not achieve successful recanalization [6]. As unsuccessful recanalization predictably leads to poor patient prognosis, it is important to identify the factors associated with unsuccessful recanalization. Factors associated with such unsuccessful recanalization include greater age, stroke severity, occlusion due to atherosclerosis, and thrombus burden [7–9]. Nonetheless, further research is still needed to identify the factors involved in unsuccessful recanalization [7–9].

Several stroke risk scores have been developed for predicting the clinical outcome or the occurrence of stroke. The $CHADS_2$ [10], CHA_2DS_2-VASc [11], and ATRIA scores [12] are mainly used to predict thromboembolic risk and vascular outcome in atrial fibrillation (AF) patients. The Essen stroke risk score predicts vascular events in patients without AF [13]. As these stroke risk scores are mainly composed of risk factors and easily identifiable laboratory findings, they have the advantage of being able to easily predict the occurrence of stroke or prognosis.

We hypothesized that stroke risk scores would be associated with unsuccessful recanalization in patients undergoing EVT. Hence, the purpose of this study was to investigate the association between increased $CHADS_2$, CHA_2DS_2-VASc, ATRIA, and Essen scores and the results of recanalization after EVT.

2. Methods

2.1. Study Population

Our study included patients from the Selection Criteria in Endovascular Thrombectomy and Thrombolytic therapy (SECRET) registry (Clinicaltrials.gov NCT02964052). The selection criteria and the definition of included variables in this registry have been published [14]. In brief, the SECRET registry is a nationwide, multicenter registry that included patients undergoing reperfusion therapy such as EVT [14]. The SECRET registry did not establish strict inclusion or exclusion criteria for reperfusion therapy and recommended treatment according to the updated guideline at the time of treatment. Furthermore, the doctor of each institution determined whether to administer reperfusion therapy, and all patients who underwent reperfusion therapy were consecutively registered in the SECRET registry. All registered clinical and imaging information was reinvestigated and rechecked by the core laboratory after the anonymization process. The demographic data, risk factors for cardiovascular disease, medication history of prior index stroke, blood and urine laboratory examination results, time parameters for reperfusion therapy, neurologic status including severity, and image findings related to reperfusion therapy were investigated.

Between January 2012 and December 2017, we retrospectively enrolled patients who received reperfusion thrombolysis and were consecutively registered in 15 hospitals. In addition, between November 2016 and December 2017, we prospectively enrolled patients who received reperfusion thrombolysis from 13 hospitals. A total of 1231 patients who underwent reperfusion thrombolysis were included, of which 507 patients underwent EVT. Finally, 501 patients who underwent EVT were included, excluding 6 patients, for whom information about the modified thrombolysis in cerebral infarction (mTICI) grade was not acquired (Figure 1). Written informed consent was obtained from the prospectively included patients or their next caregivers. Our Institutional Review Board approved our study (Yonsei University College of Medicine, 4-2015-1196).

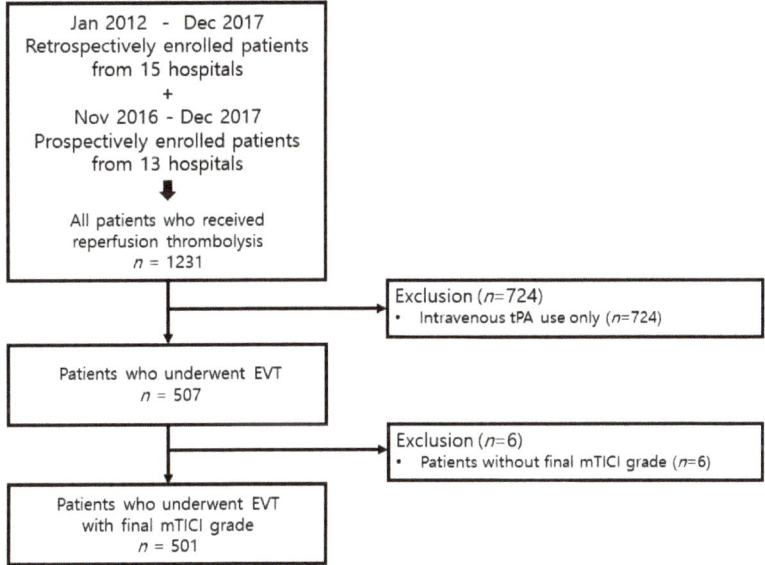

Figure 1. Patient selection strategy used in the study. tPA, tissue plasminogen activator; EVT, endovascular thrombectomy; mTICI, modified thrombolysis in cerebral infarction.

Stroke severity was defined using the National Institutes of Health Stroke Scale (NIHSS) score, and the neurologic change after 24 h of EVT was defined as the difference between the initial NIHSS score and the NIHSS score at 24 h (Initial NIHSS score—NIHSS score at 24 h = change in NIHSS score after 24 h). Therefore, if this value was positive, it means neurological improvement, 0 means no improvement, and negative means neurological worsened. Time parameters of EVT were acquired from onset-to-start of EVT (onset to puncture time) and administration of intravenous (IV) thrombolysis (tissue plasminogen activator, tPA) to start of EVT (needle to puncture time) [14]. In case of unclear symptom onset time, the last normal time (LNT) when the patient was asymptomatic was considered as the time of onset. Computed tomography (CT), CT angiography, magnetic resonance imaging (MRI), MR angiography, and digital subtraction angiography (DSA) images were acquired during the admission period.

Data related to reperfusion therapy, for example, the administration of IV thrombolysis, the total trial number of stent-retriever passes and the types of devices were investigated. Intra-arterial (IA) thrombolysis without IV tPA is defined as first-line therapy with EVT, who are contraindicated for IV tPA. Combined IV/IA thrombolysis is defined as IV tPA administration prior to EVT who could be treated with IV tPA within 4.5 h after symptom onset. The status of reperfusion therapy was investigated in the patients who underwent EVT using the final angiographic findings, including the DSA, and graded based on the mTICI grade. For the outcome parameter, a grade of mTICI 2b or 3 was defined as successful recanalization, and a grade of mTICI 0–2a was defined as unsuccessful recanalization. EVT was performed using a stent-retriever technique, a direct aspiration first pass technique (ADAPT), and the Solumbra technique. The first-line technique is based on the clinical situation of each center and each patient. If the first-line technique is unsuccessful, the second-line technique is used. Stent-retriever alone was defined as using only a stent-retriever as a first-line technique and not using ADAPT or the Solumbra technique as the second-line technique. Aspiration alone was defined as using ADAPT as a first-line technique and not using any other device as a second-line technique. The type of device used for each technique was based on operator preference (typically Solitaire FR device, Trevor stent device, and Penumbra).

2.2. The Stroke Risk Scoring Systems

We identified pre-admission $CHADS_2$, CHA_2DS_2-VASc, ATRIA, and Essen scores for each patient. The variables included in each scoring system are set according to the existing definition. The $CHADS_2$ and CHA_2DS_2-VASc scores, congestive heart failure, hypertension, age, diabetes mellitus (DM), previous stroke history, vascular diseases, and sex were included as scoring variables [10,11]. The ATRIA score included age, sex, hypertension, DM, congestive heart failure, presence of proteinuria, and kidney dysfunction (estimated glomerular filtration rate <45 mL/min per 1.73 m^2) as scoring parameters [12]. The Essen score included age, hypertension, DM, previous stroke history, myocardial infarction history, peripheral arterial occlusive disease, and other vascular diseases [13].

2.3. Statistical Analyses

Continuous variables and categorical variables were analyzed using an independent *t*-test or Mann–Whitney *U* test and the chi-square test or Fisher's exact test, respectively. Uni- and multivariable logistic regression was performed to evaluate factors for unsuccessful recanalization. Body mass index (BMI) and onset to puncture time, which are important cofounders for unsuccessful recanalization, and $p < 0.1$ (excluding age and DM, which are common overlapping variables for all stroke risk scores) from the univariable analysis were entered in multivariable analysis. The results of uni- and multivariable analyses were expressed as odds ratios (ORs) and 95% confidence intervals (CIs). Because the risk of vascular outcome increased as the stroke risk scores increased, the main outcome was defined as unsuccessful recanalization in this study. Subgroup analyses were performed, including demographic data, classical vascular risk factors, and stroke risk scores, and were dichotomized by the median values and the optimal cut off values. The interaction between unsuccessful recanalization and each subgroup was investigated with a two-tailed test in the logistic regression analyses. For the sensitivity analysis, we further analyzed all stroke risk scores for patients with AF-related stroke only.

For evaluating the predictability of $CHADS_2$, CHA_2DS_2-VASc, ATRIA, and Essen scores, receiver operating characteristic (ROC) curve analysis and area under the curve (AUC) were investigated. The AUC was calculated and the optimal cutoff values of the stroke risk scores were defined at the level with the highest Youden index (sensitivity + specificity − 1). The AUC of each stroke risk score was compared to determine whether there was a difference in the predictability of unsuccessful recanalization among the stroke risk scores. We utilized the multivariable model as the benchmark to assess the role of stroke risk scores in enhancing the risk prediction for unsuccessful recanalization in EVT patients. We compared AUCs to assess model discrimination and calculated net reclassification improvement (NRI) and the integrated discrimination improvement (IDI). All statistical analyses were performed using SPSS (version 25.0, IBM Corp., Chicago, IL, USA) and open-source statistical package R version 3.6.3 (R Project for Statistical Computing, Vienna, Austria). All variables needed a $p < 0.05$ to be considered statistically significant.

3. Results

3.1. Study Population

A total of 501 patients were included in this study. Patient demographics and information on risk factors and variables are summarized in Table 1. Of the 501 patients receiving EVT, 234 patients (46.7%) were female, and the mean age was 76.2 ± 13.3 years. The median value of the NIHSS scores of all patients was 15 (10–19, interquartile range (IQR)). IV thrombolysis was administered to 202 patients (40.3%), and the mean value of the onset to needle time was 119.9 ± 97.3 min. In all patients who underwent EVT, the mean value of the onset to puncture time was 354.6 ± 440.0 min, the mean value of the needle to puncture time was 78.7 ± 50.8 min, stent-retriever alone was used in 371 patients (74.0%), aspiration alone in 25 patients (4.9%), and combined stent-retriever and aspiration in 90 patients (17.9%). Among the patients who underwent stent-retriever alone and combined stent-retriever/aspiration, information about the stent device was obtained from 440 patients: the Solitaire FR device was used in 377 (85.6%) patients, the Trevor stent device in 58 (13.1%) patients, and both stent devices in only 5 (1.1%) patients. The mean value of the number of stent-retriever passes was 2.1 ± 1.9. Among the patients who underwent aspiration alone and combined stent-retriever/aspiration, aspiration device information was obtained from 92 patients: the Penumbra aspiration system was used in 55 (59.7%) patients and an intermediate catheter device in 37 (40.2%) patients.

Among all included patients, 410 (81.8%) patients achieved successful recanalization (mTICI $\geq$ 2b). The onset to recanalization measured only for patients who successfully recanalized (mTICI 2b/3) was 429.5 ± 481.4 min.

3.2. Association of Stroke Risk Scores with Recanalization Status

In the successful recanalization group, the proportion of patients with DM was lower (53.1% vs. 70.3%, $p = 0.004$), and there were more patients with coronary disease (31.2% vs. 17.5%, $p = 0.013$). Patients in the successful recanalization group had lower initial NIHSS scores (median 15 (IQR 10–19) vs. median 17 (IQR 12–20.5), $p = 0.020$) and the change in NIHSS scores after 24 h was greater (Initial NIHSS score—NIHSS score at 24 h, median 5 (IQR 0–10) vs. median 0 (IQR −2–3), $p < 0.001$) than those in the unsuccessful recanalization group. Combined IA/IV thrombolysis was significantly associated with successful recanalization ($p = 0.030$). In patients who administration of tPA prior to EVT, the time interval of the needle to puncture was significantly shorter in the successful recanalization group (111.8 $\pm$ 50.1 vs. 73.6 $\pm$ 49.1, $p < 0.001$). The stent-retriever alone was associated with successful recanalization ($p = 0.035$). However, aspiration alone ($p = 0.035$) was associated with unsuccessful recanalization. In patients who received stent-retrievers, the number of stent passes was significantly lower in the successful recanalization group (2.9 $\pm$ 2.8 vs. 2.0 $\pm$ 1.6, $p = 0.002$). In laboratory tests, both initial glucose level after admission (152.9 $\pm$ 54.3 mg/dL vs. 140.2 $\pm$ 49.7 mg/dL, $p = 0.042$) and fasting glucose level after admission (148.8 $\pm$ 52.9 mg/dL vs. 128.9 $\pm$ 46.9 mg/dL, $p = 0.002$) were lower in the successful recanalization group. All stroke risk scores were significantly lower in the successful recanalization group (CHADS$_2$ score; median 2 (IQR 1–3) vs. 3 (IQR 2–3), $p < 0.001$) (CHA$_2$DS$_2$VASc score; median 3 (IQR 2–4) vs. 4 (IQR 3–5), $p = 0.002$) (ATRIA score; median 7 (IQR 3–9) vs. 9 (IQR 6–10), $p = 0.002$) (Essen score; median 3 (IQR 2–4) vs. 4 (IQR 3–4), $p = 0.034$) (Table 1).

Table 1. Clinical and imaging characteristics according to the degree of recanalization.

	Total (n = 501)	Unsuccessful Recanalization mTICI ≤ 2a (n = 91)	Successful Recanalization mTICI 2b/3 (n = 410)	p-Value
Age, years, mean (SD)	76.2 ± 13.3	78.7 ± 14.1	75.6 ± 13.0	0.059
Female, (%)	234 (46.7%)	46 (50.6%)	188 (45.9%)	0.486
BMI (kg/m^2), mean (SD)	20.6 ± 4.1	20.3 ± 4.8	20.6 ± 4.0	0.519
Vascular risk factors				
Hypertension, (%)	376 (75.1%)	74 (81.3%)	302 (73.7%)	0.163
Diabetes mellitus, (%)	282 (56.3%)	64 (70.3%)	218 (53.2%)	0.004
Hypercholesterolemia, (%)	217 (43.3%)	37 (40.7%)	180 (43.9%)	0.654
Current smoking, (%)	83 (16.6%)	19 (20.9%)	64 (15.6%)	0.286
eGFR < 60 mL/min, (%)	243 (48.5%)	51 (56.0%)	192 (46.8%)	0.140
Comorbidities				
Atrial fibrillation (%)	265 (52.9%)	51 (56.0%)	214 (52.2%)	0.583
Heart failure, (%)	43 (8.6%)	11 (12.1%)	32 (7.8%)	0.266
Coronary disease, (%)	144 (28.7%)	16 (17.6%)	128 (31.2%)	0.013
Peripheral artery disease, (%)	17 (3.4%)	6 (6.6%)	11 (2.7%)	0.123
Previous infarction, (%)	118 (23.6%)	23 (25.3%)	95 (23.2%)	0.771
Previous hemorrhage, (%)	27 (5.4%)	7 (7.7%)	20 (4.9%)	0.413
Medication before admission				
Prior antiplatelet therapy, (%)	156 (31.1%)	29 (31.9%)	127 (31.0%)	0.967
Prior anticoagulant therapy, (%)	88 (17.6%)	12 (13.2%)	76 (18.5%)	0.053
Prior statin therapy, (%)	152 (30.3%)	21 (23.1%)	131 (32.0%)	0.124
Initial NIHSS score, median (IQR)	15 (10–19)	17 (12–20.5)	15 (10–19)	0.020
Change in NIHSS score after 24 h, median (IQR)	4 (0–9)	0 (−2–3)	5 (0–10)	<0.001
Treatment				
IA thrombolysis without IV tPA, (%)	299 (59.7%)	64 (70.3%)	235 (57.3%)	0.030
Combined IV/IA thrombolysis *, (%)	202 (40.3%)	27 (29.7%)	175 (42.7%)	0.030
Stent-retriever alone, (%)	371 (74.1%)	52 (57.1%)	319 (77.8%)	<0.001
Aspiration alone, (%)	25 (5.0%)	9 (9.9%)	16 (3.9%)	0.035
Combined stent-retriever/aspiration **, (%)	90 (18.0%)	15 (16.5%)	75 (18.3%)	0.521
Number of stent-retriever passes, mean (SD)	2.1 ± 1.9	2.9 ± 2.8	2.0 ± 1.6	0.002
Onset to puncture, min, mean (SD)	354.6 ± 440.0	370.1 ± 293.5	351.1 ± 466.6	0.621
LNT-to-puncture time (within 6 h)	350 (69.9%)	60 (65.9%)	290 (70.7%)	0.438
Arterial occlusion site				
Any ICA, (%)	94 (18.8%)	16 (17.6%)	78 (19.0%)	0.865
MCA, (%)	127 (25.4%)	18 (19.8%)	109 (26.6%)	0.224
ACA, (%)	7 (1.4%)	1 (1.1%)	6 (1.5%)	>0.99
PCA, (%)	8 (1.6%)	1 (1.1%)	7 (1.7%)	0.259
V-B, (%)	40 (8.0%)	10 (11.0%)	30 (7.3%)	0.340
Tandem lesion	24 (4.8%)	5 (5.5%)	19 (4.6%)	0.939
Stroke etiology				0.380
Cardioembolic	270 (53.9%)	49 (53.9%)	221 (53.9%)	
Large artery atherosclerosis	83 (16.6%)	19 (20.9%)	64 (15.6%)	
Undetermined or others	148 (29.5%)	23 (25.3%)	125 (30.5%)	
Laboratory results				
Initial glucose †, mg/dL	145.3 ± 51.4	152.9 ± 54.3	140.2 ± 49.7	0.042
Fasting glucose ‡, mg/dL	135.5 ± 51.7	148.8 ± 52.9	128.9 ± 46.9	0.002
Pre-admission stroke risk score, score, median (IQR)				
CHADS$_2$ score	2.1 ± 1.0	3 (2–3)	2 (1–3)	<0.001
CHA$_2$DS$_2$VASc score	3.4 ± 1.6	4 (3–5)	3 (2–4)	0.002
ATRIA score	6.7 ± 3.6	9 (6–10)	7 (3–9)	0.002
Essen score	3.3 ± 1.4	4 (3–4)	3 (2–4)	0.034

mTICI, modified thrombolysis in cerebral infarction; SD, standard deviation; BMI, body mass index; eGFR, estimated glomerular filtration rate; National Institutes of Health Stroke Scale, NIHSS; IQR, interquartile range; tPA, tissue plasminogen activator; IA, int; IV, intravenous; LNT, last normal time; ICA, internal carotid artery; MCA, middle cerebral artery; ACA, anterior cerebral artery; PCA, posterior cerebral artery; V-B, vertebro-basilar. * administration of intravenous tissue plasminogen activator prior to endovascular thrombectomy; ** cases in which stent-retriever and aspiration were performed simultaneously or sequentially. † The glucose level test was performed at the time of the first admission to the emergency room. ‡ The glucose level test was performed after 8 h of fasting after admission.

In univariable logistic regression analysis, age, DM, coronary disease, initial NIHSS score, combined IA/IV thrombolysis, stent-retriever alone, aspiration alone, number of stent-retriever passes, and stroke risk scores were associated with unsuccessful recanalization, as shown in Table S1. In multivariable logistic regression analysis, all stroke risk scores were predictive of unsuccessful recanalization along with BMI, onset to puncture time, coronary disease, initial NIHSS score, combined IA/IV thrombolysis, stent-retriever alone, aspiration alone, and the number of stent-retriever passes (CHADS$_2$ score: OR 1.551, 95% CI 1.198–2.009, p = 0.001; CHA$_2$DS$_2$VASc score: OR 1.269, 95% CI 1.080–1.492, p = 0.004; ATRIA score: OR 1.089, 95% CI 1.011–1.174, p = 0.024; and Essen score: OR 1.469, 95% CI 1.167–1.849, p = 0.001) (Table 2).

Table 2. Multivariable analysis for stroke risk score associated with the unsuccessful recanalization among 501 patients with endovascular thrombectomy.

Variables	CHADS$_2$ OR (95% CI)	p-Value	CHA$_2$DS$_2$VASc OR (95% CI)	p-Value	ATRIA OR (95% CI)	p-Value	Essen OR (95% CI)	p-Value
BMI, per-1-kg/m^2 increase	0.994 (0.936–1.055)	0.836	1.007 (0.947–1.071)	0.986	1.003 (0.943–1.066)	0.937	0.986 (0.928–1.047)	0.612
Coronary disease	0.372 (0.200–0.691)	0.002	0.383 (0.206–0.710)	0.002	0.380 (0.205–0.704)	0.002	0.251 (0.126–0.499)	<0.001
Initial NIHSS score, per 1-score increase	1.015 (0.977–1.055)	0.448	1.017 (0.979–1.057)	0.424	1.016 (0.978–1.056)	0.412	1.017 (0.978–1.056)	0.376
IV thrombolysis								
IA thrombolysis without IV tPA	Reference		Reference		Reference		Reference	
Combined IA/IV thrombolysis *	0.647 (0.382–1.094)	0.104	0.654 (0.388–1.105)	0.113	0.674 (0.399–1.140)	0.142	0.625 (0.370–1.055)	0.079
EVT parameters								
Stent-retriever alone	0.528 (0.302–0.924)	0.025	0.547 (0.313–0.957)	0.035	0.512 (0.294–0.892)	0.018	0.536 (0.307–0.939)	0.029
Aspiration alone	2.966 (1.048–8.394)	0.041	3.344 (1.183–9.453)	0.023	3.142 (1.122–8.880)	0.029	2.887 (1.024–8.140)	0.045
Number of stent-retriever passes, per-1-passes increase	1.267 (1.124–1.428)	<0.001	1.274 (1.131–1.436)	<0.001	1.275 (1.132–1.436)	<0.001	1.267 (1.124–1.427)	<0.001
Onset to puncture, per 1-min increase	1.000 (0.999–1.001)	0.992	1.000 (1.000–1.001)	0.992	1.000 (1.000–1.001)	0.935	1.000 (1.000–1.001)	0.980
Risk scoring score								
Per-1-point increase	1.551 (1.198–2.009)	0.001	1.269 (1.080–1.492)	0.004	1.105 (1.027–1.188)	0.007	1.469 (1.167–1.849)	0.001

OR, odds ratio; CI, confidence interval; BMI, body mass index; National Institutes of Health Stroke Scale, NIHSS; IV, intravenous; IA, intra-arterial; tPA, tissue plasminogen activator; EVT, endovascular thrombectomy; * administration of intravenous tissue plasminogen activator prior to endovascular thrombectomy.

In subgroup analysis, the association of unsuccessful recanalization was stratified by age, sex, comorbidities, NIHSS score, treatment factor (LNT, combined IA/IV thrombolysis), and stroke risk scores. A subgroup of patients with DM (p for interaction = 0.003), IA alone (p for interaction = 0.023), CHA$_2$DS$_2$VASc score ≥ 4 (p for interaction = 0.022), ATRIA score ≥ 8 (p for interaction = 0.017), CHADS$_2$ score ≥ 3 (p for interaction < 0.001), CHA$_2$DS$_2$VASc score ≥ 5 (p for interaction < 0.001), ATRIA score ≥ 9 (p for interaction = 0.001), and Essen score ≥ 4 (p for interaction = 0.009) were significantly associated with unsuccessful recanalization (Figure 2).

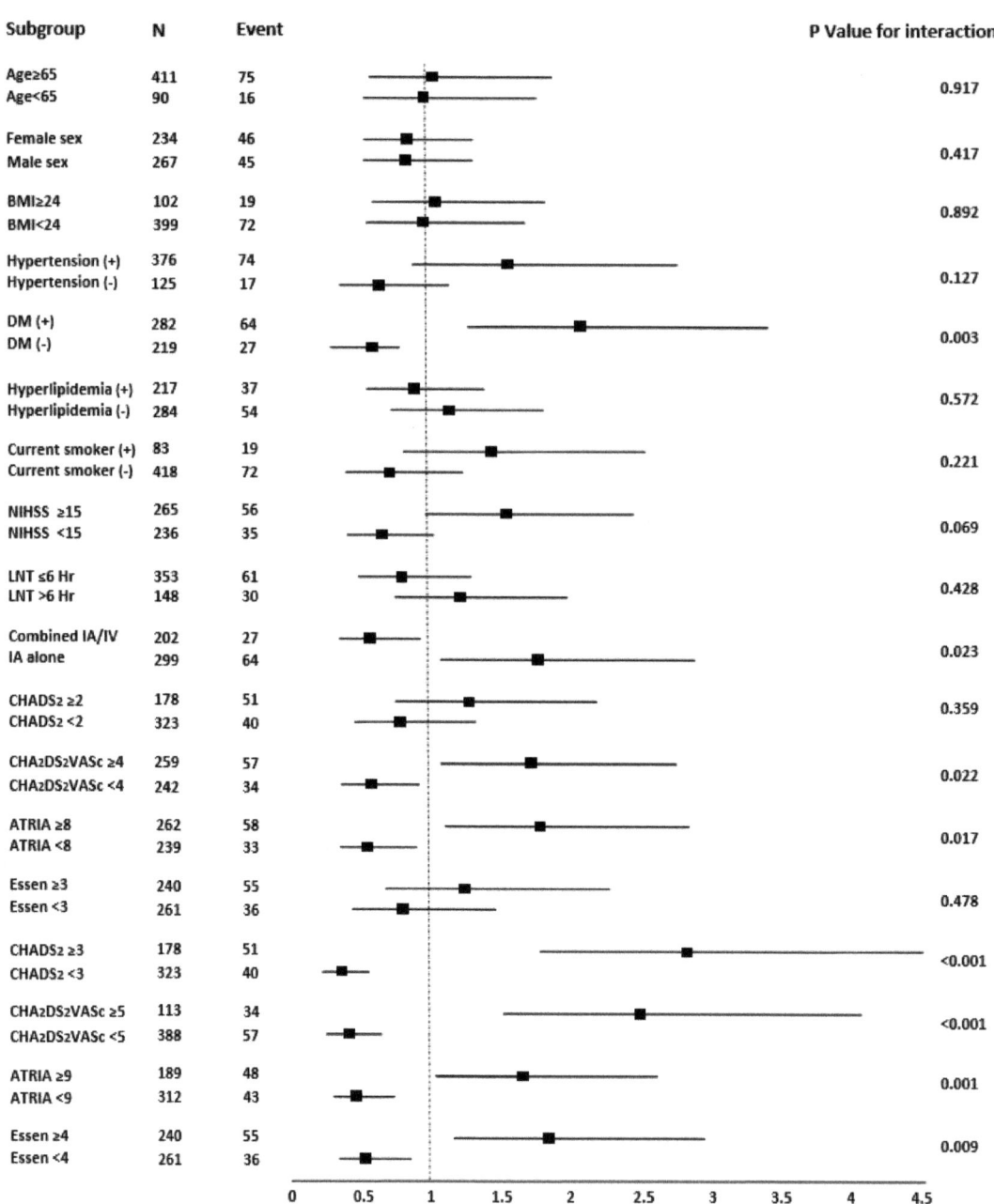

Figure 2. Forest plots of unadjusted odds ratios for unsuccessful recanalization (mTICI ≤ 2a) in patients with endovascular thrombectomy. BMI, body mass index; NIHSS, National Institutes of Health Stroke Scale; LNT, last normal time; IA, intra-arterial; IV, intra-venous; ORs, odds ratios; mTICI, modified thrombolysis in cerebral infarction.

In the comparison with AF-related stroke, there were significantly fewer patients with DM (72.1% vs. 53.6%, $p = 0.042$) and more patients with stent-retriever alone (51.2%

vs. 80.1%, $p < 0.001$) in the successful recanalization group. Moreover, patients in the successful recanalization group had lower initial NIHSS scores (median 15 (IQR 10–19) vs. median 17 (IQR 12–20.5), $p = 0.020$) and the change in NIHSS scores after 24 h was greater (Initial NIHSS score—NIHSS score at 24 h, median 5 (IQR 1–10) vs. median 0 (IQR −1–2), $p < 0.001$) than those in the unsuccessful recanalization group. An increase in the number of stent-retriever passes was associated with unsuccessful recanalization (3.3 ± 3.0 vs. 2.0 ± 1.5, $p = 0.007$). In laboratory tests, fasting glucose after admission (146.24 ± 50.3 mg/dL vs. 128.4 ± 51.9 mg/dL, $p = 0.044$) were lower in the successful recanalization group. The $CHADS_2$, CHA_2DS_2VASc, ATRIA, and Essen scores were significantly lower in the successful recanalization group ($CHADS_2$ score; median 2 (IQR 2–3) vs. 3 (IQR 2–3), $p < 0.001$) (CHA_2DS_2VASc score; median 4 (IQR 3–4] vs. 5 (IQR 4–5.5], $p = 0.003$) (ATRIA score; median 8 (IQR 6–9) vs. 9 (IQR 7.5–10), $p = 0.033$) (Essen score; median 4 (IQR 3–4) vs. 3 (IQR 3–4), $p = 0.043$). The above results are summarized in Table S2. In multivariable logistic regression analysis, the $CHADS_2$, CHA_2DS_2VASc, and Essen scores were associated with unsuccessful recanalization along with BMI, coronary disease, the initial NIHSS score, combined IA/IV thrombolysis, stent-retriever alone, aspiration alone, and number of stent-retriever passes ($CHADS_2$ score: OR 1.787, 95% CI 1.173–2.725, $p = 0.007$; CHA_2DS_2VASc score: OR 1.354, 95% CI 1.049–1.747, $p = 0.020$; and Essen score: OR 1.635, 95% CI 1.093–2.448, $p = 0.017$) (Table S3).

3.3. Comparison of Stroke Risk Scores for Unsuccessful Recanalization

Figure 3 shows the ROC curves of all stroke risk scores for unsuccessful recanalization. The AUC, optimal cutoff value, sensitivity, specificity, positive predictive value, and negative predictive value of each stroke risk score are presented in Table 3.

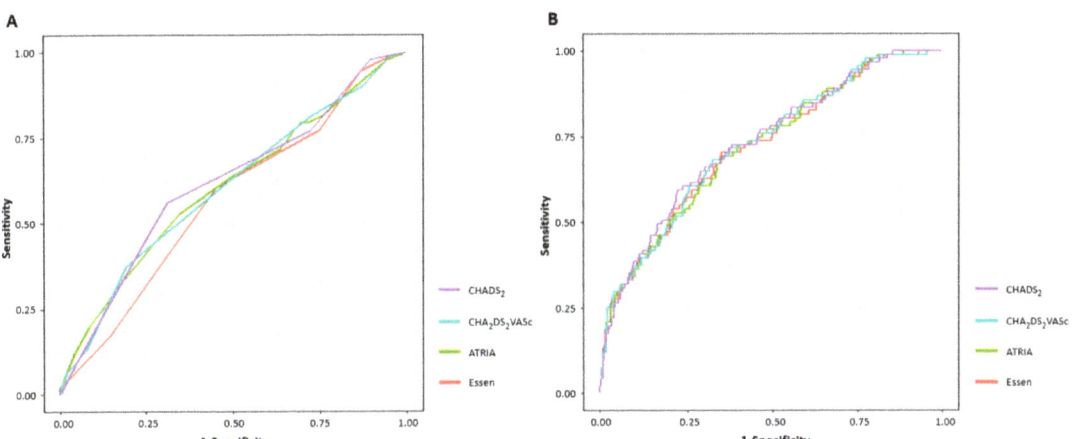

Figure 3. Receiver operating characteristic curve analyses of unsuccessful recanalization based on stroke risk scores. (**A**) Univariable ROC analysis (**B**) Multivariable ROC analysis. ROC, receiver operating characteristic.

Among stroke risk scores, the $CHADS_2$ score had the highest AUC value. However, in pairwise comparisons of the AUC, only the $CHADS_2$ and Essen scores were significantly different (AUC of $CHADS_2$ score; 0.618, 95% CI 0.554–0.681 vs. AUC of Essen score; 0.569, 95% CI 0.506–0.632, $p = 0.002$) (Table S4). Similarly, even when ROC curve analysis was performed on AF-related stroke only, the $CHADS_2$ score had the highest AUC value, and only the $CHADS_2$ and Essen scores were significantly different (AUC of $CHADS_2$ score; 0.666, 95% CI 0.570–0.761 vs. AUC of Essen score; 0.595, 95% CI 0.502–0.687, $p = 0.006$) (Table S5).

Table 3. Receiver operating characteristic (ROC) curve analysis of risk scores for the probability of an unsuccessful recanalization.

	AUC	Optimal Cutoff	Diagnostic Sensitivity	Diagnostic Specificity	PPV	NPV
$CHADS_2$ score	0.618	2.5	0.560	0.690	0.287	0.876
CHA_2DS_2VASc score	0.602	4.5	0.374	0.807	0.301	0.853
ATRIA score	0.605	8.5	0.528	0.656	0.254	0.862
Essen score	0.569	3.5	0.549	0.604	0.862	0.229

AUC, area under the curve; PPV, positive predictive value; NPV, negative predictive value.

The continuous-based NRI was significantly improved after the addition of each stroke risk score ($CHADS_2$ score: $p = 0.010$, CHA_2DS_2VASc score: $p = 0.023$, ATRIA score: $p = 0.035$, Essen score: $p = 0.005$). The IDI also showed improved risk classification after the addition of the $CHADS_2$ score ($p = 0.014$) or the ATRIA score ($p = 0.015$). Overall, the best model for prediction of unsuccessful recanalization after EVT was the $CHADS_2$ score, with the addition of the multivariable model (Table S6).

4. Discussion

The key finding of this study was that the pre-admission $CHADS_2$, CHA_2DS_2VASc, ATRIA, and Essen scores were associated with unsuccessful recanalization after EVT. The probability of unsuccessful recanalization increased as the stroke risk scores increased. The CHADS2 score had the highest AUC among all stroke risk scores, although the CHADS2 score differed significantly only from the Essen score.

Previous studies have proven the relationship between stroke risk scores and the clinical outcome of stroke. $CHADS_2$, CHA_2DS_2-VASc, and ATRIA scores are simple to obtain and are useful tools for estimating the thromboembolic risk and clinical outcomes in patients with AF [15–18]. The Essen score is a simple clinical score that was derived to predict the 1-year risk of recurrent ischemic stroke after ischemic stroke based on the presence of prior vascular comorbidities [13,19]. Unlike the purpose for which the stroke risk scores were developed, the stroke risk scores have been used as a predictor of various outcomes in various patient groups [15,20,21]. Our results are meaningful in that they provide additional information that $CHADS_2$, CHA_2DS_2-VASc, ATRIA, and Essen scores were correlated with unsuccessful recanalization in patients undergoing EVT, as well as thromboembolic risk and clinical outcome. All stroke risk scores were associated with unsuccessful recanalization even in AF-related stroke patients.

Hypertension and DM have a common weighting factor for all stroke risk scores, and DM, in particular, is known to affect recanalization after IV thrombolysis [22,23]. Although DM and fasting hyperglycemia are also known to affect clinical outcomes after EVT [24,25], there is still insufficient evidence that DM and initial and fasting hyperglycemia influence recanalization after EVT [26,27]. Our results showed that DM, initial, and fasting glucose levels were associated with unsuccessful recanalization. Factors other than hypertension and DM were weighted differently for each stroke risk score. Compared with the $CHADS_2$ score, the CHA_2DS_2-VASc score has a higher weighting for age and includes the components of sex and vascular diseases; the ATRIA score has a higher weighting for age and includes the components of sex and chronic renal disease, while the Essen score also has a higher weighting for age and sex, similarly to the other scores, along with weighting for vascular disease and current smoking. Each additional component of these scores has been reported as a predictor of stroke severity or outcome [28]. The ATRIA and CHA_2DS_2-VASc scores were reported to outperform the $CHADS_2$ score in predicting stroke outcome in patients with AF [17,28]. However, unlike previous studies that investigated the relationship between the stroke risk scores and stroke outcome, we found that the $CHADS_2$ score shows better performance in predicting recanalization than the CHA_2DS_2-VASc and ATRIA scores in EVT patients. This may be because sex, chronic kidney disease, and vascular disease weighted by the CHA_2DS_2-VASc and ATRIA scores did not differ with recanalization, and there were more patients with coronary disease in the successful recanalization group in our dataset. As the Essen score is a risk-scoring tool for the prediction of recurrent stroke and combined cerebrovascular events in patients with non-AF, there have been a few studies comparing the performance of the Essen score with that of the $CHADS_2$ score [13]. A recent observational study of the prediction for vascular outcome in stroke patients with AF found no significant difference in the performance between the $CHADS_2$ and Essen scores [21]. In contrast, the $CHADS_2$ score showed significantly better performance than the Essen score in our study. Even when only AF-related stroke patients were analyzed, the Essen score could significantly predict unsuccessful recanalization, although its performance was worse than that of the $CHADS_2$ score. Presumably, as in the case of CHA_2DS_2-VASc and ATRIA scores, this could be attributed to the observation that peripheral artery disease and current smoking weighted by the Essen score did not differ according to recanalization, and there were more patients with coronary disease in the recanalization group in our dataset. Therefore, unlike previous studies on patients with AF stroke, the ATRIA and CHA_2DS_2-VASc scores likely did not outperform and the Essen score likely underperformed compared to the $CHADS_2$ score. The significance of this result suggests that most of the factors related to unsuccessful recanalization in EVT patients overlap with most factors related to the occurrence of stroke in AF patients. Therefore, these different factors should be taken into account when creating a new scoring system that predicts recanalization after EVT. An existing pre-admission stroke risk score or suitable new scoring system can be used in addition to the current image-based patient's selection system, which can contribute to lower recanalization failure rates by appropriately selecting patients.

Limitations

First, although some of the patients included in our study were prospectively included and the registry itself consecutively included stroke patients who received reperfusion therapy, we performed a retrospective evaluation. Therefore, there may be selection bias, l and the possibility of a causal relationship cannot be concluded. Second, this registry is a nationwide observational registry that reflects real-world evidence; however, there may be a selection bias because it is not a randomized controlled study. To reduce the selection bias, we consecutively included patients eligible for EVT according to the valid guidelines [1,29,30]. Third, because our registry enrolled only the Korean population, it is difficult to generalize our findings to all races.

5. Conclusions

The pre-admission $CHADS_2$, CHA_2DS_2VASc, ATRIA, and Essen scores were associated with unsuccessful recanalization after EVT. Therefore, these results suggest that stroke risk scores, especially the $CHADS_2$ score, could predict recanalization in stroke patients undergoing EVT.

Supplementary Materials: The following supporting information can be downloaded at: https://www.mdpi.com/article/10.3390/jcm11010274/s1, Table S1: Univariate logistic regression analysis of the risk of an unsuccessful recanalization; Table S2: Clinical and imaging characteristics according to the degree of recanalization (Only atrial fibrillation-related stroke); Table S3: Multivariate analysis for stroke risk score associated with the unsuccessful recanalization among atrial fibrillation-related stroke with endovascular thrombectomy; Table S4: Comparison of the area under curve (AUC) of each stroke risk score by two. (Univariate ROC analysis); Table S5: Comparison of area under the curve (AUC) of each stroke risk score by two in AF-related stroke. (Univariate ROC analysis); Table S6: Receiver-operating characteristics curve analysis (area under curve), net reclassification improvement, and integrated discrimination improvement of predictive models for unsuccessful recanalization in endovascular thrombectomy patients.

Author Contributions: Conceptualization, T.-J.S. and H.S.N.; methodology, H.J.K., T.-J.S. and H.S.N.; data acquisition, M.-S.P., J.Y., Y.D.K., H.P., B.M.K., O.Y.B., H.C.K., E.H., D.J.K., J.H., J.K.C., K.-Y.L., H.S.L., D.H.S., H.-Y.C., S.-I.S., J.-H.H., J.Y.L., J.-H.B., G.S.K., W.-K.S., J.-W.C., S.H.K., S.W.H., J.H.P., J.K., Y.H.J., H.-J.C., S.H.A., S.I.L., K.-D.S., Y.C. and on behalf of the SECRET study Investigators; writing—original draft preparation, H.J.K. and T.-J.S.; writing—review and editing, H.J.K., T.-J.S. and H.S.N. All authors have read and agreed to the published version of the manuscript.

Funding: This work was supported by the Basic Science Research Program through the National Research Foundation of Korea (NRF) funded by the Ministry of Education (NRF-2021R1F1A1048113). The funders had no role in study design, data collection and analysis, decision to publish, or preparation of the manuscript.

Institutional Review Board Statement: The SECRET study was conducted according to the guidelines of the Declaration of Helsinki and approved by the Institutional Review Board of the Yonsei University College of Medicine, 4-2015-1196.

Informed Consent Statement: Informed consent was obtained from all subjects involved in the SECRET study.

Data Availability Statement: The data presented in this study are available on request from the corresponding authors. The data are not publicly available due to privacy.

Conflicts of Interest: The authors declare no conflict of interest.

References

1. Ko, S.-B.; Park, H.-K.; Kim, B.M.; Heo, J.H.; Rha, J.-H.; Kwon, S.U.; Kim, J.S.; Lee, B.-C.; Suh, S.H.; Jung, C.; et al. 2019 Update of the Korean Clinical Practice Guidelines of Stroke for Endovascular Recanalization Therapy in Patients with Acute Ischemic Stroke. *J. Stroke* **2019**, *21*, 231–240. [CrossRef] [PubMed]
2. Berkhemer, O.A.; Fransen, P.S.; Beumer, D.; van den Berg, L.A.; Lingsma, H.F.; Yoo, A.J.; Schonewille, W.J.; Vos, J.A.; Nederkoorn, P.J.; Wermer, M.J.H.; et al. A Randomized Trial of Intraarterial Treatment for Acute Ischemic Stroke. *N. Engl. J. Med.* **2015**, *372*, 11–20. [CrossRef] [PubMed]
3. Campbell, B.C.; Mitchell, P.J.; Kleinig, T.J.; Dewey, H.M.; Churilov, L.; Yassi, N.; Yan, B.; Dowling, R.J.; Parsons, M.W.; Oxley, T.J.; et al. Endovascular Therapy for Ischemic Stroke with Perfusion-Imaging Selection. *N. Engl. J. Med.* **2015**, *372*, 1009–1018. [CrossRef]
4. Albers, G.W.; Marks, M.P.; Kemp, S.; Christensen, S.; Tsai, J.P.; Ortega-Gutierrez, S.; McTaggart, R.A.; Torbey, M.T.; Kim-Tenser, M.; Leslie-Mazwi, T.; et al. Thrombectomy for Stroke at 6 to 16 Hours with Selection by Perfusion Imaging. *N. Engl. J. Med.* **2018**, *378*, 708–718. [CrossRef]
5. Nogueira, R.G.; Jadhav, A.P.; Haussen, D.C.; Bonafe, A.; Budzik, R.F.; Bhuva, P.; Yavagal, D.R.; Ribo, M.; Cognard, C.; Hanel, R.A.; et al. Thrombectomy 6 to 24 Hours after Stroke with a Mismatch between Deficit and Infarct. *N. Engl. J. Med.* **2018**, *378*, 11–21. [CrossRef]
6. Flottmann, F.; Leischner, H.; Broocks, G.; Nawabi, J.; Bernhardt, M.; Faizy, T.D.; Deb-Chatterji, M.; Thomalla, G.; Fiehler, J.; Brekenfeld, C. Recanalization Rate per Retrieval Attempt in Mechanical Thrombectomy for Acute Ischemic Stroke. *Stroke* **2018**, *49*, 2523–2525. [CrossRef] [PubMed]
7. Gralla, J.; Burkhardt, M.; Schroth, G.; El-Koussy, M.; Reinert, M.; Nedeltchev, K.; Slotboom, J.; Brekenfeld, C. Occlusion Length Is a Crucial Determinant of Efficiency and Complication Rate in Thrombectomy for Acute Ischemic Stroke. *Am. J. Neuroradiol.* **2008**, *29*, 247–252. [CrossRef]
8. Heider, D.M.; Simgen, A.; Wagenpfeil, G.; Dietrich, P.; Yilmaz, U.; Mühl-Benninghaus, R.; Roumia, S.; Faßbender, K.; Reith, W.; Kettner, M. Why we fail: Mechanisms and co-factors of unsuccessful thrombectomy in acute ischemic stroke. *Neurol. Sci.* **2020**, *41*, 1547–1555. [CrossRef]
9. Leischner, H.; Flottmann, F.; Hanning, U.; Broocks, G.; Faizy, T.D.; Deb-Chatterji, M.; Bernhardt, M.; Brekenfeld, C.; Buhk, J.-H.; Gellissen, S.; et al. Reasons for failed endovascular recanalization attempts in stroke patients. *J. NeuroInterv. Surg.* **2019**, *11*, 439–442. [CrossRef]
10. Gage, B.F.; Waterman, A.D.; Shannon, W.; Boechler, M.; Rich, M.W.; Radford, M.J. Validation of clinical classification schemes for predicting stroke: Results from the National Registry of Atrial Fibrillation. *JAMA* **2001**, *285*, 2864–2870. [CrossRef]
11. Lip, G.Y.; Nieuwlaat, R.; Pisters, R.; Lane, D.A.; Crijns, H.J. Refining clinical risk stratification for predicting stroke and thromboembolism in atrial fibrillation using a novel risk factor-based approach: The euro heart survey on atrial fibrillation. *Chest* **2010**, *137*, 263–272. [CrossRef]
12. Singer, D.E.; Chang, Y.; Borowsky, L.H.; Fang, M.C.; Pomernacki, N.K.; Udaltsova, N.; Reynolds, K.; Go, A.S. A New Risk Scheme to Predict Ischemic Stroke and Other Thromboembolism in Atrial Fibrillation: The ATRIA Study Stroke Risk Score. *J. Am. Heart Assoc.* **2013**, *2*, e000250. [CrossRef]

13. Weimar, C.; Diener, H.C.; Alberts, M.J.; Steg, P.G.; Bhatt, D.L.; Wilson, P.W.; Mas, J.L.; Röther, J. The Essen stroke risk score predicts recurrent cardiovascular events: A validation within the REduction of Atherothrombosis for Continued Health (REACH) registry. *Stroke* **2009**, *40*, 350–354. [CrossRef]
14. Kim, Y.D.; Heo, J.H.; Yoo, J.; Park, H.; Kim, B.M.; Bang, O.Y.; Kim, H.C.; Han, E.; Kim, D.J.; Heo, J.; et al. Improving the Clinical Outcome in Stroke Patients Receiving Thrombolytic or Endovascular Treatment in Korea: From the SECRET Study. *J. Clin. Med.* **2020**, *9*, 717. [CrossRef]
15. Topaz, G.; Pereg, D.; Shuvy, M.; Mausbach, S.; Kimiagar, I.; Telman, G.; Kitay-Cohen, Y.; Vorobeichik, D.; Shlomo, N.; Tanne, D. Pre-admission CHA2DS2-VASc score and outcome of patients with acute cerebrovascular events. *Int. J. Cardiol.* **2017**, *244*, 277–281. [CrossRef] [PubMed]
16. Kim, D.; Chung, J.W.; Kim, C.K.; Ryu, W.S.; Park, E.S.; Lee, S.H.; Yoon, B.W. Impact of CHADS(2) Score on Neurological Severity and Long-Term Outcome in Atrial Fibrillation-Related Ischemic Stroke. *J. Clin. Neurol.* **2012**, *8*, 251–258. [CrossRef] [PubMed]
17. Aspberg, S.; Chang, Y.; Atterman, A.; Bottai, M.; Go, A.S.; Singer, D.E. Comparison of the ATRIA, CHADS2, and CHA2DS2-VASc stroke risk scores in predicting ischaemic stroke in a large Swedish cohort of patients with atrial fibrillation. *Eur. Heart J.* **2016**, *37*, 3203–3210. [CrossRef]
18. Tanaka, K.; Yamada, T.; Torii, T.; Furuta, K.; Matsumoto, S.; Yoshimura, T.; Takase, K.; Wakata, Y.; Nakashima, N.; Kira, J.; et al. Pre-admission CHADS2, CHA2DS2-VASc, and R2CHADS2 Scores on Severity and Functional Outcome in Acute Ischemic Stroke with Atrial Fibrillation. *J. Stroke Cerebrovasc. Dis. Off. J. Natl. Stroke Assoc.* **2015**, *24*, 1629–1635. [CrossRef] [PubMed]
19. Weimar, C.; Goertler, M.; Röther, J.; Ringelstein, E.B.; Darius, H.; Nabavi, D.G.; Kim, I.H.; Benemann, J.; Diener, H.C. Predictive value of the Essen Stroke Risk Score and Ankle Brachial Index in acute ischaemic stroke patients from 85 German stroke units. *J. Neurol. Neurosurg. Psychiatry* **2008**, *79*, 1339–1343. [CrossRef]
20. Puurunen, M.K.; Kiviniemi, T.; Schlitt, A.; Rubboli, A.; Dietrich, B.; Karjalainen, P.; Nyman, K.; Niemelä, M.; Lip, G.Y.; Airaksinen, K.J. CHADS2, CHA2DS2-VASc and HAS-BLED as predictors of outcome in patients with atrial fibrillation undergoing percutaneous coronary intervention. *Thromb. Res.* **2014**, *133*, 560–566. [CrossRef]
21. Yu, I.; Song, T.J.; Kim, B.J.; Heo, S.H.; Jung, J.M.; Oh, K.M.; Kim, C.K.; Yu, S.; Park, K.Y.; Kim, J.M.; et al. CHADS2, CHA2DS2-VASc, ATRIA, and Essen stroke risk scores in stroke with atrial fibrillation: A nationwide multicenter registry study. *Medicine* **2021**, *100*, e24000. [CrossRef]
22. Tang, H.; Zhang, S.; Yan, S.; Liebeskind, D.S.; Sun, J.; Ding, X.; Zhang, M.; Lou, M. Unfavorable neurological outcome in diabetic patients with acute ischemic stroke is associated with incomplete recanalization after intravenous thrombolysis. *J. NeuroInterv. Surg.* **2016**, *8*, 342–346. [CrossRef] [PubMed]
23. Aoki, J.; Kimura, K.; Morita, N.; Harada, M.; Nagahiro, S. Diabetes mellitus inhibits complete recanalization in patients with middle cerebral artery occlusion. *Neurol. Res.* **2019**, *41*, 60–67. [CrossRef]
24. Wnuk, M.; Popiela, T.; Drabik, L.; Brzegowy, P.; Lasocha, B.; Wloch-Kopec, D.; Pulyk, R.; Jagiella, J.; Wiącek, M.; Kaczorowski, R.; et al. Fasting Hyperglycemia and Long-term Outcome in Patients with Acute Ischemic Stroke Treated with Mechanical Thrombectomy. *J. Stroke Cerebrovasc. Dis.* **2020**, *29*, 104774. [CrossRef] [PubMed]
25. Borggrefe, J.; Glück, B.; Maus, V.; Onur, Ö.; Abdullayev, N.; Barnikol, U.; Kabbasch, C.; Fink, G.R.; Mpotsaris, A. Clinical Outcome After Mechanical Thrombectomy in Patients with Diabetes with Major Ischemic Stroke of the Anterior Circulation. *World Neurosurg.* **2018**, *120*, e212–e220. [CrossRef] [PubMed]
26. Arnold, M.; Mattle, S.; Galimanis, A.; Kappeler, L.; Fischer, U.; Jung, S.; De Marchis, G.M.; Gralla, J.; Mono, M.-L.; Brekenfeld, C.; et al. Impact of Admission Glucose and Diabetes on Recanalization and Outcome after Intra-Arterial Thrombolysis for Ischaemic Stroke. *Int. J. Stroke* **2014**, *9*, 985–991. [CrossRef] [PubMed]
27. Kim, J.T.; Jahan, R.; Saver, J.L. Impact of Glucose on Outcomes in Patients Treated With Mechanical Thrombectomy: A Post Hoc Analysis of the Solitaire Flow Restoration With the Intention for Thrombectomy Study. *Stroke* **2016**, *47*, 120–127. [CrossRef]
28. Lane, D.A.; Lip, G.Y. Use of the CHA(2)DS(2)-VASc and HAS-BLED Scores to Aid Decision Making for Thromboprophylaxis in Nonvalvular Atrial Fibrillation. *Circulation* **2012**, *126*, 860–865. [CrossRef]
29. Powers, W.J.; Derdeyn, C.P.; Biller, J.; Coffey, C.S.; Hoh, B.L.; Jauch, E.C.; Johnston, K.C.; Johnston, S.C.; Khalessi, A.A.; Kidwell, C.S.; et al. 2015 American Heart Association/American Stroke Association Focused Update of the 2013 Guidelines for the Early Management of Patients with Acute Ischemic Stroke Regarding Endovascular Treatment: A Guideline for Healthcare Professionals from the American Heart Association/American Stroke Association. *Stroke* **2015**, *46*, 3020–3035.
30. Fiehler, J.; Cognard, C.; Gallitelli, M.; Jansen, O.; Kobayashi, A.; Mattle, H.P.; Muir, K.W.; Mazighi, M.; Schaller, K.; Schellinger, P.D. European Recommendations on Organisation of Interventional Care in Acute Stroke (EROICAS). *Int. J. Stroke Off. J. Int. Stroke Soc.* **2016**, *11*, 701–716. [CrossRef]

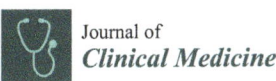

Article

Advanced Neuroimaging Preceding Intravenous Thrombolysis in Acute Ischemic Stroke Patients Is Safe and Effective

Klearchos Psychogios [1,2,*], Apostolos Safouris [1,2], Odysseas Kargiotis [1], Georgios Magoufis [1], Athina Andrikopoulou [1], Ermioni Papageorgiou [1], Maria Chondrogianni [1,2], Georgios Papadimitropoulos [1], Eftihia Polyzogopoulou [3], Stavros Spiliopoulos [4], Elias Brountzos [4], Elefterios Stamboulis [1], Sotirios Giannopoulos [2] and Georgios Tsivgoulis [2]

1. Acute Stroke Unit, Metropolitan Hospital, Ethnarhou Makariou 9, 18547 Piraeus, Greece; safouris@yahoo.com (A.S.); kargiody@gmail.com (O.K.); magoufisgeorge1@icloud.com (G.M.); andriathi@yahoo.gr (A.A.); erminapapageorgiou@yahoo.gr (E.P.); mariachondrogianni@hotmail.gr (M.C.); ge.papadim@gmail.com (G.P.); lstam@med.uoa.gr (E.S.)
2. Second Department of Neurology, National & Kapodistrian University of Athens, School of Medicine, "Attikon" University Hospital, 12462 Athens, Greece; sgiannop@uoi.gr (S.G.); tsivgoulisgiorg@yahoo.gr (G.T.)
3. Emergency Medicine Clinic, National & Kapodistrian University of Athens, School of Medicine, "Attikon" University Hospital, 12462 Athens, Greece; effiepol@med.uoa.gr
4. Second Department of Radiology, Interventional Radiology Unit, "ATTIKON" University General Hospital, 12462 Athens, Greece; stavspiliop@med.uoa.gr (S.S.); eliasbrountzos@gmail.com (E.B.)
* Correspondence: apsychoyio@yahoo.gr; Tel.: +30-(210)480-9788 or +30-(697)340-7804

Abstract: Advanced neuroimaging is one of the most important means that we have in the attempt to overcome time constraints and expand the use of intravenous thrombolysis (IVT). We assessed whether, and how, the prior use of advanced neuroimaging (AN), and more specifically CT/MR perfusion post-processed with RAPID software, regardless of time from symptoms onset, affected the outcomes of acute ischemic stroke (AIS) patients who received IVT. Methods. We retrospectively evaluated consecutive AIS patients who received intravenous thrombolysis monotherapy (without endovascular reperfusion) during a six-year period. The study population was divided into two groups according to the neuroimaging protocol used prior to IVT administration in AIS patients (AN+ vs. AN−). Safety outcomes included any intracranial hemorrhage (ICH) and 3-month mortality. Effectiveness outcomes included door-to-needle time, neurological status (NIHSS-score) on discharge, and functional status at three months assessed by the modified Rankin Scale (mRS). Results. The rate of IVT monotherapy increased from ten patients per year ($n = 29$) in the AN− to fifteen patients per year ($n = 47$) in the AN+ group. Although the onset-to-treatment time was longer in the AN+ cohort, the two groups did not differ in door-to-needle time, discharge NIHSS-score, symptomatic ICH, any ICH, 3-month favorable functional outcome (mRS-scores of 0–1), 3-month functional independence (mRS-scores of 0–2), distribution of 3-month mRS-scores, or 3-month mortality. Conclusion. Our pilot observational study showed that the incorporation of advanced neuroimaging in the acute stroke chain pathway in AIS patients increases the yield of IVT administration without affecting the effectiveness and safety of the treatment.

Keywords: acute stroke; intravenous thrombolysis; perfusion imaging; CT perfusion; MR perfusion; RAPID

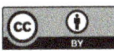

1. Introduction

Intravenous thrombolysis (IVT) with alteplase in acute ischemic stroke (AIS) administered within the first 4.5 hours following symptom onset remains the mainstay of acute reperfusion therapies [1–3]. Despite tissue plasminogen activator (tPA) effectiveness, only a small number of AIS patients worldwide benefit from IVT [4,5]. Short therapeutic time window, strict inclusion and exclusion criteria of the pivotal randomized controlled clinical trials (RCTs), as well as health care system disparities, such as public awareness on how to act in case of stroke symptoms, organization of emergency medical services, and the paucity of organized stroke centers in rural areas [6], have been significant barriers to overcome. Nevertheless, off-label use of IVT [7,8] is increasingly incorporated in the everyday clinical practice of many stroke practitioners.

Advanced neuroimaging may help us overcome time constraints and expand the implementation of acute reperfusion therapies [9]. CT and MR perfusion with automated post-processing software (RAPID, iSchemaView, Menlo Park, CA, USA) have proven effective in recent RCTs, for both mechanical thrombectomy candidates in the late time window (6–24 h) [10,11] and for IVT (4.5–9 h and wake-up patients) [12–14]. Advanced neuroimaging provides a "brain physiology snapshot in time" that can guide decisions for recanalization therapies in clinical practice [15]. Numerous stroke centers and stroke units worldwide have incorporated the use of CT and MR perfusion in their acute therapeutic pathways.

In view of the former considerations, we assessed the differences in the use of IVT monotherapy and the outcomes of the AIS patients with or without the use of advanced neuroimaging.

2. Materials and Methods

We retrospectively evaluated consecutive AIS patients who received IVT admitted to our European Stroke Organization certified stroke unit. We also participate in the SITS (Safe Implementation of Thrombolysis in Stroke) and RES-Q (Registry of Stroke Care Quality) international registries [16,17]. Patients were included if they fulfilled the following criteria: (1) aged over 18 years old; (2) clinically diagnosed with AIS with a measurable neurologic deficit on the National Institute of Health Stroke Scale (NIHSS) presenting within the 4.5 h window from symptom onset; (3) AIS patients were considered eligible for the extended time window of 4.5–9 h if they presented after 4.5 h and sooner than 9 h from last-seen-well (late window patients), according to the clinical and neuroimaging inclusion criteria of the EXTEND trial [10]; (4) AIS patients who woke up with symptoms of stroke («wake-up stroke») were treated according to the WAKE-UP trial [18] protocol; and (5) AIS patients treated with IVT monotherapy. All patients with large vessel occlusion (LVO) who underwent mechanical thrombectomy were excluded. Transient ischemic attacks and stroke mimics were excluded from the current study based on clinical and neuroimaging criteria.

The study population was divided into two different groups according to the neuroimaging protocol used on admission and prior to IVT administration in AIS patients (with prior Advanced Neuroimaging (AN+) vs. without prior advanced neuroimaging (AN−)). Of note, the neuroimaging protocol was modified in our center on December 2017 after the introduction of perfusion imaging (with RAPID software) and on August 2018 after the publication of the WAKE-UP trial. Patients in the first study group (AN−) underwent baseline emergent neurovascular imaging using either non-contrast-enhanced computed tomography (NCCT), with or without CT angiography (CTA), or magnetic resonance imaging (MRI) with magnetic resonance angiography based on the treating physician's decision. Patients in the second study group (AN+) underwent NCCT/CTA/computed tomography perfusion (CTA/CTP) or magnetic resonance angiography/magnetic resonance perfusion (MRA/MRP) unless they presented certain contraindications (e.g., renal insufficiency, severe allergic reactions to iodinised agents, etc.). CT perfusion was performed using two continuous 2.5 cm slabs, starting at the level of the circle of Willis for most patients, lower for those presenting with symptoms suggesting posterior fossa ischemia, and higher for those presenting with symptoms suggestive of cortical ischemia. Ischemic core (rCBF < 30%), critically hypoperfused ischemic region (Tmax > 6 s), and mismatch volume corresponding to ischemic penumbra, were estimated by using RAPID as previously described [19]. The hyperdense vessel sign (HVS), a highly specific marker of arterial obstruction [20], was identified on non-contrast CT if the lumen of any, non-calcified, intracranial artery appeared denser than adjacent or equivalent contralateral arteries. Clot length was quantified based on CT angiography by using standard methodology [21]. The LVO was defined as the occlusion of the internal carotid artery (ICA), basilar artery (BA), and the first segment of the Middle Cerebral Artery (MCA-M1). CT/MR findings were interpreted and extracted independently by experienced neurologists or neuroradiologists that were blinded to clinical outcomes.

The following parameters were recorded for all included patients: (1) demographic characteristics; (2) history of vascular risk factors (diabetes mellitus, hypertension, current smoking, hypercholesterolemia, coronary artery disease, peripheral artery disease, congestive heart failure, and valvular disease) as previously described [22]; (3) prior history of stroke or Transient Ischemic Attack (TIA); (4) laboratory test values on admission (total platelet count, glucose, and low-density lipoprotein (LDL) levels); and (5) admission systolic and diastolic blood pressures, measured using automated blood pressure cuffs. Stroke severity was assessed with the NIHSS (National Institute of Health Stroke Scale) score at admission, 2 h and 24 h post IVT, and at discharge. Safety outcomes included prevalence of symptomatic intracranial hemorrhage (sICH), prevalence of any intracranial hemorrhage in the 24-h post thrombolysis neuroimaging studies, and 3-month mortality. sICH was defined using standard SITS registry definitions (local or remote parenchymatous hemorrhage type 2 combined with an NIHSS-score increase of >4 points or leading to death\22–36 h) [14]. Any intracranial hemorrhage was recorded according to the ECASS criteria [23]. Effectiveness outcomes included door-to-needle time, neurological improvement at 24 h and on discharge, and functional status at discharge and at 3 months by using the modified Rankin Scale (mRS). Functional independence (FI) and favorable functional outcome (FFO) were defined as an mRS-score of 0–2 or an mRS-score of 0–1 at 3 months, respectively. Stroke severity and functional outcome (mRS) at discharge and at 3 months were assessed by certified vascular neurologists as previously described [24].

All follow-up evaluations occurred at 90 ± 10 days from symptom onset at the Stroke Outpatient Clinic of our institution as previously described [25]. The evaluation of the mRS-score was performed by certified vascular neurologists who were unaware of the neuroimaging protocol that was implemented at baseline.

Statistical Analysis

All binary variables were presented as percentages, while continuous variables were presented with their corresponding mean values and standard deviations (SDs), in cases of normal distributions, or as medians with interquartile ranges (IQRs) in cases of skewed distributions. Statistical comparisons between the two groups were performed using the unpaired t test, Mann–Whitney U-test, χ^2 test, and Fisher exact test, as appropriate. The distribution of the 3-month mRS scores between patients treated before and after RAPID implementation was compared using the Cochran–Mantel–Haenszel test and the univariable/multivariable ordinal logistic regression (shift analysis).

All efficacy and safety outcomes of interest were further assessed in univariable and multivariable binary logistic regression models adjusting for the a priori defined confounders of the age and baseline NIHSS-score. The final variables that were independently associated in the multivariable logistic and the ordinal regression analyses with the outcome of interest, were selected using an alpha value of 0.05 and adjusted associations were provided as odds ratios (ORs) or common odds ratios (cORs), with their corresponding 95% confidence intervals (95% CI).

All statistical analyses were conducted with the Stata Statistical Software Release 13 (StataCorp LP, College Station, TX, USA).

3. Results

A total of eight hundred and nineteen patients were screened in the setting of an acute stroke code between February 2015 and January 2021. The complete flowchart of our study is shown in Figure 1. Three hundred and seventy-seven patients were screened before December 2017 (AN implementation) and twenty-six received IVT, whereas four hundred and forty-two were screened after December 2017 and fifty patients among them received IVT (three of them were not screened with prior AN due to contraindications).

Our final cohort was comprised of 76 AIS patients who received IVT throughout the entire study period. All patients who received endovascular reperfusion therapy with mechanical thrombectomy were excluded from our analysis ($n = 71$). Twenty-nine patients received IVT without prior advanced neuroimaging (AN−) and forty-seven patients with the use of advanced neuroimaging (AN+). The rate of IVT monotherapy increased from ten patients per year in the AN− to fifteen patients per year in the AN+ group. Baseline characteristics of the two treatment groups are summarized in Table 1. Patients in the AN+ group were significantly ($p = 0.003$) older than patients in the AN− group (mean age 73 years vs. 63 years, respectively). Median admission NIHSS-scores were 4 points (IQR: 2–7) in the AN− group and 5 points (IQR: 4–9) in the AN+ group, a difference that was also significant ($p = 0.047$). The prevalence of large vessel occlusions was 17.2% in the AN− group and 19.1% in the AN+ group ($p = 0.835$). The location of stroke in posterior circulation was more frequent in the AN− group (34.5%) than in the second study group (19.1%). The median elapsed time between symptom onset (or last-seen-well) to initiation of IVT was significantly longer in the second group (198 min (IQR: 151–240)) in AN+ vs. 121 min ((IQR: 130–220) in AN−; $p < 0.001$), whereas the door-to-needle time was almost identical between the two groups (median 44 min (IQR: 36–60)) in AN− vs. 45 min ((IQR: 30–61) in AN+; $p = 0.956$). The rate of patients treated according to the EXTEND trial or WAKE-UP protocol was significantly higher in the second study group (23.4% vs. 3.4%; $p = 0.020$). All patients were treated with alteplase, except for four patients in the AN+ with large vessel occlusions who were treated with tenecteplase.

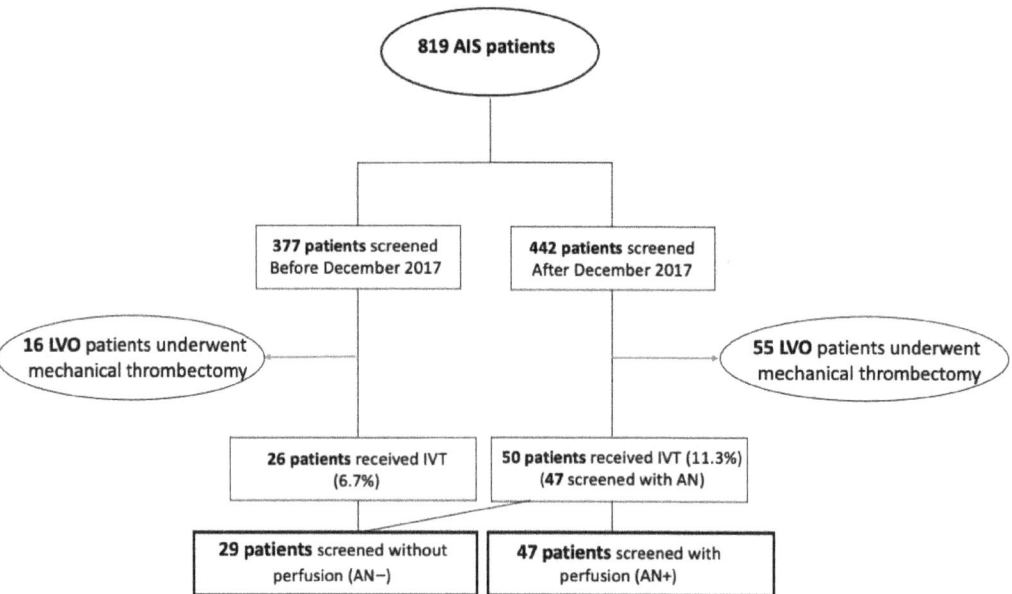

Figure 1. Flowchart of the study population. Acute Ischemic Stroke, AIS; Large vessel occlusion, LVO; intravenous thrombolysis, IVT; Advanced Neuroimaging, AN.

Table 1. Baseline characteristics in patients treated before and after the implementation of advanced neuroimaging.

Baseline Characteristics	AN− (n = 29)	AN+ (n = 47)	p-Value
Age, years (mean, SD)	63 ± 16	73 ± 13	0.003
Weight, kg (mean, SD)	82 ± 18	80 ± 21	0.631
Smoking (%)	27.6%	25.5%	0.850
Hypertension (%)	72.4%	57.4%	0.189
Diabetes (%)	31.0%	17.0%	0.154
Hypercholesterolemia (%)	27.6%	42.6%	0.189
Prior stroke (%)	3.4%	4.3%	0.861
Prior TIA (%)	0.0%	6.4%	0.165
Congestive heart failure (%)	3.0%	0.0%	0.200
Valvular disease (%)	6.9%	0.0%	0.068
Coronary artery disease (%)	10.3%	4.3%	0.298
Peripheral Arterial Disease (%)	3.4%	6.4%	0.578
Extended window 4.5–9 h (%)	0.0%	14.9%	0.029
Wake up stroke (%)	3.4%	8.5%	0.387
Extended window or wake up	3.4%	23.4%	0.020
NIHSS-score on admission, points (median, IQR)	4 (2–7)	5 (4–9)	0.047
Systolic BP on admission, mmHg (mean ± SD)	152 ± 34	153 ± 21	0.837
Diastolic BP on admission, mmHg (mean ± SD)	80 ± 15	82 ± 14	0.549
Platelet count on admission, $\times 10^9$/L (mean ± SD)	267 ± 152	228 ± 83	0.477
LDL on admission, mg/dL (mean ± SD)	137.5 ± 49	129.5 ± 34	0.554
Glucose on admission, mg/dL (mean ± SD)	129 ± 39	129 ± 39	0.174
Onset-to-imaging time, min (median, IQR)	105 (87.5–161)	160 (120–202.5)	0.011
Door-to-needle time, min (median, IQR)	43.5 (36–60)	45 (30–61)	0.956
Onset-to-treatment time (median, IQR)	121 (110–153)	197.5 (151–240)	<0.001
ASPECTS (median, IQR)	10 (9–10)	10 (9–10)	0.278
Duration of Hospitalization (median, IQR)	10 (8–18)	9.5 (5–16.5)	0.725
Location of stroke in the left hemisphere (%)	43.2%	56.8%	0.564
Location of stroke in posterior circulation (%)	34.5%	19.1%	0.199
Hyperdense vessel sign in CT (%)	3.6%	4.3%	0.870
MR imaging (%)	6.9%	10.6%	0.584
Thrombus length, mm (median, IQR)	8.5 (5.75–14)	12 (9–20)	0.053
Large Vessel occlusion (%)	17.2%	19.1%	0.835
Medium Vessel Occlusion (%)	44.8%	40.4%	0.706

Blood pressure, BP; National Institute of Health Stroke Scale, NIHSS; interquartile range, IQR; Alberta Stroke Program Early CT score, ASPECTS; standard deviation, SD.

The neuroimaging characteristics are summarized in Tables 1 and 2. The median thrombus length tended to be higher in the AN+ group (12 vs. 9 mm, $p = 0.053$). The median ASPECTS score and the presence of a hyperdense vessel sign were similar across the study groups. MR imaging was performed in 6.9% of AN− and 10.3% of AN+ patients ($p = 0.584$). In patients who underwent perfusion imaging, the mean ischemic core volume was calculated at 2.1 ± 1.2 mL and the mean volume of critical hypoperfusion was 16.3 ± 4.0 mL (Table 2).

Table 2. Neuroimaging characteristics of patients treated after the implementation of perfusion imaging.

Mean ischemic core volume (rCBF < 30%) (mean ± SD) (mL)	2.1 ± 1.2
Mean volume of critical hypo perfusion (Tmax > 6 s) (mean ± SD) (mL)	16.3 ± 4
Mean mismatch volume (mean ± SD) (mL)	13.5 ± 3.3

Table 3 summarizes the effectiveness and the safety outcomes in the two patient groups. There was only one missing 3-month follow-up evaluation in each treatment group. Neurological status assessed by NIHSS at 2 h, 24 h, and at hospital discharge was similar between the two groups. The rates of sICH (3.4% vs. 0%; $p = 0.2$) and any intracranial hemorrhage (6.9% vs. 10.6%; $p = 0.584$) were similar between the two groups. The rates of 3-month favorable functional outcome (75% vs. 78.3%; $p = 0.746$), 3-month functional independence (82.1% vs. 89.1%; $p = 0.394$), and 3-month mortality (0% vs. 4.3%; $p = 0.263$) did not differ between the two groups either. A secondary analysis restricted to the patients in the early time window shows similar results (Supplemental Table S1).

Table 3. Outcomes in patients treated before and after the implementation of AN.

Outcomes	AN− (n = 29)	AN+ (n = 47)	p-Value
Any Hemorrhagic transformation (%)	6.9%	10.6%	0.584
Symptomatic Intracranial Hemorrhage (%)	3.4%	0.0%	0.200
NIHSS-score 2 h, points (median, IQR)	2 (0.5–3.5)	3 (1–5.25)	0.230
NIHSS 24 h, points (median, IQR)	1 (0–4)	1.5 (0–4)	0.697
Discharge NIHSS (median, IQR)	0 (0–2.5)	0 (0–3)	0.977
3-month mRS-score, points (median, IQR)	2 (1–4)	3 (1–5)	0.614 ***
3-month Functional Independence (%) *	82.1%	89.1%	0.394
3-month Favorable Functional Outcome (%) **	75.0%	78.3%	0.746
3-month Mortality (%)	0.0%	4.3%	0.263

National Institute of Health Stroke Scale, NIHSS. * mRS-scores of 0–2. ** mRS-scores of 0–1. *** Cochran–Mantel–Haenszel test.

The distribution of 3-month mRS-scores was similar between the two groups (p for Cochran–Mantel–Haenszel test: 0.466). Table 4 shows the univariable and multivariable associations of the neuroimaging protocol with safety and efficacy outcomes in multivariable logistic regression models adjusting for the age and admission NIHSS-score. There was no association between the advanced neuroimaging protocol and any ICH (crude OR 1.60, 95% CI: 0.29–8.88; p = 0.586), functional independence at three months (crude OR 1.78, 95% CI: 0.47–6.8; p = 0.398), and favorable functional outcome at three months (crude OR 1.20, 95% CI: 0.40–3.63; p = 0.747). In adjusted analysis AN was associated with better functional independence at 3 months (adjusted OR 12.89, 95% CI: 1.47–113; p = 0.021).

Table 4. Univariable and multivariable binary logistic regression analyses evaluating the association of the use of advanced neuroimaging in acute stroke chain pathway with outcomes.

Outcomes	Crude OR (95% CI)	p-Value	Adjusted * OR (95% CI)	p-Value
Any ICH	1.60 (0.29, 8.88)	0.586	1.30 (0.21, 8.01)	0.840
Functional Independence at 3 months	1.78 (0.47, 6.80)	0.398	12.89 (1.47, 113.00)	0.021
Favorable Functional Outcome at 3 months	1.20 (0.40, 3.63)	0.747	1.97 (0.54, 7.17)	0.304

Odds ratio, OR; confidence intervals, CI. * Adjusted for the age and baseline NIHSS score.

4. Discussion

Our pilot observational single-center study showed that the shift in our clinical practice, with the incorporation of advanced neuroimaging in AIS patients, increases the yield of IVT administration by approximately 50% without major effectiveness and safety repercussions. On the contrary, all comparisons showed that it is equally safe, and even in a population with more negative prognostic factors (higher admission NIHSS-score, older age, longer thrombus), we documented a trend towards better functional outcomes without any delays in door-to-needle time. Better outcomes in patients with prior AN possibly reflect the comparison between different study periods and the accumulating experience of the stroke team through the years. It might also encompass the more favorable prognosis of patients treated in the extended time window, already proven by large clinical trials [12]. However, this result should be treated with caution given the large confidence intervals due to our small study sample and the fact that it was not demonstrated in the crude analysis as well.

Almost 25% of patients in the advanced neuroimaging group were treated based on neuroimaging criteria (either extended time window 4.5–9 h or wake-up strokes, see Figure 2) and this further substantiates our previous observations [20]. Considering that the extra time needed to perform the CT perfusion and to acquire the RAPID templates is at least ten min, it is striking that the median door-to-needle time was only one min longer in the advanced neuroimaging group compared to the median door-to-needle time in the standard neuroimaging group. This observation reflects the interplay of many other important key factors: the acquired experience of the personnel who are involved in the acute stroke chain, the increased use of perfusion imaging particularly in "borderline" cases (e.g., stroke mimics) [26] that otherwise would necessitate two different imaging modalities (CT and MRI), and the fact that the clinical decision in most cases was made immediately after the non-contrast CT and IVT could be initiated in the radiology department before completion of the perfusion imaging.

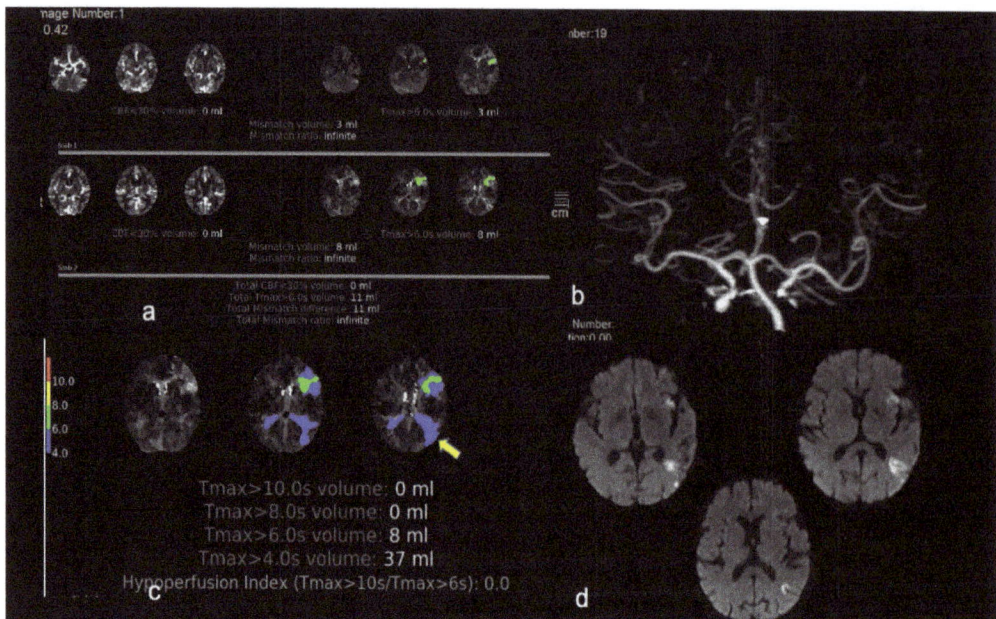

Figure 2. This is an illustrative case of a patient fulfilling both neuroimaging and clinical EXTEND eligibility criteria who was treated successfully with intravenous thrombolysis in the extended time window. An 80-year-old woman was transferred from an island to the emergency department 5 h after an acute onset of expressive aphasia, mild right facial paresis, and mild right upper arm paresis (NIHSS score 9 points). (**a**) Her CT-perfusion mismatch map post-processed with RAPID software demonstrated a hypoperfused region of 11 mL in the Broca's area (shown in green) and no area of reduced cerebral blood flow, resulting in a 11 mL mismatch difference (infinite mismatch ratio). (**b**,**c**) CT angiogram revealed no large vessel occlusion. The patient fulfilled all EXTEND eligibility criteria; IVT with alteplase started 5 h and 45 min after symptom onset with partial resolution of symptoms at the end of tPA infusion (NIHSS-score of 6 points). (**d**) Repeat MRI at 24 h demonstrated a small insular infarct and another acute infarct in the left temporoparietal region which was captured in the Tmax maps of initial perfusion imaging as Tmax > 4 s prolongation (c/arrow). The patient's mRS-score at three months was 0.

The present study investigated the effect of advanced neuroimaging on IVT monotherapy. Patients who received endovascular reperfusion therapy were excluded from our analyses. Consequently, our cohort included predominantly mild to moderate severity strokes with a small ischemic core and penumbra volumes or patients with LVO who responded to IVT with successful reperfusion and did not need further endovascular treatment. This probably induces a selection bias by excluding AIS patients with a more "unfavorable prognosis". Previous studies [27,28] that served as pilot studies for the major MT RCTs, have underscored the feasibility of this physiologic imaging approach in cases with LVO-attributed ischemic stroke. Major RCTs that also used the same approach in the early time window [29,30] showed even greater treatment effects, substantially enhancing the use of this approach in clinical practice.

The use of perfusion imaging in AIS patients who present in the first 4.5 h after symptoms onset is still controversial. In our cohort, patients who did not present with a favorable profile (based on neuroimaging criteria) in the early time window, were still offered tPA according to current recommendations. The majority of these patients (n = 19) had no ischemic core or had only hypoperfusion that did not meet the Tmax > 6 s typical criteria of the penumbra. Some of these patients (4/19, 21%) had a "benign oligemia" profile with Tmax prolongation > 4 s, but with either ongoing clinical symptoms or symptoms in partial resolution. This could be due to technical issues (lesion outside the selected slabs when

CT perfusion was used), lacunar infarcts [31], spontaneous recanalization before imaging, or small lesions in the posterior circulation [32] where CT perfusion has lower sensitivity. However, it may also imply that among the "benign oligemia" regions, there might exist grey zones close to the Tmax 6 s threshold delay that correspond more to critical hypoperfused areas, and which, if left untreated, may lead to permanent neurological deficits. Indeed, the DEFUSE study [33] showed that among patients who did not experience early reperfusion, Tmax > 4 s threshold was more accurate in predicting final infarct volume. Even though Tmax > 6 s has been proven to be the best perfusion measurement marker in predicting clinical outcome [34,35] after successful recanalization, infarct growth is perhaps a more complex process influenced by many clinical and pathological factors.

Based on current knowledge, perfusion imaging may not be critical for therapeutic decisions in the early time window by excluding patients with large ischemic core or those with no or minimal perfusion deficit. For instance, the "too good to treat" pattern [36] of small distal perfusion lesions with no vessel occlusion, needs to be studied in larger populations and with more potent thrombolytic agents, including tenecteplase. Even though time since last-seen-well is a poor proxy for perfusion status, we are far from changing the paradigm of IVT administration and endovascular treatment in the early time window from time-based to imaging-based. Nevertheless, in the era of precision medicine and shared decision-making [37], perfusion imaging may still provide additional support to the clinician: for instance, to communicate the decisions with the patient and the patient proxies, strengthen the diagnostic confidence by excluding stroke mimics, accelerate the processes in fast-progressors, and possibly, predict prognosis.

Certain limitations of the present pilot study need to be acknowledged including the single-center retrospective design and analysis of a prospectively maintained patient database, the relatively small sample size, the lack of randomization, and blinding in the evaluation of clinical outcomes. In addition, a major limitation is the heterogeneity induced by the comparison of data from different time periods where practices and experiences of the involved personnel are changing and protocols are reviewed and updated periodically.

5. Conclusions

In conclusion, the implementation of advanced neuroimaging in unselected AIS patients receiving reperfusion monotherapy with IVT, results in an increase of tPA administration rates without delaying door-to-needle time and without raising safety or effectiveness concerns.

Supplementary Materials: The following are available online at https://www.mdpi.com/article/10.3390/jcm10132819/s1, Table S1: Outcomes in patients treated before and after the implementation of AN, confined in patients treated with IVT during the early time window.

Author Contributions: Conceptualization, K.P. and G.T.; writing—original draft preparation, K.P. and G.T.; writing—review and editing, K.P., A.S., O.K., G.M., A.A., Ermioni Papageorgiou (E.P.), M.C., G.P., Eftihia Polyzogopoulou (E.P.), S.S., E.B., E.S., S.G. and G.T.; visualization, G.T.; supervision, K.P. and G.T. All authors have read and agreed to the published version of the manuscript.

Funding: This research received no external funding.

Institutional Review Board Statement: Ethical review and approval were waived for this study as per current Greek law regarding retrospective studies of anonymized standard care data. No Internal Review Board approval and no written consent were required but patients were informed of their participation and offered the possibility to withdraw.

Informed Consent Statement: Informed consent was obtained regarding the use of imaging data.

Data Availability Statement: The data presented in this study are available on request from the corresponding author. The data are not publicly available due to privacy.

Conflicts of Interest: The authors declare no conflict of interest.

References

1. Berge, E.; Whiteley, W.; Audebert, H.; De Marchis, G.M.; Fonseca, A.C.; Padiglioni, C.; de la Ossa, N.P.; Strbian, D.; Tsivgoulis, G.; Turc, G. European Stroke Organisation (ESO) guidelines on intravenous thrombolysis for acute ischaemic stroke. *Eur. Stroke J.* **2021**, *6*, 1–62. [CrossRef] [PubMed]
2. Powers, W.J.; Rabinstein, A.A.; Ackerson, T.; Adeoye, O.M.; Bambakidis, N.C.; Becker, K.; Biller, J.; Brown, M.; Demaerschalk, B.M.; Hoh, B.; et al. Guidelines for the Early Management of Patients with Acute Ischemic Stroke: 2019 Update to the 2018 Guidelines for the Early Management of Acute Ischemic Stroke: A Guideline for Healthcare Professionals from the American Heart Association/American Stroke Association. *Stroke* **2019**, *50*, e344–e418. [CrossRef] [PubMed]
3. Tsivgoulis, G.; Kargiotis, O.; Alexandrov, A.V. Intravenous thrombolysis for acute ischemic stroke: A bridge between two centuries. *Expert Rev. Neurother.* **2017**, *17*, 819–837. [CrossRef]
4. Eissa, A.; Krass, I.; Levi, C.; Sturm, J.; Ibrahim, R.; Bajorek, B. Understanding the reasons behind the low utilisation of thrombolysis in stroke. *Australas. Med. J.* **2013**, *6*, 152–167. [CrossRef]
5. De Sousa, D.A.; Von Martial, R.; Abilleira, S.; Gattringer, T.; Kobayashi, A.; Gallofré, M.; Fazekas, F.; Szikora, I.; Feigin, V.; Caso, V.; et al. Access to and delivery of acute ischaemic stroke treatments: A survey of national scientific societies and stroke experts in 44 European countries. *Eur. Stroke J.* **2019**, *4*, 13–28. [CrossRef]
6. Soto-Cámara, R.; González-Santos, J.; González-Bernal, J.; Trejo-Gabriel-Galán, J.M. Factors associated with a rapid call for assistance for patients with ischemic stroke. *Emergencias* **2020**, *32*, 33–39.
7. Tsivgoulis, G.; Kargiotis, O.; De Marchis, G.; Kohrmann, M.; Sandset, E.C.; Karapanayiotides, T.; de Sousa, D.A.; Sarraj, A.; Safouris, A.; Psychogios, K.; et al. Off-label use of intravenous thrombolysis for acute ischemic stroke: A critical appraisal of randomized and real-world evidence. *Ther. Adv. Neurol. Disord.* **2021**, *14*, 1756286421997368. [CrossRef]
8. Tsivgoulis, G.; Safouris, A.; Alexandrov, A.V. Safety of intravenous thrombolysis for acute ischemic stroke in specific conditions. *Expert Opin. Drug Saf.* **2015**, *14*, 845–864. [CrossRef]
9. Tsivgoulis, G.; Katsanos, A.H.; Schellinger, P.D.; Köhrmann, M.; Caso, V.; Palaiodimou, L.; Magoufis, G.; Arthur, A.; Fischer, U.; Alexandrov, A.V. Advanced Neuroimaging in Stroke Patient Selection for Mechanical Thrombectomy. *Stroke* **2018**, *49*, 3067–3070. [CrossRef] [PubMed]
10. Nogueira, R.G.; Jadhav, A.P.; Haussen, D.C.; Bonafe, A.; Budzik, R.F.; Bhuva, P.; Yavagal, D.R.; Ribo, M.; Cognard, C.; Hanel, R.A.; et al. Thrombectomy 6 to 24 Hours after Stroke with a Mismatch between Deficit and Infarct. *N. Engl. J. Med.* **2018**, *378*, 11–21. [CrossRef]
11. Albers, G.W.; Marks, M.P.; Kemp, S.; Christensen, S.; Tsai, J.P.; Ortega-Gutierrez, S.; McTaggart, R.A.; Torbey, M.T.; Kim-Tenser, M.; Leslie-Mazwi, T.; et al. Thrombectomy for Stroke at 6 to 16 Hours with Selection by Perfusion Imaging. *N. Engl. J. Med.* **2018**, *378*, 708–718. [CrossRef]
12. Ma, H.; Campbell, B.C.V.; Parsons, M.W.; Churilov, L.; Levi, C.R.; Hsu, C.; Kleinig, T.J.; Wijeratne, T.; Curtze, S.; Dewey, H.M.; et al. Thrombolysis guided by perfusion imaging up to 9 hours after onset of stroke. *N. Engl. J. Med.* **2019**, *380*, 1795–1803. [CrossRef] [PubMed]
13. Campbell, B.C.V.; Ma, H.; Ringleb, P.A.; Parsons, M.W.; Churilov, L.; Bendszus, M.; Levi, C.R.; Hsu, C.; Kleinig, T.J.; Fatar, M.; et al. Extending thrombolysis to 4·5–9 h and wake-up stroke using perfusion imaging: A systematic review and meta-analysis of individual patient data. *Lancet* **2019**, *394*, 139–147. [CrossRef]
14. Thomalla, G.; Boutitie, F.; Ma, H.; Koga, M.; Ringleb, P.; Schwamm, L.H.; Wu, O.; Bendszus, M.; Bladin, C.F.; Campbell, B.C.V.; et al. Intravenous alteplase for stroke with unknown time of onset guided by advanced imaging: Systematic review and meta-analysis of individual patient data. *Lancet* **2020**, *396*, 1574–1584. [CrossRef]
15. Hill, M.D.; Goyal, M.; Demchuk, A.M.; Fisher, M. Ischemic Stroke Tissue-Window in the New Era of Endovascular Treatment. *Stroke* **2015**, *46*, 2332–2334. [CrossRef] [PubMed]
16. Tsivgoulis, G.; Kargiotis, O.; Rudolf, J.; Komnos, A.; Tavernarakis, A.; Karapanayiotides, T.; Ellul, J.; Katsanos, A.H.; Giannopoulos, S.; Gryllia, M.; et al. Intravenous thrombolysis for acute ischemic stroke in Greece: The Safe Implementation of Thrombolysis in Stroke registry 15-year experience. *Ther. Adv. Neurol. Disord.* **2018**, *11*, 1756286418783578. [CrossRef] [PubMed]
17. Tsivgoulis, G.; Goyal, N.; Mikulik, R.; Sharma, V.K.; Katsanos, A.H.; Zand, R.; Paliwal, P.R.; Roussopoulou, A.; Volny, O.; Pandhi, A.; et al. Eligibility for mechanical thrombectomy in acute ischemic stroke: A phase IV multi-center screening log registry. *J. Neurol. Sci.* **2016**, *371*, 96–99. [CrossRef]
18. Thomalla, G.; Simonsen, C.Z.; Boutitie, F.; Andersen, G.; Berthezene, Y.; Cheng, B.; Cheripelli, B.; Cho, T.-H.; Fazekas, F.; Fiehler, J.; et al. MRI-Guided Thrombolysis for Stroke with Unknown Time of Onset. *New Engl. J. Med.* **2018**, *379*, 611–622. [CrossRef]
19. Psychogios, K.; Magoufis, G.; Safouris, A.; Kargiotis, O.; Katsanos, A.H.; Spiliopoulos, S.; Papageorgiou, E.; Palaiodimou, L.; Brountzos, E.; Stamboulis, E.; et al. Eligibility for intravenous thrombolysis in acute ischemic stroke patients presenting in the 4.5–9 h window. *Neuroradiology* **2020**, *62*, 733–739. [CrossRef]
20. Mair, G.; Boyd, E.V.; Chappell, F.M.; Von Kummer, R.; Lindley, R.I.; Sandercock, P.; Wardlaw, J.M.; IST-3 Collaborative Group. Sensitivity and Specificity of the Hyperdense Artery Sign for Arterial Obstruction in Acute Ischemic Stroke. *Stroke* **2015**, *46*, 102–107. [CrossRef]
21. Riedel, C.H.; Jensen, U.; Rohr, A.; Ulmer, S.; Tietke, M.; Alfke, K.; Jansen, O. Assessment of thrombus in acute stroke using ultra-thin slice nonenhanced CT reconstructions. *Stroke* **2010**, *41*, 1659–1664. [CrossRef]

22. Psychogios, K.; Palaiodimou, L.; Katsanos, A.H.; Magoufis, G.; Safouris, A.; Kargiotis, O.; Spiliopoulos, S.; Papageorgiou, E.; Theodorou, A.; Voumvourakis, K.; et al. Real-world comparative safety and efficacy of tenecteplase versus alteplase in acute ischemic stroke patients with large vessel occlusion. *Ther. Adv. Neurol. Disord.* **2021**, *14*, 1756286420986727. [CrossRef]
23. Fiorelli, M.; Bastianello, S.; Von Kummer, R.; Del Zoppo, G.J.; Larrue, V.; Lesaffre, E.; Ringleb, A.P.; Lorenzano, S.; Manelfe, C.; Bozzao, L. Hemorrhagic Transformation Within 36 Hours of a Cerebral Infarct: Relationships with early clinical deterioration and 3-month outcome in the European Cooperative Acute Stroke Study I (ECASS I) cohort. *Stroke* **1999**, *30*, 2280–2284. [CrossRef] [PubMed]
24. Goyal, N.; Tsivgoulis, G.; Pandhi, A.; Dillard, K.; Katsanos, A.H.; Magoufis, G.; Chang, J.J.; Zand, R.; Hoit, D.; Safouris, A.; et al. Admission hyperglycemia and outcomes in large vessel occlusion strokes treated with mechanical thrombectomy. *J. NeuroInterv. Surg.* **2018**, *10*, 112–117. [CrossRef] [PubMed]
25. Tsivgoulis, G.; Goyal, N.; Katsanos, A.H.; Malhotra, K.; Ishfaq, M.F.; Pandhi, A.; Frohler, M.T.; Spiotta, A.M.; Anadani, M.; Psychogios, M.; et al. Intravenous thrombolysis for large vessel or distal occlusions presenting with mild stroke severity. *Eur. J. Neurol.* **2020**, *27*, 1039–1047. [CrossRef] [PubMed]
26. Psychogios, K.; Kargiotis, O.; Safouris, A.; Magoufis, G.; Gelagoti, M.; Bonakis, A.; Stamboulis, E.; Tsivgoulis, G. Perfusion imaging averting intravenous thrombolysis in stroke mimics. *Neurol. Sci.* **2021**, *10*, 2591–2594. [CrossRef] [PubMed]
27. Turk, A.S.; Nyberg, E.M.; Chaudry, M.I.; Turner, R.D.; Magarik, J.A.; Nicholas, J.S.; Holmstedt, C.A.; Chalela, J.A.; Hays, A.; Lazaridis, C.; et al. Utilization of CT perfusion patient selection for mechanical thrombectomy irrespective of time: A comparison of functional outcomes and complications. *J. NeuroInterv. Surg.* **2012**, *5*, 518–522. [CrossRef]
28. Turk, A.; Magarik, J.A.; Chaudry, I.; Turner, R.D.; Nicholas, J.; Holmstedt, C.A.; Chalela, J.; Hays, A.; Lazaridis, C.; Jauch, E.; et al. CT perfusion-guided patient selection for endovascular treatment of acute ischemic stroke is safe and effective. *J. NeuroInterv. Surg.* **2011**, *4*, 261–265. [CrossRef]
29. Campbell, B.; Mitchell, P.J.; Kleinig, T.; Dewey, H.M.; Churilov, L.; Yassi, N.; Yan, B.; Dowling, R.J.; Parsons, M.W.; Oxley, T.; et al. Endovascular Therapy for Ischemic Stroke with Perfusion-Imaging Selection. *New Engl. J. Med.* **2015**, *372*, 1009–1018. [CrossRef]
30. Saver, J.L.; Goyal, M.; Bonafe, A.; Diener, H.-C.; Levy, E.I.; Pereira, V.M.; Albers, G.W.; Cognard, C.; Cohen, D.J.; Hacke, W.; et al. Stent-Retriever Thrombectomy after Intravenous t-PA vs. t-PA Alone in Stroke. *New Engl. J. Med.* **2015**, *372*, 2285–2295. [CrossRef]
31. Rudilosso, S.; Urra, X.; Román, L.S.; Laredo, C.; López-Rueda, A.; Amaro, S.; Oleaga, L.; Chamorro, Á. Perfusion Deficits and Mismatch in Patients with Acute Lacunar Infarcts Studied with Whole-Brain CT Perfusion. *AJNR Am. J. Neuroradiol.* **2015**, *36*, 1407–1412. [CrossRef] [PubMed]
32. Ostman, C.; Garcia-Esperon, C.; Lillicrap, T.; Tomari, S.; Holliday, E.; Levi, C.; Bivard, A.; Parsons, M.W.; Spratt, N.J. Multi-modal Computed Tomography Increases the Detection of Posterior Fossa Strokes Compared to Brain Non-contrast Computed Tomography. *Front. Neurol.* **2020**, *11*, 588064. [CrossRef]
33. Olivot, J.-M.; Mlynash, M.; Thijs, V.N.; Kemp, S.; Lansberg, M.G.; Wechsler, L.; Bammer, R.; Marks, M.P.; Albers, G.W. Optimal Tmax Threshold for Predicting Penumbral Tissue in Acute Stroke. *Stroke* **2009**, *40*, 469–475. [CrossRef] [PubMed]
34. Bivard, A.; Levi, C.; Spratt, N.; Parsons, M. Perfusion CT in Acute Stroke: A Comprehensive Analysis of Infarct and Penumbra. *Radiology* **2013**, *267*, 543–550. [CrossRef] [PubMed]
35. Wheeler, H.M.; Mlynash, M.; Inoue, M.; Tipirneni, A.; Liggins, J.; Zaharchuk, G.; Straka, M.; Kemp, S.; Bammer, R.; Lansberg, M.G.; et al. Early Diffusion-Weighted Imaging and Perfusion-Weighted Imaging Lesion Volumes Forecast Final Infarct Size in DEFUSE 2. *Stroke* **2013**, *44*, 681–685. [CrossRef]
36. Bivard, A.; Lou, M.; Levi, C.R.; Krishnamurthy, V.; Cheng, X.; Aviv, R.I.; McElduff, P.; Lin, L.; Kleinig, T.; O'Brien, B.; et al. Too good to treat? ischemic stroke patients with small computed tomography perfusion lesions may not benefit from thrombolysis. *Ann. Neurol.* **2016**, *80*, 286–293. [CrossRef] [PubMed]
37. Tikkinen, K.A.O.; Guyatt, G.H. Understanding of research results, evidence summaries and their applicability—not critical appraisal—are core skills of medical curriculum. *BMJ Evid. Based Med.* **2021**. [CrossRef]

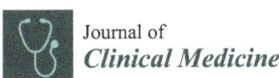

Article

Low Hypoperfusion Intensity Ratio Is Associated with a Favorable Outcome Even in Large Ischemic Core and Delayed Recanalization Time

Jang-Hyun Baek [1,2], Young Dae Kim [2,3], Ki Jeong Lee [2,4], Jin Kyo Choi [2,5], Minyoul Baik [2], Byung Moon Kim [6], Dong Joon Kim [6], Ji Hoe Heo [2,3] and Hyo Suk Nam [2,3,*]

1. Department of Neurology, Kangbuk Samsung Hospital, Sungkyunkwan University School of Medicine, Seoul 10450, Korea; janghyun.baek@gmail.com
2. Department of Neurology, Severance Hospital, Yonsei University College of Medicine, Seoul 03722, Korea; neuro05@yuhs.ac (Y.D.K.); juno8263@gmail.com (K.J.L.); jksnail85@yuhs.ac (J.K.C.); minyoulbaik@yuhs.ac (M.B.); jhheo@yuhs.ac (J.H.H.)
3. Integrative Research Institute for Cerebral and Cardiovascular Diseases, Yonsei University College of Medicine, Seoul 03722, Korea
4. Department of Neurology, National Health Insurance Service Ilsan Hospital, Ilsan 10444, Korea
5. Department of Neurology, Seoul Medical Center, Seoul 02053, Korea
6. Department of Radiology, Severance Hospital, Yonsei University College of Medicine, Seoul 03722, Korea; bmoon21@hanmail.net (B.M.K.); djkimmd@yuhs.ac (D.J.K.)
* Correspondence: hsnam@yuhs.ac; Tel.: +822-2228-1617; Fax: +822-393-0705

Abstract: In ischemic brain tissue, hypoperfusion severity can be assessed using the hypoperfusion intensity ratio (HIR). We evaluated the link between HIR and clinical outcomes after successful recanalization by endovascular treatment. We retrospectively reviewed 162 consecutive patients who underwent endovascular treatment for intracranial large vessel occlusion. The HIR was calculated using an automated software program, with initial computed tomography perfusion images. The HIR was compared between patients with and without favorable outcomes. To observe the modifying effect of the HIR on the well-known major outcome determinants, regression analyses were performed in the low and high HIR groups. The median HIR value was significantly lower in patients with a favorable outcome, with an optimal cut-off point of 0.54. The HIR was an independent factor for a favorable outcome in a specific multivariable model and was significantly correlated with the Alberta Stroke Program Early Computed Tomography Score (ASPECTS). In contrast to the high HIR group, the low HIR group showed that ASPECTS and onset-to-recanalization time were not independently associated with a favorable outcome. Finally, the low HIR group had a more favorable outcome even in cases with an unfavorable ASPECTS and onset-to-recanalization time. The HIR could be useful in predicting outcomes after successful recanalization.

Keywords: hypoperfusion; collaterality; stroke; outcome; thrombectomy

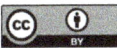

1. Introduction

Hypoperfusion severity and duration are important factors affecting the clinical outcome of patients with acute ischemic stroke who undergo endovascular treatment (EVT). Collateral status is a commonly used method that reflects hypoperfusion severity. Robust collateral flow is associated with smaller ischemic core lesions and slower progression, which may lead to improved clinical outcomes [1–4]. Moreover, time windows for EVT eligibility can be determined based on the collateral status. Patients with better collateral flow may have a more favorable outcome, even in cases in which recanalization is delayed [5].

Hypoperfusion severity can be assessed directly using the hypoperfusion intensity ratio (HIR) [6]. The HIR reflects the proportion of the critically hypoperfused lesion ($T_{max} > 10$ s) in the whole hypoperfused lesion (e.g., $T_{max} > 6$ s) on perfusion images [7,8].

The HIR correlates well with the quality of the collateral status and is considered a quantitative marker of the collateral status [7,9,10]. Furthermore, the HIR has been reported to be significantly associated with initial stroke severity, target mismatch profile, and infarct growth [6–8,11]. Based on the collateral nature of the HIR, we assumed that the clinical outcome after EVT may be affected by the HIR, as in the case of the collateral status.

Accordingly, we hypothesized that a low HIR is associated with a favorable outcome, even in patients with a lower Alberta Stroke Program Early Computed Tomography Score (ASPECTS) or longer onset-to-recanalization time in patients who achieved recanalization through EVT.

2. Materials and Methods

2.1. Participants

We retrospectively reviewed consecutive patients with acute stroke who underwent EVT for intracranial large artery occlusion in the anterior circulation between January 2016 and April 2020. All patients had been registered to a prospectively maintained registry of a tertiary stroke center. EVT was considered for patients who met the following criteria: (1) Computed tomography (CT) angiography-confirmed, endovascularly accessible intracranial occlusions associated with neurological symptoms; (2) in the earlier study period, within 8 h from stroke onset; patients within 8–12 h were also considered if they had an ASPECTS ≥ 7; (3) the eligibility criteria of the Diffusion and Perfusion Imaging Evaluation for Understanding Stroke Evolution 3 (DEFUSE 3) and DWI or CTP Assessment with Clinical Mismatch in the Triage of Wake-Up and Late Presenting Strokes Undergoing Neurointervention with Trevo (DAWN) trials were applied to patients within 6–24 h from stroke onset; and (4) initial National Institutes of Health Stroke Scale (NIHSS) score ≥ 4. We also preferably performed EVT for patients with a premorbid modified Rankin Scale (mRS) score ≤ 3. Patients eligible for intravenous tissue plasminogen activator treatment were treated with 0.9 mg/kg tissue plasminogen activator. EVT procedures were performed under local anesthesia. In most cases, a stent retriever was used as the front-line EVT modality and a balloon-guiding catheter was routinely used. The detailed procedure is described elsewhere [12].

We included patients with intracranial large vessel occlusion, which was defined as occlusion of the intracranial internal carotid artery or middle cerebral artery M1 or proximal M2 segment, and those in whom the occlusion was successfully recanalized by EVT. Successful recanalization was defined as modified Thrombolysis in Cerebral Infarction grade 2b or 3.

2.2. Imaging and Clinical Data

All patients underwent CT as soon as they arrived at the hospital. The pretreatment CT scan included non-contrast CT images, CT angiography, and CT perfusion images. To obtain the HIR, hypoperfusion lesion volumes were quantitatively assessed from CT perfusion images using an automated software (RAPID, iSchemaView, Menlo Park, CA, USA). The lesion volume was measured by a stroke neurologist without any manual correction. The HIR was calculated as the ratio of the lesion volume with $T_{max} > 10$ s to $T_{max} > 6$ s [7].

Data on all variables used in this study were collected from the prospective registry of patients with acute stroke. The functional outcome was assessed based on the mRS score at 3 months after stroke onset and was primarily evaluated by stroke neurologists during the patient's routine clinical follow-up at 3 months ± 2 weeks. If a patient was unable to present to the follow-up appointment, a stroke neurologist or a trained nurse interviewed the patient or their family via telephone to determine the mRS score using a standard questionnaire. A favorable outcome was defined as an mRS score of 0–2. Intracerebral hemorrhage (ICH) was assessed on follow-up CT or magnetic resonance images obtained 24 ± 6 h after EVT. The assessment of ICH was based on the consensus of stroke neurologists, neurointerventionalists, and neuroradiologists during the regular stroke conference. The determination of ICH was immediately entered into the prospective registry. ICH was regarded as symptomatic if the patient's NIHSS score increased by ≥ 4 according to the European Cooperative Acute Stroke Study III [13].

The ASPECTS was reassessed by two independent neurointerventionalists and stroke neurologists [14], who only had access to the initial non-contrast CT images and who were completely blinded to any endovascular outcome and clinical information, except for the lesion side. The interrater agreement for the ASPECTS was good (intraclass correlation coefficient, 0.657). Discrepancies in the assessment of cases were resolved by consensus.

2.3. Statistical Analysis

Based on the study hypotheses, we performed the following analyses step by step. First, to evaluate the association between the HIR and clinical outcomes, patients were assigned to the favorable outcome group or the unfavorable outcome group. Then, (1) HIR values were compared among groups along with patient demographics, risk factors for stroke, clinical and radiological severity of stroke, and symptomatic ICH. Student's *t*-test, the Mann–Whitney *U* test, the chi-square test, and Fisher's exact test were used for group comparisons. (2) We calculated the optimal cut-off point of the HIR for a favorable outcome using the Youden index. Through the receiver operating characteristic curve analysis, the area under the curve was also calculated. (3) To quantify the association between the HIR and a favorable outcome, we performed univariable binary logistic regression analyses for a favorable outcome. Multivariable analysis was also performed to identify whether the HIR was an independent variable for a favorable outcome. Variables with a *p*-value of < 0.1 in univariable analyses were entered in the multivariable model.

Second, to evaluate whether the HIR can modify the effect of the well-established outcome determinants (the ASPECTS and onset-to-recanalization time) on clinical outcomes, the HIR was dichotomized into low and high by its optimal cut-off point for a favorable outcome. According to the low HIR group and the high HIR group, the association between the ASPECTS and a favorable outcome was analyzed by logistic regression analyses. The association between onset-to-recanalization time and a favorable outcome was also analyzed in the same way. We also plotted regression curves by combining the HIR, the ASPECTS, onset-to-recanalization time, and a favorable outcome. For this, patients were assigned to one of the four groups according to the HIR and ASPECTS: (1) the low HIR and small core (ASPECTS ≥ 8) group, (2) the low HIR and large core (ASPECTS < 8) group, (3) high HIR and small core group, and (4) the high HIR and large core group. Regression curves of onset-to-recanalization time for a favorable outcome in the respective groups were compared.

A *p*-value of < 0.05 was considered statistically significant for 95% confidence intervals (CIs). All statistical analyses were performed using R software (version 4.0.1, The R Foundation, r-project.org, Vienna, Austria).

3. Results

Of the 188 patients who underwent successful recanalization of intracranial large vessel occlusion, perfusion images of 26 (13.9%) were not analyzable due to poor quality, including motion artifacts (n = 24) and undetectable T_{max} > 6 s perfusion lesions (n = 2). A total of 162 patients (mean age, 70.7 ± 12.8 years; male, 51.9%) who met the inclusion criteria were analyzed (Figure 1). The median imaging-to-recanalization time was 126.0 min (interquartile range [IQR], 97.0–153.5). The mean lesion volumes of T_{max} > 6 s and T_{max} > 10 s were 160.8 mL (IQR, 104.2–205.2) and 80.3 mL (IQR, 30.3–136.0), respectively. The median HIR value was 0.51 (IQR, 0.29–0.68).

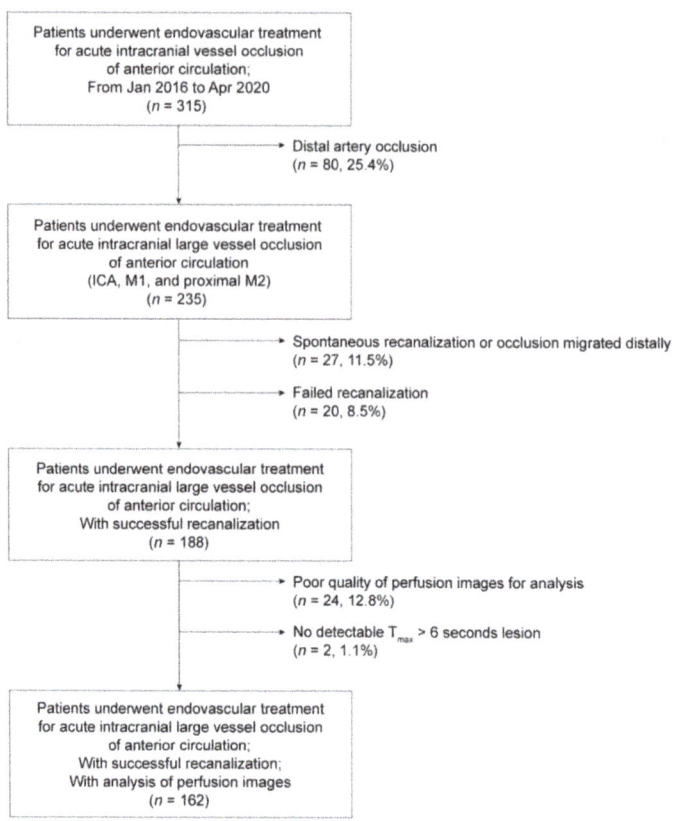

Figure 1. Patients selection flow chart.

3.1. Association between the HIR and Clinical Outcomes

Of the patients included, 85 (52.5%) patients had a favorable outcome. The median HIR value was significantly lower in patients with a favorable outcome than those with an unfavorable outcome (0.45 [IQR, 0.15–0.54] vs. 0.60 [IQR, 0.44–0.73]; $p < 0.001$; Table 1). The optimal cut-off point of the HIR for a favorable outcome was 0.54 (sensitivity, 63.6%; specificity, 74.1%). The area under the curve of the HIR to predict a favorable outcome was 0.728 (95% CI, 0.651–0.805; $p < 0.001$).

In univariable logistic regression analysis, the HIR was significantly associated with a favorable outcome (odds ratio [OR], 0.69 per 0.1; 95% CI, 0.59–0.81; $p < 0.001$; Figure 2), although it was not an independent factor for a favorable outcome after adjustment (adjusted OR [aOR], 0.84 per 0.1; 95% CI, 0.68–1.03; $p = 0.094$; Model 1 in Table 2). We found that the HIR was significantly correlated with the ASPECTS (correlation coefficient, −0.49; $p < 0.001$; Figure 3). Considering the collinearity, the HIR was independently associated with a favorable outcome in a model without the ASPECTS (aOR, 0.76 per 0.1; 95% CI, 0.62–0.92; $p = 0.006$; Model 2 in Table 2).

Table 1. Comparison of clinical variables and hypoperfusion intensity ratio between patients with and without favorable outcome.

Variables	All Patients (n = 162)	Favorable Outcome (n = 85)	Unfavorable Outcome (n = 77)	p-Value
Age	70.7 (± 12.8)	67.6 (± 12.9)	74.1 (± 11.8)	0.001
Sex, male	84 (51.9)	48 (56.5)	36 (46.8)	0.216
Hypertension	122 (75.3)	65 (76.5)	57 (74.0)	0.719
Diabetes	75 (46.3)	31 (36.5)	44 (57.1)	0.008
Hypercholesterolemia	77 (47.5)	39 (45.9)	38 (49.4)	0.659
Smoking	31 (19.1)	21 (24.7)	10 (13.0)	0.058
Coronary artery disease	29 (17.9)	19 (22.4)	11 (14.3)	0.187
Atrial fibrillation	80 (49.4)	38 (44.7)	42 (54.5)	0.211
Occlusion site				0.406
Internal carotid artery	64 (39.5)	31 (36.5)	33 (42.9)	
Middle cerebral artery	98 (60.5)	54 (63.5)	44 (57.1)	
Initial NIHSS score	15.0 [11.0; 19.8]	12.0 [7.0; 16.0]	19.0 [15.0; 20.0]	<0.001
Use of intravenous tPA	78 (48.1)	50 (58.8)	28 (36.4)	0.004
ASPECTS	7.0 [5.0; 9.0]	8.0 [7.0; 9.0]	6.0 [4.0; 7.0]	<0.001
Onset-to-recanalization, min	298.5 [197.0; 583.5]	274.0 [190.0; 434.0]	336.0 [212.0; 674.0]	0.045
Symptomatic ICH	10 (6.2)	4 (4.7)	6 (7.8)	0.520
Volume of rCBF < 30% (mm^3)	33.7 (± 53.6)	12.0 (± 21.7)	57.6 (± 66.7)	<0.001
Volume of T$_{max}$ > 6 s (mm^3)	160.8 (± 76.7)	140.4 (± 67.6)	183.2 (± 80.2)	<0.001
Hypoperfusion intensity ratio	0.51 [0.29; 0.68]	0.45 [0.15; 0.54]	0.60 [0.44; 0.73]	<0.001

Values in parentheses represent the standard deviation (±) or number of patients (%); brackets represent first and third quartiles, respectively. NIHSS, National Institutes of Health Stroke Scale; tPA, tissue plasminogen activator; ASPECTS, Alberta Stroke Program Early Computed Tomography Score; ICH, intracerebral hemorrhage; rCBF, relative cerebral blood flow.

Table 2. Multivariable analyses for a favorable outcome.

Variables	Model 1 aOR (95% CI)	p-Value	Model 2 aOR (95% CI)	p-Value
Age	0.97 (0.94–1.01)	0.153	0.98 (0.94–1.01)	0.171
Diabetes	0.95 (0.40–2.25)	0.899	0.77 (0.34–1.76)	0.531
Smoking	2.35 (0.75–7.37)	0.142	1.74 (0.59–5.14)	0.314
Initial NIHSS score	0.81 (0.74–0.89)	<0.001	0.82 (0.74–0.90)	<0.001
Use of intravenous tPA	2.72 (1.06–6.97)	0.037	2.66 (1.07–6.65)	0.036
ASPECTS	1.33 (1.10–1.61)	0.003		
Onset-to-recanalization time (per 30 min)	0.97 (0.93–1.00)	0.086	0.96 (0.93–1.00)	0.069
Hypoperfusion intensity ratio (per 0.1)	0.84 (0.68–1.03)	0.094	0.76 (0.62–0.92)	0.006

aOR, adjusted odds ratio; CI, confidence interval; NIHSS, National Institutes of Health Stroke Scale; tPA, tissue plasminogen activator; ASPECTS, Alberta Stroke Program Early Computed Tomography Score.

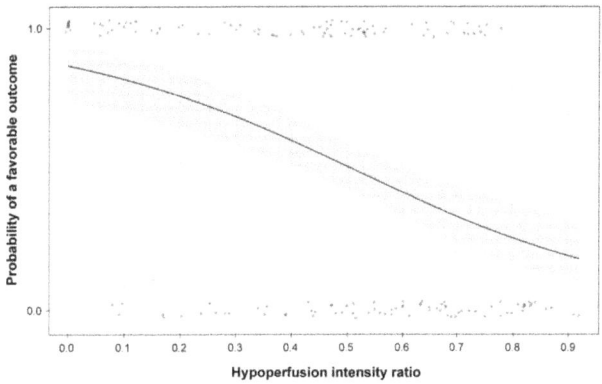

Figure 2. Association between the hypoperfusion intensity ratio and a favorable outcome.

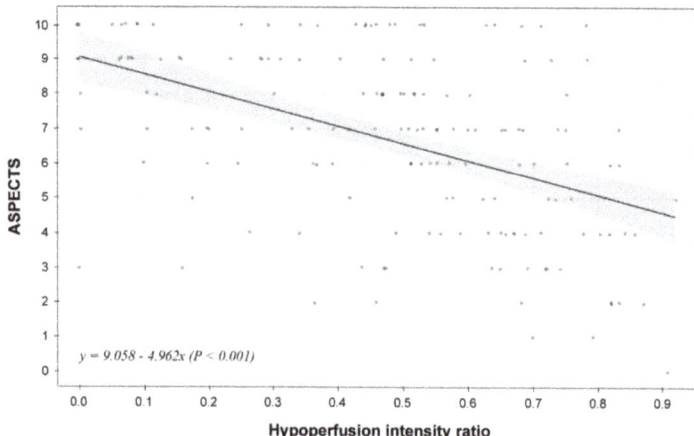

Figure 3. Association between hypoperfusion intensity ratio and Alberta Stroke Program Early CT Score (ASPECTS).

3.2. Association between the ASPECTS, Onset-To-Recanalization Time, and Clinical Outcomes According to the HIR

Based on the optimal cut-off point of the HIR for a favorable outcome, 91 (56.2%) patients were assigned to the low HIR group (HIR < 0.54). The effect of the ASPECTS and onset-to-recanalization time on a favorable outcome was different between the low and high HIR groups. In the low HIR group, only the initial NIHSS score was associated with a favorable outcome. The ASPECTS (aOR, 1.20; 95% CI, 0.92–1.56; p = 0.178) and onset-to-recanalization time (aOR, 0.97 per 30 min; 95% CI, 0.94–1.01; p = 0.194) were not significantly associated with a favorable outcome (Table 3; Figure 4A,B). In contrast, in the high HIR group, the ASPECTS was an independent factor for a favorable outcome (aOR, 1.49; 95% CI, 1.09–2.03; p = 0.012). Although onset-to-recanalization time was not independently associated with a favorable outcome (OR, 0.92 per 30 min; 95% CI, 0.79–1.07; p = 0.283) in the high HIR group, the probability of a favorable outcome decreased sharply when onset-to-recanalization time was relatively short (Figure 4B). As a whole, 3-dimensional regression planes showed that the probability of a favorable outcome was still above 20% even under the lower ASPECTS and longer onset-to-recanalization time in the low HIR group (Figure 5). In contrast, the combined probability of a favorable outcome was sharply decreased as the ASPECTS and onset-to-recanalization time changed in the high HIR group.

Table 3. Effects of the Alberta Stroke Program Early Computed Tomography Score (ASPECTS) and onset-to-recanalization time on a favorable outcome in the low hypoperfusion intensity ratio (HIR) group and the high HIR group.

Variables	Low HIR Group (n = 91) aOR (95% CI)	p-Value	High HIR Group (n = 71) aOR (95% CI)	p-Value
Age	0.96 (0.92–1.01)	0.137		
Diabetes			0.26 (0.07–1.01)	0.051
Smoking	2.70 (0.42–17.6)	0.298		
Initial NIHSS score	0.82 (0.73–0.93)	0.002	0.80 (0.68–0.95)	0.010
Use of intravenous tPA	2.34 (0.67–8.16)	0.182	4.27 (0.76–23.9)	0.098
ASPECTS	1.20 (0.92–1.56)	0.178	1.49 (1.09–2.03)	0.012
Onset-to-recanalization time (per 30 min)	0.97 (0.94–1.01)	0.194	0.92 (0.79–1.07)	0.283

aOR, adjusted odds ratio; CI, confidence interval; NIHSS, National Institutes of Health Stroke Scale; tPA, tissue plasminogen activator; ASPECTS, Alberta Stroke Program Early Computed Tomography Score.

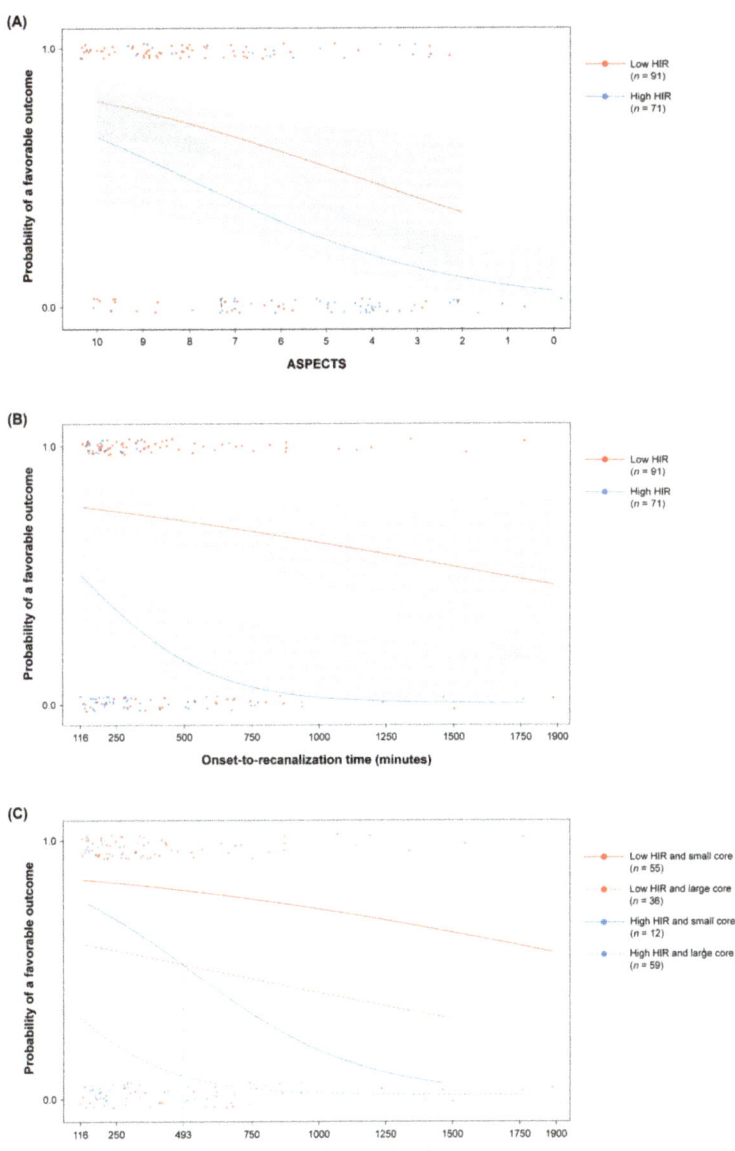

Figure 4. Influence of the Alberta Stroke Program Early CT Score (ASPECTS) and onset-to-recanalization time on clinical outcomes based on the hypoperfusion intensity ratio (HIR). (**A**) Although the ASPECTS was not significantly associated with a favorable outcome in the low HIR group ($p = 0.178$), it was an independent factor for a favorable outcome in the high HIR group ($p = 0.012$). (**B**) For patients with a high HIR, the chances of a favorable outcome sharply decrease when the onset-to-recanalization time is relatively short. (**C**) Considering both the HIR and ASPECTS, patients with a low HIR (<0.54) and small core (ASPECTS ≥ 8) have the best clinical outcome in all ranges of onset-to-recanalization time ($p < 0.05$). In contrast, patients with a high HIR (≥ 0.54) and large core (ASPECTS < 8) have the worst outcome in all ranges of onset-to-recanalization time. Patients with a high HIR and small core have a more favorable outcome than those with a low HIR and large core when onset-to-recanalization time is relatively short. However, for patients with a high HIR and small core, the chance of a favorable outcome decreases more drastically with the course of time and then finally reverses from a particular point of onset-to-recanalization time.

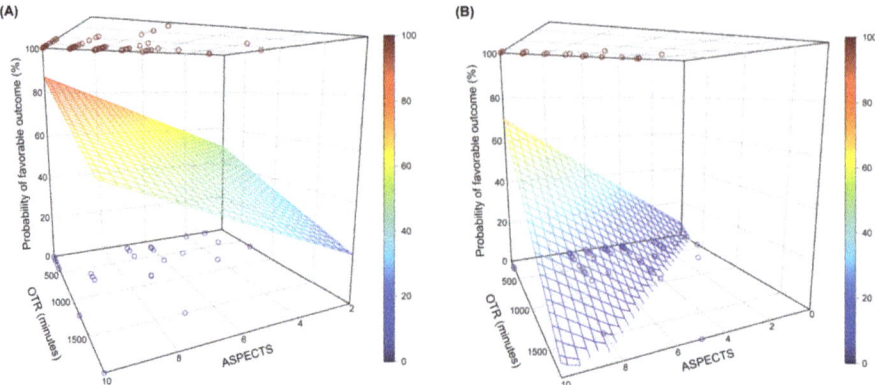

Figure 5. The probability of a favorable outcome according to Alberta Stroke Program Early CT Score (ASPECTS) and onset-to-recanalization time in the low hypoperfusion intensity ratio (HIR) group (**A**) and the high HIR group (**B**). (**A**) In the low HIR group, the probability of a favorable outcome was still above 20% even under the lower ASPECTS and longer onset-to-recanalization time. (**B**) The probability of a favorable outcome was sharply decreased as the ASPECTS and onset-to-recanalization time changed in the high HIR group.

Based on the HIR and ASPECTS, 55 (34.0%) patients had a low HIR and small core, 12 (7.4%) patients had a high HIR and small core, 36 (22.2%) patients had a low HIR and large core, and 59 (36.4%) patients had a high HIR and large core. The decreasing trend of a favorable outcome was significantly different between the groups ($p < 0.05$). Patients with a low HIR and small core had the highest probability of a favorable outcome throughout the study period, while patients with a high HIR and large core had the lowest probability. Patients with a high HIR and small core had a more favorable outcome than those with a low HIR and large core when the onset-to-recanalization time was relatively short. However, their clinical outcomes were reversed after the onset-to-recanalization time of 493 min since the probability of a favorable outcome decreased substantially in patients with a high HIR and small core (Figure 4C).

4. Discussion

In this study, we found that clinical outcomes were substantially different based on the HIR value. A low HIR led to a favorable outcome even in cases with a low ASPECTS and longer onset-to-recanalization time. In contrast, in patients with a high HIR, the ASPECTS was still important for clinical outcome. In addition, the chance of a favorable outcome drastically decreased when the onset-to-recanalization time was relatively short in the high HIR group. Although a study simply reported the association between the HIR and the clinical outcome [7], our study showed more specifically that the probability of a favorable outcome based on the onset-to-recanalization time and the ASPECTS was clearly disparate according to the HIR. The HIR might be an ancillary preprocedural marker to predict the clinical outcomes after EVT.

The collateral nature of HIR was more clearly observed in patients with a high HIR and small core. They had a more favorable outcome than patients with a large core in the shorter onset-to-recanalization time, where the clinical outcome was mainly determined by their core size. However, in the high HIR group, clinical outcome was less favorable despite a small core. Patients with good collaterals could have a favorable outcome even with a longer onset-to-recanalization time; however, the probability of a favorable outcome was substantially reduced in patients with poor collaterals [5]. In addition, the effect of rapid recanalization on a favorable outcome was deliberated in patients with good collaterals, similar to that seen in the low HIR group in our study. In the same manner, it appears that a low HIR may also have a favorable effect on infarct development and its progression. In a previous study, a high HIR was significantly associated with greater infarct growth [7,15–17]. Our study showed that the HIR alone was an independent factor for a favorable outcome in the multivariable model without considering the ASPECTS. After adjusting the ASPECTS, the HIR was not an independent factor for a favorable outcome, which would be mainly because of tight correlation between the HIR and the ASPECTS.

Specific perfusion deficit volumes—for examples, ischemic core volume (relative cerebral blood flow < 30%) and penumbral volume (T_{max} > 6 s) can be associated with clinical outcome. In fact, also in this study, ischemic core volume was independently associated with a favorable outcome, as ASPECTS does. Although such a perfusion parameter is still important in determining clinical outcome, HIR seems still valuable in clinical practice. Along with the common perfusion deficit parameters, HIR could be one of the influencing factors for clinical outcome. Based on its collateral nature, HIR might differentially affect clinical outcome even under the similar ischemic core status or onset-to-recanalization time.

Calculation of the HIR can be clinically advantageous compared to the evaluation of the collateral status, a typical marker reflecting hypoperfusion severity. First, although the assessment of collateral status is easy to perform on pretreatment CT angiography images, quantifying the collateral status are inconsistent and may be qualitative or merely categorical. Most importantly, the evaluation of the collateral status is subjective and reviewer dependent. In contrast, the HIR is more objective in nature. The use of an automated software for the calculation of the HIR can minimize the potential interrater variability and is associated with greater generalization capacity. In addition, the HIR is essentially quantitative as a continuous value, which enables quantitative analysis and can reveal subtle differences in hypoperfusion severity. Furthermore, the HIR can be assessed even in a magnetic resonance-based eligibility strategy. Typical CT angiography-based collateral assessment methods cannot be applied to time-of-flight magnetic resonance angiography. However, the HIR can be calculated with perfusion-weighted images taken using the magnetic resonance technique; thus, its use may be more generalizable. Second, based on the specific cut-off point for a favorable outcome, the HIR may constitute a clinical element that can be used to determine EVT eligibility. In a retrospective study, patients eligible for EVT had a more favorable HIR value than those ineligible for EVT [18]. The HIR may also be a dependable eligibility factor in interfacility transfer since the HIR can significantly predict future infarct growth [8]. According to the recent guidelines for EVT, perfusion imaging with lesion volume analysis has been widely performed to determine the EVT eligibility. Unlike the earlier situation where simple neuroimaging is favored, advanced neuroimaging, including software-based lesion volume analysis, has been increasingly used for EVT eligibility since the DEFUSE 3 and DAWN trials. Although lesion volume analysis is not available in all stroke centers, it is becoming increasingly popular.

In previous studies, a cut-off point of the HIR to predict a favorable functional outcome were not calculated; the cut-off points of the HIR for the collateral status and infarct growth were calculated as 0.40 and 0.50, respectively [7–9]. Most studies merely dichotomized the HIR by its median value, with a range of 0.30–0.45, to evaluate the association of the dichotomized HIR value with the fluid-attenuated inversion recovery (FLAIR) hyperintense vessel sign, infarct growth, or first-pass effect in mechanical thrombectomy [7,19–21]. In these studies, a median HIR value of <0.40 was significantly associated with a positive outcome [7]. In our study, the cut-off point of the HIR for a favorable outcome was calculated as 0.54, which was higher than the 0.40 value, although direct comparison is limited. This may be due to the fact that our study included only patients who underwent successful recanalization. Successful recanalization may give a more favorable clinical outcome in patients with higher HIR values than those with lower HIR values.

This study has several limitations. First, this study was performed retrospectively using prospectively collected data on consecutive patients diagnosed with acute ischemic stroke. The treatment eligibility criteria and protocol were revised during the study period according to the guidelines. Furthermore, the study results from a single center can limit generalizability. Although the HIR value was a rather objective finding obtained from an automated software, the cut-off point of the HIR for a favorable outcome and its significance may be limited to the specific study population. Thus, the results of this study should be interpreted with caution. Second, we evaluated the significance of the HIR only in patients who underwent successful recanalization; however, considering its collateral nature, the HIR may also influence the clinical outcomes in cases of EVT failure, because good collaterals were significantly associated with a favorable outcome even for patients in whom recanalization was unsuccessful [22]. Further studies are needed to demonstrate that the HIR could be a marker in case of EVT failure and to validate the current cut-off in that group.

5. Conclusions

The HIR was associated with clinical outcomes in patients who underwent successful recanalization using EVT. Specifically, a low HIR was associated with a favorable outcome. EVT might need to be considered for patients with a low HIR despite the relatively unfavorable ischemic core status and time profile. Further prospective studies are needed to establish the EVT eligibility criteria based on HIR.

Author Contributions: Conceptualization, H.S.N.; data curation, J.-H.B., Y.D.K., K.J.L., J.K.C., M.B., B.M.K., D.J.K., J.H.H., and H.S.N.; formal analysis, J.-H.B. and H.S.N.; funding acquisition, H.S.N.; methodology, J.-H.B. and H.S.N.; writing—original draft, J.-H.B.; writing—review and editing, J.-H.B. and H.S.N. All authors have read and agreed to the published version of the manuscript.

Funding: This research was supported by a grant from the Korea Health Technology R&D Project through the Korea Health Industry Development Institute, funded by the Ministry of Health & Welfare, Republic of Korea (HI19C0481, HC19C0028).

Institutional Review Board Statement: The study was conducted according to the guidelines of the Declaration of Helsinki, and approved by the Institutional Review Board of Severance Hospital (4-2020-1201; 14 December 2020).

Informed Consent Statement: Patient consent was waived due to the retrospective nature of the study.

Data Availability Statement: The data presented in this study are available on request from the corresponding author.

Conflicts of Interest: The authors declare no conflict of interest.

References

1. Berkhemer, O.A.; Jansen, I.G.H.; Beumer, D.; Fransen, P.S.S.; Berg, L.A.V.D.; Yoo, A.J.; Lingsma, H.F.; Sprengers, M.E.S.; Jenniskens, S.F.M.; Nijeholt, G.J.L.À.; et al. Collateral Status on Baseline Computed Tomographic Angiography and Intra-Arterial Treatment Effect in Patients With Proximal Anterior Circulation Stroke. *Stroke* **2016**, *47*, 768–776. [CrossRef] [PubMed]
2. De Havenon, A.; Mlynash, M.; Kim-Tenser, M.A.; Lansberg, M.G.; Leslie-Mazwi, T.; Christensen, S.; McTaggart, R.A.; Alexander, M.; Albers, G.; Broderick, J.; et al. Results from DEFUSE 3: Good Collaterals are Associated with Reduced Ischemic Core Growth but not Neurologic Outcome. *Stroke* **2019**, *50*, 632–638. [CrossRef]
3. Kim, B.J.; Chung, J.-W.; Park, H.-K.; Kim, J.Y.; Yang, M.-H.; Han, M.-K.; Jeong, C.; Hwang, G.; Kwon, O.-K.; Bae, H.-J. CT Angiography of Collateral Vessels and Outcomes in Endovascular-Treated Acute Ischemic Stroke Patients. *J. Clin. Neurol.* **2017**, *13*, 121–128. [CrossRef] [PubMed]
4. Elijovich, L.; Goyal, N.; Mainali, S.; Hoit, D.; Arthur, A.S.; Whitehead, M.; Choudhri, A.F. CTA Collateral Score Predicts Infarct Volume and Clinical Outcome after Endovascular Therapy for Acute Ischemic Stroke: A Retrospective Chart Review. *J. Neuro Interv. Surg.* **2016**, *8*, 559–562. [CrossRef] [PubMed]
5. Kim, B.M.; Baek, J.-H.; Heo, J.H.; Nam, H.S.; Kim, Y.D.; Yoo, J.; Kim, D.J.; Jeon, P.; Baik, S.K.; Suh, S.H.; et al. Collateral Status Affects the Onset-to-Reperfusion Time Window for Good Outcome. *J. Neurol. Neurosurg. Psychiatry* **2018**, *89*, 903–909. [CrossRef]

6. Bang, O.Y.; Saver, J.L.; Alger, J.R.; Starkman, S.; Ovbiagele, B.; Liebeskind, D.S. Determinants of the Distribution and Severity of Hypoperfusion in Patients with Ischemic Stroke. *Neurology* **2008**, *71*, 1804–1811. [CrossRef] [PubMed]
7. Olivot, J.M.; Mlynash, M.; Inoue, M.; Marks, M.P.; Wheeler, H.M.; Kemp, S.; Straka, M.; Zaharchuk, G.; Bammer, R.; Lansberg, M.G.; et al. Hypoperfusion Intensity Ratio Predicts Infarct Progression and Functional Outcome in the DEFUSE 2 Cohort. *Stroke* **2014**, *45*, 1018–1023. [CrossRef]
8. Guenego, A.; Mlynash, M.; Christensen, S.; Bs, S.K.; Heit, J.J.; Lansberg, M.G.; Albers, G.W. Hypoperfusion Ratio Predicts Infarct Growth During Transfer for Thrombectomy. *Ann. Neurol.* **2018**, *84*, 616–620. [CrossRef]
9. Guenego, A.; Fahed, R.; Albers, G.W.; Kuraitis, G.; Sussman, E.S.; Martin, B.W.; Marcellus, D.G.; Olivot, J.; Marks, M.P.; Lansberg, M.G.; et al. Hypoperfusion Intensity Ratio Correlates with Angiographic Collaterals in Acute Ischaemic Stroke with M1 Occlusion. *Eur. J. Neurol.* **2020**, *27*, 864–870. [CrossRef]
10. Wouters, A.; Dupont, P.; Christensen, S.; Norrving, B.; Laage, R.; Thomalla, G.; Albers, G.; Thijs, V.; Lemmens, R. Association Between Time From Stroke Onset and Fluid-Attenuated Inversion Recovery Lesion Intensity Is Modified by Status of Collateral Circulation. *Stroke* **2016**, *47*, 1018–1022. [CrossRef]
11. Christensen, S.; Mlynash, M.; Kemp, S.; Yennu, A.; Heit, J.J.; Marks, M.P.; Lansberg, M.G.; Albers, G.W. Persistent Target Mismatch Profile >24 Hours After Stroke Onset in DEFUSE 3. *Stroke* **2019**, *50*, 754–757. [CrossRef]
12. Baek, J.-H.; Kim, B.M.; Kang, D.-H.; Heo, J.H.; Nam, H.S.; Kim, Y.D.; Hwang, Y.-H.; Kim, Y.-W.; Kim, D.J.; Kwak, H.S.; et al. Balloon Guide Catheter Is Beneficial in Endovascular Treatment Regardless of Mechanical Recanalization Modality. *Stroke* **2019**, *50*, 1490–1496. [CrossRef]
13. Yaghi, S.; Willey, J.Z.; Cucchiara, B.; Goldstein, J.N.; Gonzales, N.R.; Khatri, P.; Kim, L.J.; Mayer, S.A.; Sheth, K.N.; Schwamm, L.H. Treatment and Outcome of Hemorrhagic Transformation After Intravenous Alteplase in Acute Ischemic Stroke: A Scientific Statement for Healthcare Professionals From the American Heart Association/American Stroke Association. *Stroke* **2017**, *48*, e343–e361. [CrossRef]
14. Barber, P.; Demchuk, A.M.; Zhang, J.; Buchan, A.M. Validity and Reliability of a Quantitative Computed Tomography Score in Predicting Outcome of Hyperacute Stroke Before Thrombolytic Therapy. *Lancet* **2000**, *355*, 1670–1674. [CrossRef]
15. Hotter, B.; Ostwaldt, A.-C.; Levichev-Connolly, A.; Rozanski, M.; Audebert, H.J.; Fiebach, J.B. Natural Course of Total Mismatch and Predictors for Tissue Infarction. *Neurology* **2015**, *85*, 770–775. [CrossRef]
16. Jeong, H.G.; Kim, B.J.; Kim, H.; Cheolkyu, J.; Moon-Ku, H.; David, S.; Liebeskind, H.-J.B. Blood Pressure Drop and Penumbral Tissue Loss in Nonrecanalized Emergent Large Vessel Oc-Clusion. *Stroke* **2019**, *50*, 2677–2684. [CrossRef]
17. Rao, V.L.; Mlynash, M.; Christensen, S.; Yennu, A.; Kemp, S.; Zaharchuk, G.; Heit, J.J.; Marks, M.P.; Lansberg, M.G.; Albers, G.W. Collateral Status Contributes to Differences Between Observed and Predicted 24-h Infarct Volumes in DEFUSE 3. *Br. J. Pharmacol.* **2020**, *40*, 1966–1974. [CrossRef]
18. Guenego, A.; Marcellus, D.G.; Martin, B.W.; Soren, C.; Gregory, W.A.; Maarten, G.L.; Michael, P.M.; Max, W.; Jeremy, J.H. Hypoperfusion Intensity Ratio is Correlated with Patient Eligibility for Thrombectomy. *Stroke* **2019**, *50*, 917–922. [CrossRef]
19. Mohammaden, M.H.; Haussen, D.C.; Pisani, L.; Al-Bayati, A.R.; Da Camara, C.P.; Bhatt, N.; Belagaje, S.R.; Liberato, B.B.; Bianchi, N.; Anderson, A.M.; et al. Baseline ASPECTS and Hypoperfusion Intensity Ratio Influence the Impact of First Pass Reperfusion on Functional Outcomes. *J. Neuro Interv. Surg.* **2021**, *13*, 124–129. [CrossRef]
20. Mahdjoub, E.; Turc, G.; Legrand, L.J.; Benzakoun, M.; Edjlali, P.; Seners, S.; Charron, W.; Ben, H.O.; Naggara, J.-F.; Meder, J.-L.; et al. Baron Do Fluid-Attenuated Inversion Recovery Vascular Hyperintensities Represent Good Col-Laterals Before Reperfusion Therapy? *AJNR Am. J. Neuroradiol.* **2018**, *39*, 77–83. [CrossRef]
21. Kufner, A.; Galinovic, I.; Ambrosi, V.; Nolte, C.H.; Endres, M.; Fiebach, J.B.; Ebinger, M. Hyperintense Vessels on FLAIR, Hemodynamic Correlates and Response to Throm-Bolysis. *AJNR Am. J. Neuroradiol.* **2015**, *36*, 1426–1430. [CrossRef] [PubMed]
22. Park, H.; Kim, B.M.; Baek, J.-H.; Kim, J.-H.; Heo, J.H.; Kim, D.J.; Nam, H.S.; Kim, Y.D. Predictors of Good Outcomes in Patients with Failed Endovascular Thrombectomy. *Korean J. Radiol.* **2020**, *21*, 582–587. [CrossRef] [PubMed]

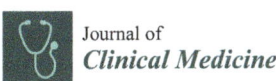

Article

Hypoperfusion Index Ratio as a Surrogate of Collateral Scoring on CT Angiogram in Large Vessel Stroke

Chun-Min Wang, Yu-Ming Chang *, Pi-Shan Sung * and Chih-Hung Chen

Department of Neurology, National Cheng Kung University Hospital, College of Medicine, National Cheng Kung University, Tainan 704, Taiwan; ro2003yes@gmail.com (C.-M.W.); lchih@mail.ncku.edu.tw (C.-H.C.)
* Correspondence: cornworldmirror@hotmail.com (Y.-M.C.); pishansung@gmail.com (P.-S.S.);
Tel.: +886-6-2353535-5481 (P.-S.S.); Fax: +886-6-2374285 (P.-S.S.)

Abstract: Background: This study was to evaluate the correlation of the hypoperfusion intensity ratio (HIR) with the collateral score from multiphase computed tomography angiography (mCTA) among patients with large vessel stroke. Method: From February 2019 to May 2020, we retrospectively reviewed the patients with large vessel strokes (intracranial carotid artery or proximal middle cerebral artery occlusion). HIR was defined as a Tmax > 10 s lesion volume divided by a Tmax > 6 s lesion volume, which was calculated by automatic software (Syngo.via, Siemens). The correlation between the HIR and mCTA score was evaluated by Pearson's correlation. The cutoff value predicting the mCTA score was evaluated by receiver operating characteristic analysis. Result: Ninety-four patients were enrolled in the final analysis. The patients with good collaterals had a smaller core volume (37.3 ± 24.7 vs. 116.5 ± 70 mL, $p < 0.001$) and lower HIR (0.51 ± 0.2 vs. 0.73 ± 0.13, $p < 0.001$) than those with poor collaterals. A higher HIR was correlated with a poorer collateral score by Pearson's correlation. ($r = -0.64$, $p < 0.001$). The receiver operating characteristic (ROC) analysis suggested that the best HIR value for predicting a good collateral score was 0.68 (area under curve: 0.82). Conclusion: HIR is a good surrogate of collateral circulation in patients with acute large artery occlusion.

Keywords: hypoperfusion index ratio; collateral circulation; collateral scoring; CTA; CTP; large vessel occlusion

1. Introduction

Evaluating pial (leptomeningeal) collateral status is of great importance in predicting the evolution of infarction [1], predicting the prognosis of acute ischemic stroke [2], and selecting eligible patients for endovascular thrombectomy (EVT) [3]. Leptomeningeal collateral flow can be assessed by conventional angiography, computed tomography angiography (CTA) (including single-phase CTA, dynamic CTA, and multiphase CTA) and magnetic resonance imaging (MRI) [4]. Different scoring systems have been proposed, and most of them are semiquantitative measures [5]. In clinical practice, multiphase CTA (mCTA) has become one of the most reliable and rapid techniques to visualize collateral circulation [6]. However, there may be potentially an interrater difference in reading the result of mCTA and obtaining collateral scores on mCTA in real-world setting.

Along with mCTA, computed tomography perfusion (CTP) plays a role in decision making regarding the management of acute stroke, especially before EVT [7]. The development of automatic postprocessing software for CTP gives physicians more quantitative and rapid measures to evaluate the infarct core and potentially salvageable tissue. Calculated by automatic software, the hypoperfusion intensity ratio (HIR) was defined as the Tmax > 10 s lesion volume (Tmax10) divided by the Tmax > 6 s lesion volume (Tmax6) [8]. The HIR has been shown to predict the rate of infarct growth and functional outcome at 90 days after stroke in the DEFUSE 2 cohort; thus, it is thought to be a clinical parameter that evaluates the degree of collateral circulation [8]. In another retrospective study, patients who met the American Heart Association guidelines for thrombectomy were more likely to have a lower HIR [9].

A recent study showed that HIR was correlated with collateral circulation in digital subtraction angiography (DSA), suggesting a cutoff value (HIR < 0.4) as the best prediction for good DSA collaterals [10]. There may be a correlation between collateral scores on mCTA and HIR, but the cutoff value of HIR for the prediction of good collaterals on mCTA may be different from the cutoff value to predict good DSA collaterals.

On the other hand, the studies above all used RAPID software (iSchemaView, Menlo Park, CA, USA) as postprocessing software. Although other software programs have been developed and have shown some degree of agreement with RAPID [11,12], no study has demonstrated that the HIR calculated by other automatic software correlates with collateral status.

In this study, we aimed to establish the association between the HIR calculated by Syngo.via and the collateral score by mCTA and determine the best cutoff value for predicting good collaterals on mCTA.

2. Materials and Methods

2.1. Patient Inclusion, Population, and Clinical Data

National Cheng Kung University Hospital (NCKUH) is a 1320-bed tertiary medical center in southern Taiwan that can provide intravenous tissue plasminogen activator injection (IV-tPA) and endovascular thrombectomy (EVT). Between 800 and 900 patients with acute ischemic stroke are admitted to our stroke ward annually. As a participating hospital of the nationwide Taiwan Stroke Registry (TSR) [13], NCKUH has been maintaining prospective stroke registries according to the TSR protocol since 2006. Our comprehensive stroke center prospectively enrolls patients who present to our hospital within 10 days after stroke onset and receive CT and/or MRI for the index stroke. The patients' demographic characteristics and medical history were recorded according to a predefined system.

In this study, we retrospectively identified consecutive patients receiving CTA and CTP scans on arrival at our emergency department for acute stroke management between February 2019 and May 2020. By assessing each patient's CTA data, we enrolled patients with occlusions in either the internal carotid artery (ICA) or the M1 and M2 branches of the middle cerebral artery (MCA). Patients without large vessel occlusion (LVO) or with occlusion in the anterior cerebral artery (ACA), posterior cerebral artery (PCA), posterior circulation, or multiple sites were excluded because the collateral scores were non applicable. The demographic data, last known well time or onset time, initial National Institutes of Health Stroke Scale (NIHSS) score, comorbidities, details of IV-tPA and/or EVT, and modified Rankin scale (mRS) at discharge, were obtained from our registry system.

All patients needed to complete written consents prior to receive brain imaging. This study was approved by the Institutional Review Board of National Cheng Kung University Hospital (B-ER-109192).

2.2. Multiphase Computed Tomography Angiography Collateral Score, Hypoperfusion Intensity Ratio, and the Eligibility of EVT

The mCTA protocol was described in a previous study [6]. In brief, three phases (peak arterial phase, peak venous phase, and late venous phase) of consecutive scanning with an interval of 8 s were obtained, allowing for time-resolved assessment. The mCTA collateral scores (range from 0 to 5) are defined as follows: Grade 5—no filling delay compared to the asymptomatic contralateral hemisphere, normal pial vessels in the affected hemisphere; Grade 4—a filling delay of one phase in the affected hemisphere, but the extent and prominence of pial vessels is the same; Grade 3—a filling delay of two phases in the affected hemisphere, or a delay of one phase with a significantly reduced number of vessels in the ischemic territory; Grade 2—a filling delay of two phases in the affected hemisphere with a significantly reduced number of vessels in the ischemic territory, or one phase delay showing regions without visible vessels; Grade 1—only a few vessels are visible in the affected hemisphere in any phase; Grade 0—no vessels visible in the affected hemisphere in any phase.

The mCTA collateral scores were independently assessed by two raters (Wang C-M and Chang Y-M). Those results with different mCTA collateral scores were further discussed at the research conference by these two raters. A final mCTA collateral score was given after discussion and agreement. An mCTA collateral score of 3 or lower indicates poor collateral status [14].

The CTP images were postprocessed by the software Syngo.via CT Neuro Perfusion (version VB30 HF03; Siemens Healthcare, Erlangen, Germany). Tmax is defined as the time to maximum of the residue function obtained by deconvolution [15]. The volume of the ischemic core, penumbra and perfusion mismatch were automatically calculated based on cerebral blood flow (<30%) and Tmax (>6 s) lesion volume. The HIR was defined as the Tmax > 10 s lesion volume divided by the Tmax > 6 s lesion volume.

The eligibility criteria of EVT at our site are mainly based on the guidelines from the American Heart Association/American Stroke Association (AHA/ASA) [16] and Taiwan Stroke Society [17]. In brief, for patients with LVO within 6 h of stroke onset and an Alberta stroke program early CT score (ASPECTS) ≥ 6, EVT was considered unless patients had poor baseline conditions, such as a pre-mRS score greater than 2, terminal cancer status, unstable vital signs or multiple comorbidities. Perfusion imaging may provide complementary information alongside CTA for neurointerventionists, especially for patients within 6 h to 24 h of last known normal. For those patients, EVT was considered case by case based on the criteria of the DAWN [18] or DEFUSE 3 trial [19].

2.3. Outcome and Statistical Analysis

The continuous variables (age, NIHSS score, time after stroke onset, HIR, mCTA collateral score, ischemic core, penumbra, and perfusion mismatch volume) are expressed as the means ± standard deviation (SD) or median, quartiles and interquartile range (IQR). The nominal variables (medical history of comorbidity and medication, occlusion sites, IV-tPA and EVT) were summarized as frequency descriptive analyses. The interrater reliability of mCTA score was measured by using Cohen's kappa coefficient.

The subjects were divided into subgroups based on the mCTA collateral score (good collaterals (scores 4–5) vs. poor collaterals (scores 0–3)). Univariate analyses were performed to compare the age, initial stroke severity assessed by initial NIHSS score, ischemic core volume, penumbra volume, perfusion mismatch volume and perfusion ratio between groups by using independent T-test or Mann–Whitney U-test; the sex, comorbidity, medication history, treatment with IV-tPA or EVT, and post-EVT TICI score between groups by using Pearson's chi-squared test. The correlation between the HIR and mCTA collateral score was calculated using Pearson's correlation. Statistical tests are considered significant at a < 0.05 level. Receiver operating characteristic (ROC) curve analysis was performed to determine an HIR threshold for predicting good collaterals, which was defined as mCTA collateral scores of 4–5.

3. Results

From February 2019 to May 2020, 341 patients with acute ischemic stroke underwent CTA and CTP at NCKUH. After excluding those without LVO ($n = 153$), those with stroke in the posterior circulation and PCA territory ($n = 56$), those in the ACA territory ($n = 9$), those with bilateral or multiple occlusion sites ($n = 3$) and those with poor image quality (e.g., failure to be processed by software, poorly enhanced vessels, severe motion artifacts, etc.) or missing data ($n = 26$), 94 patients were enrolled in the final analysis (male/female: $n = 59/36$) (Figure 1). The mean age was 72 (SD: 12.9, range: 30–94), and the median NIHSS score was 21 (IQR: 14–27). The occlusion sites were at the ICA ($n = 23$), M1 ($n = 42$) and M2 ($n = 29$). The median HIR was 0.65 (IQR: 0.47–0.74), and the median mCTA score was 4 (IQR: 2–4). The mCTA score showed substantial agreement between the two raters with a kappa value of 0.64.

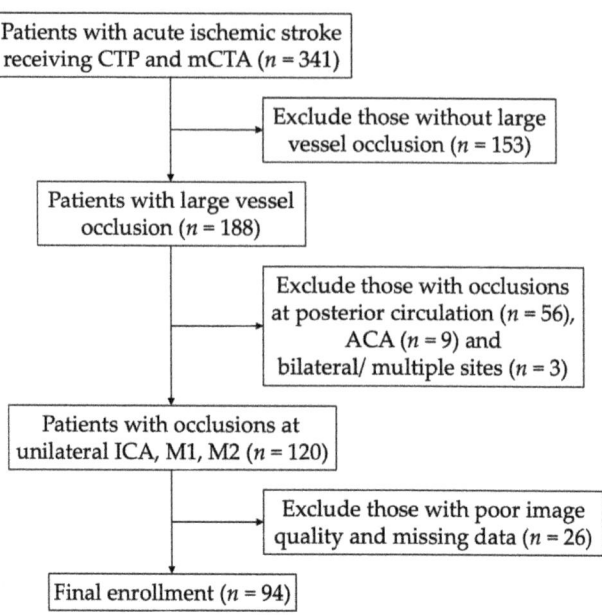

Figure 1. The flow chart of enrollment. CTP, computed topography perfusion; mCTA, multiphase computed topographic angiography; ACA anterior cerebral artery; ICA, internal carotid artery; M1/M2, M1, and M2 segments of the middle cerebral artery.

There were no significant differences in age, sex, history of hypertension, diabetes mellitus, coronary artery disease, congestive heart failure, prior antiplatelet or anticoagulant use, or tobacco use between patients with good and poor collaterals (Table 1). The patients with good collaterals had significantly lower stroke severity (median NIHSS = 14, IQR: 10–21) than those with poor collaterals (median NIHSS = 25, IQR: 21–30, $p < 0.001$). There were also more patients with good collaterals receiving IV-tPA (44.2% versus 16.7%, $p = 0.004$). There were no significant differences in the percentage of patients receiving EVT between the two groups.

Table 1. Demographic characteristics of patients with poor collaterals (score 0–3) and good collaterals (score 4–5) based on multiphase CT angiography collateral score in acute ischemic stroke.

Characteristics	All ($n = 94$)	Poor Collaterals ($n = 42$)	Good Collaterals ($n = 52$)	p Value
Age (years) (mean (SD))	71.9 (12.9)	73.0 (11.3)	71.0 (14.1)	0.439
Male	55 (58.5%)	23 (54.8%)	32 (61.5%)	0.507
Medical history				
Hypertension	71 (75.5%)	32 (76.2%)	39 (75%)	0.894
Diabetes Mellitus	35 (37.2%)	15 (35.7%)	20 (38.5%)	0.784
Hyperlipidemia	64 (68.1%)	25 (59.5%)	39 (75%)	0.110
Atrial fibrillation	42 (44.7%)	24 (57.1%)	18 (34.6%)	0.029
Coronary artery disease	19 (20.2%)	12 (28.6%)	7 (13.5%)	0.070

Table 1. Cont.

Characteristics	All (n = 94)	Poor Collaterals (n = 42)	Good Collaterals (n = 52)	p Value
Congestive heart failure	10 (10.6%)	7 (16.7%)	3 (5.8%)	0.088
Prior AP	25 (26.9%)	11 (26.2%)	14 (26.9%)	0.936
Prior AC	13 (13.8%)	7 (16.7%)	6 (11.5%)	0.474
Smoker	24 (25.8%)	7 (16.7%)	17 (33.3%)	0.095
Initial NIHSS (median (IQR))	20.5 (14–27)	25 (21–30)	14 (10–21)	<0.001
Lesion site				0.021
ICA	23 (24.5%)	11 (26.2%)	12 (23.1%)	
M1	42 (44.7%)	24 (57.1%)	18 (34.6%)	
M2	29 (30.9%)	7 (16.7%)	22 (42.3%)	
Initial SBP (mmHg) (median (IQR))	152.5 (137.75–171.25)	154 (137–180)	151.5 (137.5–167.75)	0.451
IV-tPA	30 (31.9%)	7 (16.7%)	23 (44.2%)	0.004
EVT	32 (34.0%)	12 (28.6%)	20 (38.5%)	0.314
Onset to ER (median (IQR))	154 (61–311.75)	172.5 (123–277.75)	111.50 (37.5–364.25)	0.050
Onset to CTP (median (IQR))	40.50 (23.75–75.25)	30.50 (20–49.5)	52 (31.50–82.75)	0.005

NIHSS, National Institutes of Health Stroke Scale; ICA, internal carotid artery; M1/M2, M1, and M2 segments of the middle cerebral artery; EVT, endovascular thrombectomy; CTP, computed tomography perfusion.

The patients with good collaterals had smaller cores (37.3 ± 24.7 vs. 116.5 ± 70 mL, $p < 0.001$) and Tmax6 (120 ± 64.9 vs. 203.5 ± 88 mL, $p < 0.001$) and Tmax10 volumes (59.2 ± 31.1 vs. 152 ± 82.6 mL, $p < 0.001$) and lower HIRs (0.51 ± 0.2 vs. 0.73 ± 0.13, $p < 0.001$), as well as lower mRS scores (2 (IQR: 1–3.75) vs. 5 (IQR: 2–6), $p = 0.02$) at discharge (Table 2).

Table 2. Core volume, Tmax > 6- and 10-s lesion volume, hypoperfusion index ratio (HIR) and modified Rankin scale (mRS) at discharge in patients with poor collaterals (score 0–3) and good collaterals (score 4–5) based on the multiphase CT angiography collateral score.

Characteristics	All (n = 94)	Poor Collaterals (n = 42)	Good Collaterals (n = 52)	p Value
Core volume (mL) (SD)	72.7 (63.7)	116.5 (70.0)	37.3 (24.7)	<0.001
Tmax > 6 volume (mL) (SD)	157.3 (86.4)	203.5 (88.0)	120.0 (64.9)	<0.001
Tmax > 10 volume (mL) (SD)	100.7 (75.2)	152.0 (82.6)	59.2 (31.1)	<0.001
HIR (SD)	0.61 (0.20)	0.73 (0.13)	0.51 (0.20)	<0.001
Discharge mRS (IQR)	4 (1.25–5)	5 (2–6)	2 (1–3.75)	0.021

HIR, hypoperfusion intensity ratio.

A higher HIR was correlated with a poorer collateral score by Pearson's correlation ($r = -0.64$, $p < 0.001$) (Figure 2). The ROC analysis suggested that the best value for predicting a good collateral score was 0.68, with a sensitivity of 0.76, specificity of 0.81, and area under the curve of 0.82 (Figure 3).

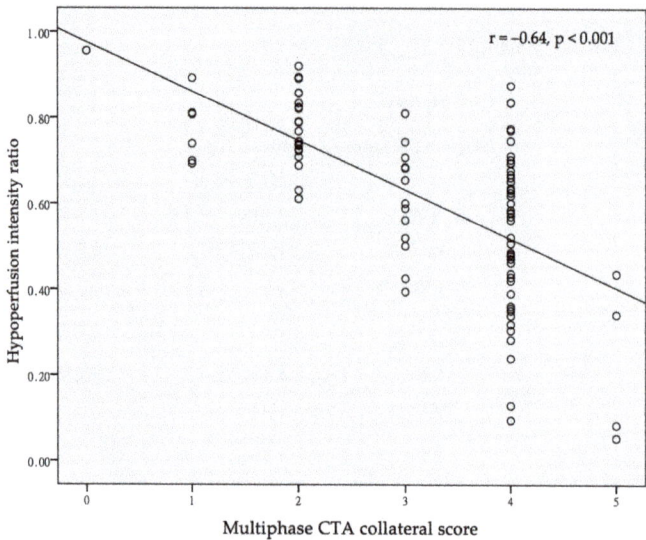

Figure 2. Scatter plot of hypoperfusion index (HIR) and multiphase CT angiography (mCTA) collateral score. Pearson's r = −0.64, $p < 0.001$.

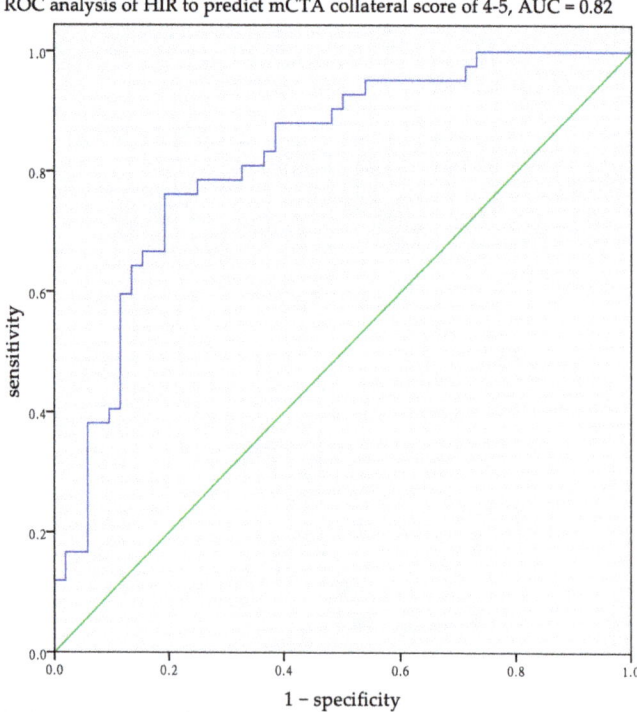

Figure 3. Receiver operating characteristic (ROC) analysis of the hypoperfusion index (HIR) to predict good collateral by multiphase CT angiography (mCTA) collateral score (4 or 5). The best predicted value of HIR was 0.68, with a sensitivity of 76%, specificity of 81% and area under curve (AUC) of 0.82.

4. Discussion

Our study found that the HIR is correlated with the mCTA collateral score in patients with acute occlusions at the ICA, M1, or M2 segment of the MCA, with 0.68 being the best value that predicts a good collateral score by Syngo.via CT Neuro Perfusion software.

In clinical practice, we may evaluate collateral status directly via CTA, and the collateral scores were correlated with clinical outcomes, even with reperfusion by IV-tPA and EVT [2,20,21]. However, there are some pitfalls in scoring the collateral status from CTA. It is somehow subjective and rater-dependent, and the raters need to be trained to reduce the interrater variability. Objective automatic software may be helpful in the clinical scenario of managing acute ischemic stroke. HIR, automatically calculated by software, is defined as Tmax10 divided by Tmax6. Tmax6 was shown to predict penumbra well in a previous study [22], while Tmax10 was found to represent the most endangered tissue with extremely delayed perfusion [23]. HIR may be considered a quantitative measure of collateral blood flow to the brain as "tissue-level collaterals". One previous study demonstrated that HIR was correlated with collateral circulation in DSA in patients during EVT [10]. Another analysis of the SWIFT PRIME study also showed that collateral status was correlated with relative blood volume and HIR by using RAPID software [24]. Our findings confirm the concept of using HIR as an indicator for collateral circulation even with a different software package and provide a particular cutoff value of HIR to predict good collateral status by using Syngo.via software.

In the study mentioned above [8], the ROC analysis showed that an HIR > 0.4 had a sensitivity of 0.66 and a specificity of 0.70 for predicting poor collateral flow. Another study [10] also revealed that an HIR < 0.403 best predicted good angiographic collaterals with a sensitivity of 0.79 and specificity of 0.56. Both reports used RAPID software. We found that the cutoff value for predicting good collaterals in mCTA was 0.68 by using Syngo.via software. This may result from the different algorithms of image processing and chosen parameters in different software packages. A study reported that the infarct core predicted by Syngo.via will meet good agreement with RAPID if changing the parameters to CBV < 1.2 mL/100 mL and applying an additional smoothing filter [12], while another study suggested that the predicted volume of the infarct core calculated by Syngo.via could be concordant with RAPID if the relative cerebral blood flow threshold is changed to <20% [25]. In the same study, when analyzed as a subgroup, in patients with LVOs (ICA and M1 occlusion), there was no statistically significant difference between the calculated values for the core and hypoperfusion volumes. To the best of our knowledge, there have been no studies comparing and correlating the Tmax10 or HIR of the two software packages. Further study is warranted to correlate the HIR acquired by different software programs. Despite some difference in predicted volume of core and penumbra, Syngo.via and RAPID software showed high concordance in correctly triaging patients into "go or no-go" for EVT in real-world settings [26].

Potential delay may exist between activating the thrombectomy team and the actual reperfusion time. Better collateral circulation may extend the survival period of the penumbra. A study showed that patients with good collaterals had a smaller infarct core and higher mismatch ratio in ICA and M1/M2 occlusion and within 12 h of stroke onset [27]. Interestingly, in the DEFUSE 3 cohort, good collaterals were associated with reduced ischemic core growth but not neurologic outcome in the late therapeutic window [28]. Another study also showed that in patients with LVO who underwent endovascular intervention, collateral status was strongly associated with MCA territory final infarct volumes but not correlated with favorable outcomes at discharge [24]. The authors' explanation was that good collaterals preserved the watershed area of the ACA/MCA and MCA/PCA but had no influence on certain critical brain regions (such as the precentral gyrus and the posterior limb of the internal capsule), which have larger impacts on functional independence. On the other hand, in the DEFUSE 2 cohort, final infarction volume increased in association with HIR quartiles as well as infarct growth regardless of reperfusion. After adjusting for the factor of early reperfusion, a favorable outcome was still associated with a low HIR [8].

Therefore, by using HIR as a surrogate for "tissue-level collateral assessment", a stroke neurologist may have additional information to accelerate the patient selection of EVT and predict the outcome. If our result is further validated in other independent database, multiphase CTA may not be necessary in most of the cases because the HIR could already represent the collateral status and even correlate prognosis better. Patients could benefit from reduced exposure of radiation and contrast medium, and we may save more time during pre-EVT evaluation.

There were some limitations of our study. First, this was a retrospective observational study in a single medical center, and sampling bias was inevitable, although we collected consecutive acute stroke patients who received CTA/CTP. Second, despite the specific definition, the mCTA score is a subjective scoring system that may have interrater differences, and there are different scoring systems for collaterals in CTA [29], which are not fully comparable. Third, we only included patients with acute stroke and large vessel occlusion patients. Those with occlusion sites other than the ICA or MCA were excluded; thus, the correlation of the mCTA score and HIR may not be reliable at other occlusion sites or in post-acute stage of stroke. Fourth, the proportion of patients undergoing EVT was comparable between good and poor collaterals in our study. This may be due to the higher proportion of M2 occlusion in patients with good collaterals, and EVT in patients with M2 occlusions is optional at our sites. Fifth, the sensitivity and specificity of this threshold by Syngo.via has not been validated in other independent database. Furthermore, the chronic stenosis of large vessels, old stroke and poor cardiac output tremendously affect the image quality of CTP. Therefore, the above conditions may interfere with the relationship between collateral status and HIR. Last but not least, this study was performed in an Eastern Asian population; thus, extrapolating our findings to other ethnicities must be done with caution.

5. Conclusions

In our study, we found that a lower HIR correlates with a good mCTA collateral core in patients with occlusions in the ICA and M1 and M2 segments of the MCA. The best cutoff value of HIR is 0.68 to predict good collaterals by Syngo.via. The HIR is a good surrogate of tissue-level collateral status, even in different automatic software packages. However, the best HIR cutoff value to predict good collaterals may be adjusted by different software programs.

Author Contributions: Conceptualization, C.-M.W., Y.-M.C. and P.-S.S.; methodology: C.-M.W. and Y.-M.C.; software, C.-M.W.: validation: C.-M.W., P.-S.S. and C.-H.C.; formal analysis, C.-M.W. and P.-S.S.; investigation, P.-S.S.; resources, P.-S.S.; data curation, C.-M.W. and Y.-M.C.; writing—original draft preparation, C.-M.W.; writing—review and editing, C.-M.W. and P.-S.S.; visualization, C.-H.C.; supervision, P.-S.S.; project administration, P.-S.S.; funding acquisition, Y.-M.C. and P.-S.S. All authors have read and agreed to the published version of the manuscript.

Funding: This work received grants from National Cheng Kung University Hospital (Grant numbers: NCKUH-10902039 and NCKUH-11003022) and the Ministry of Science and Technology of Taiwan via contract MOST 108-2321-B-006-024–MY2. The funding source was not involved in any of the study processes or the writing of this manuscript. This research had no relationship with industry and pharmaceutical companies.

Institutional Review Board Statement: The study was conducted according to the guidelines of the Declaration of Helsinki, and approved by the This study was approved by the Institutional Review Board of National Cheng Kung University Hospital (B-ER-109192).

Informed Consent Statement: All patients needed to complete written consents prior to receive brain imaging. Informed consent was waived due to retrospective analysis of imaging study and was approved by the institutional review board of National Cheng Kung University Hospital.

Data Availability Statement: The data was available upon reasonable email request.

Acknowledgments: We thank the staff of the stroke center of National Cheng Kung University Hospital for their support.

Conflicts of Interest: The authors declare no conflict of interest.

References

1. Christoforidis, G.A.; Mohammad, Y.; Kehagias, D.; Avutu, B.; Slivka, A.P. Angiographic assessment of pial collaterals as a prognostic indicator following intra-arterial thrombolysis for acute ischemic stroke. *Am. J. Neuroradiol.* **2005**, *26*, 1789–1797. [PubMed]
2. Gerber, J.C.; Petrova, M.; Krukowski, P.; Kuhn, M.; Abramyuk, A.; Bodechtel, U.; Dzialowski, I.; Engellandt, K.; Kitzler, H.; Pallesen, L.P. Collateral state and the effect of endovascular reperfusion therapy on clinical outcome in ischemic stroke patients. *Brain Behav.* **2016**, *6*, e00513. [CrossRef] [PubMed]
3. Woo, H.G.; Jung, C.; Sunwoo, L.; Bae, Y.J.; Choi, B.S.; Kim, J.H.; Kim, B.J.; Han, M.-K.; Bae, H.-J.; Jung, S. Dichotomizing level of pial collaterals on multiphase CT angiography for endovascular treatment in acute ischemic stroke: Should it be refined for 6-hour time window? *Neurointervention* **2019**, *14*, 99. [CrossRef] [PubMed]
4. McVerry, F.; Liebeskind, D.; Muir, K. Systematic review of methods for assessing leptomeningeal collateral flow. *Am. J. Neuroradiol.* **2012**, *33*, 576–582. [CrossRef] [PubMed]
5. Piedade, G.S.; Schirmer, C.M.; Goren, O.; Zhang, H.; Aghajanian, A.; Faber, J.E.; Griessenauer, C.J. Cerebral collateral circulation: A review in the context of ischemic stroke and mechanical thrombectomy. *World Neurosurg.* **2019**, *122*, 33–42. [CrossRef]
6. Menon, B.K.; d'Esterre, C.D.; Qazi, E.M.; Almekhlafi, M.; Hahn, L.; Demchuk, A.M.; Goyal, M. Multiphase CT angiography: A new tool for the imaging triage of patients with acute ischemic stroke. *Radiology* **2015**, *275*, 510–520. [CrossRef]
7. Demeestere, J.; Wouters, A.; Christensen, S.; Lemmens, R.; Lansberg, M.G. Review of perfusion imaging in acute ischemic stroke: From time to tissue. *Stroke* **2020**, *51*, 1017–1024. [CrossRef]
8. Olivot, J.M.; Mlynash, M.; Inoue, M.; Marks, M.P.; Wheeler, H.M.; Kemp, S.; Straka, M.; Zaharchuk, G.; Bammer, R.; Lansberg, M.G. Hypoperfusion intensity ratio predicts infarct progression and functional outcome in the DEFUSE 2 Cohort. *Stroke* **2014**, *45*, 1018–1023. [CrossRef]
9. Guenego, A.; Marcellus, D.G.; Martin, B.W.; Christensen, S.; Albers, G.W.; Lansberg, M.G.; Marks, M.P.; Wintermark, M.; Heit, J.J. Hypoperfusion intensity ratio is correlated with patient eligibility for thrombectomy. *Stroke* **2019**, *50*, 917–922. [CrossRef]
10. Guenego, A.; Fahed, R.; Albers, G.W.; Kuraitis, G.; Sussman, E.S.; Martin, B.W.; Marcellus, D.G.; Olivot, J.M.; Marks, M.P.; Lansberg, M.G. Hypoperfusion intensity ratio correlates with angiographic collaterals in acute ischaemic stroke with M1 occlusion. *Eur. J. Neurol.* **2020**, *27*, 864–870. [CrossRef]
11. Austein, F.; Riedel, C.; Kerby, T.; Meyne, J.; Binder, A.; Lindner, T.; Huhndorf, M.; Wodarg, F.; Jansen, O. Comparison of perfusion CT software to predict the final infarct volume after thrombectomy. *Stroke* **2016**, *47*, 2311–2317. [CrossRef]
12. Koopman, M.S.; Berkhemer, O.A.; Geuskens, R.R.; Emmer, B.J.; van Walderveen, M.A.; Jenniskens, S.F.; van Zwam, W.H.; van Oostenbrugge, R.J.; van der Lugt, A.; Dippel, D.W. Comparison of three commonly used CT perfusion software packages in patients with acute ischemic stroke. *J. Neurointerventional Surg.* **2019**, *11*, 1249–1256. [CrossRef] [PubMed]
13. Hsieh, C.-Y.; Wu, D.P.; Sung, S.-F. Registry-based stroke research in Taiwan: Past and future. *Epidemiol. Health* **2018**, *40*, e2018004. [CrossRef]
14. García-Tornel, A.; Carvalho, V.; Boned, S.; Flores, A.; Rodríguez-Luna, D.; Pagola, J.; Muchada, M.; Sanjuan, E.; Coscojuela, P.; Juega, J. Improving the evaluation of collateral circulation by multiphase computed tomography angiography in acute stroke patients treated with endovascular reperfusion therapies. *Intervig. Neurol.* **2016**, *5*, 209–217. [CrossRef] [PubMed]
15. Calamante, F.; Christensen, S.; Desmond, P.M.; Østergaard, L.; Davis, S.M.; Connelly, A. The physiological significance of the time-to-maximum (Tmax) parameter in perfusion MRI. *Stroke* **2010**, *41*, 1169–1174. [CrossRef]
16. Powers, W.J.; Rabinstein, A.A.; Ackerson, T.; Adeoye, O.M.; Bambakidis, N.C.; Becker, K.; Biller, J.; Brown, M.; Demaerschalk, B.M.; Hoh, B. Guidelines for the early management of patients with acute ischemic stroke: 2019 update to the 2018 guidelines for the early management of acute ischemic stroke: A guideline for healthcare professionals from the American Heart Association/American Stroke Association. *Stroke* **2019**, *50*, e344–e418. [PubMed]
17. Tang, S.; Tsai, L.; Chen, C.; Lee, C.; Wang, K.; Lai, Y. Taiwan Stroke Society guideline for endovascular thrombectomy in acute ischemic stroke patients. *J. Stroke* **2019**, *1*, 77–89.
18. Nogueira, R.G.; Jadhav, A.P.; Haussen, D.C.; Bonafe, A.; Budzik, R.F.; Bhuva, P.; Yavagal, D.R.; Ribo, M.; Cognard, C.; Hanel, R.A. Thrombectomy 6 to 24 hours after stroke with a mismatch between deficit and infarct. *N. Engl. J. Med.* **2018**, *378*, 11–21. [CrossRef]
19. Albers, G.W.; Marks, M.P.; Kemp, S.; Christensen, S.; Tsai, J.P.; Ortega-Gutierrez, S.; McTaggart, R.A.; Torbey, M.T.; Kim-Tenser, M.; Leslie-Mazwi, T. Thrombectomy for stroke at 6 to 16 hours with selection by perfusion imaging. *N. Engl. J. Med.* **2018**, *378*, 708–718. [CrossRef]
20. Arenillas, J.F.; Cortijo, E.; García-Bermejo, P.; Levy, E.I.; Jahan, R.; Liebeskind, D.; Goyal, M.; Saver, J.L.; Albers, G.W. Relative cerebral blood volume is associated with collateral status and infarct growth in stroke patients in SWIFT PRIME. *J. Cereb. Blood Flow Metab.* **2018**, *38*, 1839–1847. [CrossRef]
21. Wufuer, A.; Wubuli, A.; Mijiti, P.; Zhou, J.; Tuerxun, S.; Cai, J.; Ma, J.; Zhang, X. Impact of collateral circulation status on favorable outcomes in thrombolysis treatment: A systematic review and meta-analysis. *Exp. Ther. Med.* **2018**, *15*, 707–718. [CrossRef] [PubMed]
22. Olivot, J.-M.; Mlynash, M.; Thijs, V.N.; Kemp, S.; Lansberg, M.G.; Wechsler, L.; Bammer, R.; Marks, M.P.; Albers, G.W. Optimal Tmax threshold for predicting penumbral tissue in acute stroke. *Stroke* **2009**, *40*, 469–475. [CrossRef] [PubMed]
23. Mlynash, M.; Lansberg, M.G.; De Silva, D.A.; Lee, J.; Christensen, S.; Straka, M.; Campbell, B.C.; Bammer, R.; Olivot, J.-M.; Desmond, P. Refining the definition of the malignant profile: Insights from the DEFUSE-EPITHET pooled data set. *Stroke* **2011**, *42*, 1270–1275. [CrossRef] [PubMed]

24. Al-Dasuqi, K.; Payabvash, S.; Torres-Flores, G.A.; Strander, S.M.; Nguyen, C.K.; Peshwe, K.U.; Kodali, S.; Silverman, A.; Malhotra, A.; Johnson, M.H. Effects of collateral status on infarct distribution following endovascular therapy in large vessel occlusion stroke. *Stroke* **2020**, *51*, e193–e202. [CrossRef]
25. Bathla, G.; Limaye, K.; Policeni, B.; Klotz, E.; Juergens, M.; Derdeyn, C. Achieving comparable perfusion results across vendors. The next step in standardizing stroke care: A technical report. *J. Neurointerventional Surg.* **2019**, *11*, 1257–1260. [CrossRef]
26. Bathla, G.; Ortega-Gutierrez, S.; Klotz, E.; Juergens, M.; Zevallos, C.B.; Ansari, S.; Ward, C.E.; Policeni, B.; Samaniego, E.; Derdeyn, C. Comparing the outcomes of two independent computed tomography perfusion softwares and their impact on therapeutic decisions in acute ischemic stroke. *J. Neurointerventional Surg.* **2020**, *12*, 1028–1032. [CrossRef]
27. Xia, Q.; Wang, X.; Zhang, Z.; Fang, Q.; Hu, C. Relationship between CT angiography-derived collateral status and CT perfusion-derived tissue viability. *Clin. Radiol.* **2019**, *74*, 956–961. [CrossRef]
28. de Havenon, A.; Mlynash, M.; Kim-Tenser, M.A.; Lansberg, M.G.; Leslie-Mazwi, T.; Christensen, S.; McTaggart, R.A.; Alexander, M.; Albers, G.; Broderick, J. Results from DEFUSE 3: Good collaterals are associated with reduced ischemic core growth but not neurologic outcome. *Stroke* **2019**, *50*, 632–638. [CrossRef]
29. Seker, F.; Potreck, A.; Möhlenbruch, M.; Bendszus, M.; Pham, M. Comparison of four different collateral scores in acute ischemic stroke by CT angiography. *J. Neurointerventional Surg.* **2016**, *8*, 1116–1118. [CrossRef]

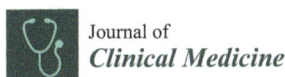

Article

Novel Estimation of Penumbra Zone Based on Infarct Growth Using Machine Learning Techniques in Acute Ischemic Stroke

Yoon-Chul Kim [1], Hyung Jun Kim [2], Jong-Won Chung [2], In Gyeong Kim [2], Min Jung Seong [3], Keon Ha Kim [3], Pyoung Jeon [3], Hyo Suk Nam [4], Woo-Keun Seo [2], Gyeong-Moon Kim [2] and Oh Young Bang [2,*]

[1] Clinical Research Institute, Samsung Medical Center, School of Medicine, Sungkyunkwan University, Seoul 06351, Korea; yoonckim1@gmail.com
[2] Department of Neurology, Samsung Medical Center, School of Medicine, Sungkyunkwan University, Seoul 06351, Korea; khhhj7@naver.com (H.J.K.); neurocjw@gmail.com (J.-W.C.); smcingyeong@naver.com (I.G.K.); mcastenosis@gmail.com (W.-K.S.); kimgm@skku.edu (G.-M.K.)
[3] Department of Radiology, Samsung Medical Center, School of Medicine, Sungkyunkwan University, Seoul 06351, Korea; m.seong@samsung.com (M.J.S.); somatom.kim@samsung.com (K.H.K.); pyoung.jeon@samsung.com (P.J.)
[4] Department of Neurology, Yonsei University, Seoul 03722, Korea; hsnam@yuhs.ac
* Correspondence: neuroboy50@naver.com; Tel.: +82-2-3410-3599

Received: 19 May 2020; Accepted: 22 June 2020; Published: 24 June 2020

Abstract: While the penumbra zone is traditionally assessed based on perfusion–diffusion mismatch, it can be assessed based on machine learning (ML) prediction of infarct growth. The purpose of this work was to develop and validate an ML method for the prediction of infarct growth distribution and volume, in cases of successful (SR) and unsuccessful recanalization (UR). Pre-treatment perfusion-weighted, diffusion-weighted imaging (DWI) data, and final infarct lesions annotated from day-7 DWI from patients with middle cerebral artery occlusion were utilized to develop and validate two ML models for prediction of tissue fate. SR and UR models were developed from data in patients with modified treatment in cerebral infarction (mTICI) scores of 2b–3 and 0–2a, respectively. When compared to manual infarct annotation, ML-based infarct volume predictions resulted in an intraclass correlation coefficient (ICC) of 0.73 (95% CI = 0.31–0.91, $p < 0.01$) for UR, and an ICC of 0.87 (95% CI = 0.73–0.94, $p < 0.001$) for SR. Favorable outcomes for mismatch presence and absence in SR were 50% and 36%, respectively, while they were 61%, 56%, and 25%, respectively, for the low, intermediate, and high infarct growth groups. The presented method can offer novel and alternative insights into selecting patients for recanalization therapy and predicting functional outcome.

Keywords: stroke; ischemia; machine learning; cerebral infarction

1. Introduction

Measurement of ischemic core and penumbra volumes in acute ischemic stroke provides clinicians with important clues for predicting clinical response after successful recanalization (SR) and selecting patients for treatments, such as intravenous thrombolysis and endovascular therapy (EVT) [1–3]. Diffusion-weighted imaging (DWI) and perfusion-weighted imaging (PWI) in magnetic resonance imaging (MRI) are neuroimaging modalities that can visualize the location and extent of ischemic stroke lesions with high sensitivity and specificity. The target mismatch criteria help determine patient selection for EVT and are evaluated using DWI and PWI lesion volumes [2].

Besides measurement of the PWI–DWI mismatch zone, estimation of infarct growth would provide a direct approach to the prediction of penumbra areas and the final infarct lesion volume [4].

There have been conflicting results on whether mismatch volume predicts infarct growth volume. It was reported that the infarct growth volume was greater than the mismatch volume, and half of the patients without target mismatch suffered from infarct growth regardless of the revascularization [5,6], while a recent randomized trial of EVT showed a good correlation between the predicted infarct volume and the 27-h infarct volume in target mismatch patients [7]. A clinical trial with a serial MRI study reported that ischemic lesion volume increased, by various degrees, from baseline to 12 weeks in untreated patients [8].

Machine learning (ML) has emerged as a promising methodology in acute stroke neuroimaging to predict ischemic stroke growth by interpolation of shape representations [9], and to predict the voxel-based tissue outcome [10,11] and the clinical outcome [12]. In particular, an ML method, referred to as fully automated stroke tissue estimation using random forest classifiers (FASTER) [13], showed potential to accurately predict final lesion volumes in cases of SR and unsuccessful recanalization (UR). However, the study did not investigate the performance of ML-based infarct growth estimation in comparison with target mismatch based on PWI–DWI mismatch volume and did not evaluate the prediction of clinical outcomes according to ML-based infarct growth estimation.

In the present study, we investigated the feasibility of an ML-based tissue outcome prediction technique using features derived from DWI and PWI data. Based on the ML method, we evaluated the performance of predicting final infarct volumes and infarct growth in the SR and UR cases. We also investigated how well the selection based on the ML-predicted infarct growth volume corresponded with the target mismatch classification in actual infarct growth and functional outcome distributions.

2. Materials and Methods

2.1. Patients

This study included patients who were admitted to a university medical center between 5 June 2005 and 31 December 2016. The study inclusion criteria were as follows: (1) symptomatic middle cerebral artery (MCA) occlusion, (2) MRI scan including DWI and PWI sequences prior to treatment and including DWI at 7 days after symptom onset, and (3) baseline MRI within 6 h of symptom onset.

Patients were divided into two groups: UR and SR. The UR group consisted of patients with modified treatment in cerebral infarction (mTICI) scores of 0–2a. The SR group consisted of patients with mTICI scores of 2b–3. For patients treated with EVT, the mTICI score was determined based on post procedural digital subtraction angiography (DSA), and for patients treated with intravenous (IV) tissue plasminogen activator (tPA), it was determined based on 24 h MRI and MR angiography (MRA).

The UR group was divided into the UR development and UR external validation groups, and the SR group was divided into the SR development and SR external validation groups. All patients in the SR group underwent EVT. The development/validation division criterion was based on the chronology of acute ischemic stroke occurrence: The UR and SR development groups corresponded to stroke onset dates prior to 31 December 2010 and 31 December 2011, respectively.

Demographic information including age and sex, baseline National Institutes of Health Stroke Scale (NIHSS) scores, and the 90-day modified Rankin Scale (mRS) scores were collected. The baseline NIHSS score is used to quantify the impairment due to a stroke and ranges from no symptoms at all (0) to the most severe stroke (42). The 90-day mRS score is used to assess clinical outcome and ranges from no symptoms at all (0) to death (6). Radiologic information, such as time interval from symptom onset to MRI, was obtained from electronic medical records.

All patients or patient guardians provided informed consent for inclusion before they participated in the study. The study was conducted in accordance with the Declaration of Helsinki, and the protocol was approved by the institutional review board of the Samsung Medical Center (IRB no. 2016-08-064).

2.2. Data Acquisition

MRI data were acquired on a 3T scanner system (Philips Achieva, Best, the Netherlands). DWI sequence parameters were as follows: repetition time = 3 s, echo time = 81–88 ms, number of slices = 22, image matrix size = 256 × 256, pixel spacing = 0.9375 mm × 0.9375 mm, and spacing between slices = 6.5 mm. The apparent diffusion coefficient (ADC) was calculated in a pixel-by-pixel manner from DWI acquired with b = 0 and b = 1000 s/mm^2. The PWI sequence was based on the commonly used T2*-weighted dynamic susceptibility contrast with the injection of a bolus of extracellular gadolinium contrast agent, and the parameters were as follows: repetition time = 1.5–1.7 s, echo time = 35 ms, number of slices = 22, spacing between slices = 6.5 mm, echo train length = 67, number of frames = 50, image matrix = 256 × 256, pixel spacing = 0.9375 mm × 0.9375 mm, and spacing between slices = 6.5 mm.

2.3. ADC/rTTP and Data Preprocessing

Typically, ADC and time-to-maximum (Tmax) are used to determine diffusion and perfusion lesion volumes, respectively. A recent study suggested that relative time to peak (rTTP) > 4.5 s was empirically identical to Tmax (>6 s) in determining perfusion lesion volume and resulted in > 90% accuracy, when compared with the conventional Tmax (>6 s) [14]. Notably, in the present study we used the statistics of rTTP as features for ML training, as opposed to a previous study, which used the statistics of Tmax, cerebral blood flow (CBF), cerebral blood volume (CBV), and time to peak (TTP) values as features for ML training [13]. Tmax, CBF, and CBV calculations involve numerical deconvolution with arterial input function (AIF), which is known to be sensitive to image artifacts and the choice of region of interest in major cerebral arteries [15]. The present study only considered the calculation of rTTP (i.e., the TTP delay relative to the contralateral region) for the extraction of PWI-related imaging features, and it did not consider estimating the AIF and performing numerical deconvolution. We sought to evaluate the correspondence between the rTTP-derived PWI lesion volume and the Tmax-derived PWI lesion volume, and the rTTP > 4.5 s volume showed Pearson correlation coefficient of 0.84 with the Tmax > 6 s volume in the subjects considered in the study (Figure A1).

Baseline DWI/ADC, PWI, and day-7 DWI images were co-registered using Statistical Parametric Mapping (SPM) 12 [16]. The rTTP maps from baseline PWI data were automatically calculated as follows. At each voxel, the MR signal was converted to contrast agent concentration, and TTP was measured from the concentration curve. Median TTP values were computed from the right and left hemispheric regions, respectively. The hemisphere with the lower median TTP value was defined as the contralateral region, and the median TTP value in this region served as the baseline TTP. The rTTP maps were calculated by voxel-wise subtraction of the baseline TTP from TTP values.

The midsagittal plane in the axial brain slice was automatically estimated after determining the optimal values of the translation and rotation parameters. The parameter values were used to identify the midline of an image. The midline helped to identify the correct location of a symmetric contralateral voxel, given a stroke lesion voxel, when feature extraction was performed for ML model development.

2.4. ML Model Development

A schematic of the presented ML method is illustrated in Figure 1B, in comparison with the traditional approach based on the PWI/DWI target mismatch (Figure 1A).

Feature extraction was conducted as follows. Seven consecutive axial slices covering the brain tissue in the MCA territory were considered for feature extraction. All the voxels in the tissue of the lesion hemisphere were considered as candidates, where the infarct voxels were labeled as "1", and the non-infarct voxels were labeled as "0". For training, to avoid class imbalance issues, we set the number of infarct voxels to be equal to the number of non-infarct voxels. For each candidate voxel, we considered its neighborhood as 5 × 5 × 3 voxels surrounding the candidate voxel. From the ADC values of the neighborhood, a set of 12 features was computed, consisting of range, mean, median, min, max, standard deviation (SD), skew, kurtosis, 10th percentile, 25th percentile, 75th percentile, and 90th percentile. Another set of 12 features was computed from the rTTP values in the neighborhood. These 24 features were also computed from a neighborhood of the voxel in the contralateral hemisphere. Hence, the number of features was 24 × 2 = 48. For the UR model, the dimensions of (# of samples) × (# of features) in the training dataset were 297,192 × 48, which provided the input for the UR model. For the SR model, the dimensions in the training dataset were 193,510 × 48, which provided the input for the SR model. Binary infarct masks, manually delineated while referring to the day-7 DWI images, were obtained from all the datasets using the ITK-SNAP software [17]. The output class labels for supervised ML were obtained from the binary infarct masks.

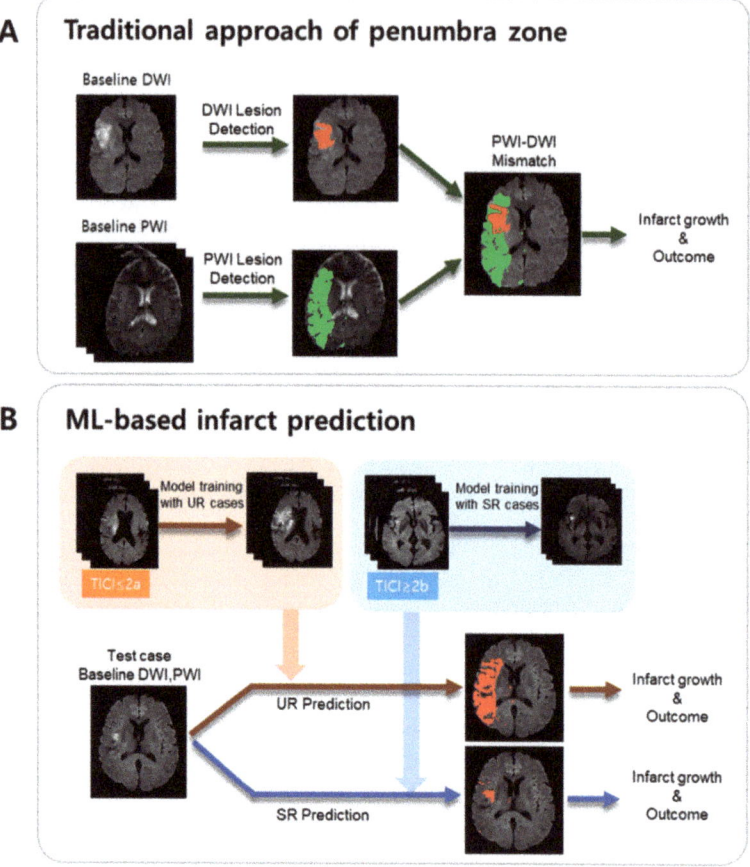

Figure 1. Schematics of two approaches for the estimation of final infarct volume and functional outcome. (**A**) Traditional approach of penumbra zone estimation. (**B**) Machine learning (ML)-based infarct prediction.

With the training dataset, a five-fold cross-validation was performed to evaluate the performance of the UR and SR models. The splitting in the cross-validation folds was constructed on the basis of patients rather than voxels. The assignment of patients to each fold was performed randomly. The ML model of the random forest classifier, provided by the Python scikit-learn module, was used for cross-validation [18]. After hyperparameter selection of the model using a random search, the mean and SD of cross-validation accuracy was computed for each model.

2.5. External Validation

For external validation, we used baseline DWI and PWI images from the 12 UR and the 27 SR patients. Candidate voxels were chosen, and for each candidate voxel, the feature extraction procedures were performed in the same manner as those for the model development. For each voxel, the extracted features were input to the trained UR and SR models to result in a tissue outcome probability score p, where $p \geq 0.5$ indicated an infarct voxel, and $p < 0.5$ indicated a non-infarct voxel. After processing all the candidate voxels, we obtained binary infarct prediction maps for both the UR and SR cases. The final infarct volume was calculated as the number of predicted infarct voxels multiplied by the voxel volume. Two final infarct volumes were calculated: one for the UR case and the other for the SR case.

For the UR (or SR) patient group, the final infarct volumes from the UR (or SR) model were compared with the final infarct volumes from the manually annotated day-7 DWI infarct masks. The Dice similarity coefficient (i.e., Dice score) was computed for each patient to evaluate the overlap between the ML predicted infarct mask and the manually segmented day-7 DWI infarct mask.

2.6. Mismatch and Infarct Growth Estimation

Target mismatch classification requires information on baseline diffusion and perfusion lesion volumes. We computed the Tmax > 6 s volume (i.e., perfusion lesion volume), the Tmax > 10 s volume (i.e., severe ischemic lesion volume), and the ischemic core volume based on the ADC < 600×10^{-6} mm^2/s threshold. Target mismatch criteria were defined as (1) a perfusion lesion volume to ischemic core volume ratio of 1.8 or more, (2) a difference between perfusion lesion volume and ischemic core volume of 15 mL or more, (3) the ischemic core volume less than 70 mL, and (4) the Tmax > 10 s volume less than 100 mL.

Actual infarct growth volume was calculated as the difference between the day-7 final infarct volume and the baseline diffusion lesion volume (i.e., ischemic core volume). The day-7 final infarct volume was measured after manual segmentation of the infarct lesions. Predicted infarct growth volume was calculated as the difference between the SR (or UR) predicted infarct volume and the baseline diffusion lesion volume. The SR (or UR) patients were categorized into tertiles according to the predicted infarct growth volume.

The percentage of favorable functional outcome was evaluated for the patient groups with and without target mismatch and for the patient groups categorized into tertiles based on SR (or UR) predicted infarct growth. Favorable functional outcome was defined as a 90-day mRS score of ≤ 1.

2.7. Statistical Analysis

We conducted statistical analysis using the R software package (R Foundation for Statistical Computing, Vienna, Austria). Descriptive demographics, and clinical and radiological data are shown as mean ± SDs, numbers, or median and interquartile ranges. An unpaired two-sample Student's t-test was performed to determine if the development and external validation data were significantly different in terms of age, NIHSS score, lesion volume, or onset to MRI time. A p-value < 0.05 was considered statistically significant. The intraclass correlation coefficient (ICC) and its 95% confidence interval (CI) were computed between the two infarct volume measurements. A p-value < 0.05 was considered to identify a statistically significant correlation, given the null hypothesis of no relationship between the two measurements. Bland–Altman analysis was performed by computing the mean difference and 95% limits of agreement (LOA) between the two volume measurements.

2.8. Data Statement

The datasets in the present study are not publicly available since they have private patient information. The de-identified data are available from the corresponding author upon request after approval of the institutional review board of Samsung Medical Center.

3. Results

A total of 102 patients satisfied the criteria of < 6 h stroke onset to MRI time, MCA occlusion, and baseline NIHSS score of ≥ 4. Of 102 patients, 40 patients had an mTICI score of 0–2a (comprising the UR group), and 62 patients had an mTICI score of 2b–3 (comprising the SR group). A total of 10 patients were excluded, since their image data were problematic in terms of (1) severe motion artifacts in PWI data ($n = 8$), (2) susceptibility artifact near frontal brain regions ($n = 1$), and (3) infarcts detected in unexpected locations on day-7 DWI, which were related to stroke recurrence or procedural complications ($n = 1$). Hence, out of 92 patients, the final numbers of SR and UR patients were 56 and 36, respectively (Table 1). In both the SR and UR groups, there were no statistically significant differences in age, male sex, baseline NIHSS score, onset to MRI time, baseline DWI and PWI lesion volumes, and day-7 DWI lesion volumes between the development and external validation groups, except for the baseline NIHSS score between the UR development and external validation groups (Table 1).

Table 1. Patient characteristics for machine learning (ML) model development and external validation.

	SR (mTICI 2b–3)			UR (mTICI 0–2a)		
	Development	External Validation	p-value	Development	External Validation	p-value
Number of patients	29	27	-	24	12	-
Age (years), mean ± SD	63 ± 13	67 ± 11	0.17	64 ± 14	67 ± 18	0.62
Male sex, n (%)	19 (66)	15 (56)	0.46	17 (71)	7 (58)	0.49
NIHSS score at baseline *	15 (11–18)	16 (10–20)	0.84	13 (9–18)	18 (15–19)	0.03
Onset to MRI time (m) *	131 (99–173)	97 (70–140)	0.20	187 (113–225)	138 (124–216)	0.75
DWI lesion vol (mL), initial *	15 (6–33)	11 (5–28)	0.88	9 (5–18)	15 (6–38)	0.58
PWI lesion vol (mL), initial *	93 (59–133)	104 (72–146)	0.73	83 (53–143)	96 (81–125)	0.93
DWI lesion vol (mL), day-7 *	17 (8–57)	21 (14–79)	0.20	61 (32–118)	124 (84–173)	0.12
Mode of treatment						
No, n (%)	0 (0)	0 (0)	-	4 (17)	0 (0)	-
IV tPA only, n (%)	0 (0)	0 (0)	-	1 (4)	3 (25)	-
EVT ± IV tPA, n (%)	29 (100)	27 (100)	-	19 (79)	9 (75)	-

* Median (IQR), Abbreviations: SR, successful recanalization; UR, unsuccessful recanalization; mTICI, modified treatment in cerebral infarction; SD, standard deviation; NIHSS, National Institutes of Health Stroke Scale; IQR, interquartile range; MRI, magnetic resonance imaging; DWI, diffusion-weighted imaging; PWI, perfusion-weighted imaging; IV, intravenous; tPA, tissue plasminogen activator; EVT, endovascular treatment.

For the UR model, the five-fold cross-validation resulted in a mean accuracy (SD) of 74.6% (2.5%) and a 95% CI of 69.8%–79.4%. For the SR model, the five-fold cross-validation resulted in a mean accuracy (standard deviation) of 76.4% (6.5%) and a 95% CI of 63.7%–89.2%.

Final infarct predictions using the UR and SR models are shown for four different cases (Figure 2; patient A: UR with large infarct growth; patient B: SR with small infarct growth; patient C: UR with small infarct growth; and patient D: SR with large infarct growth). The large differences between the UR-predicted and SR-predicted volumes were observed in both patients A and B, but the failure of revascularization led to the large final infarct volume (243 mL) and unfavorable outcome (90-day mRS = 5) in patient A, whereas the success of revascularization led to the small final infarct volume (4 mL) and favorable outcome (90-day mRS = 0) in patient B. Regarding the actual infarct growth, patient A's (239 mL) was significantly larger than patient C's (28 mL), while patient D's (69 mL) was significantly larger than patient B's (3 mL). All four cases had target mismatch and showed substantial differences in infarct growth volume, regardless of recanalization status.

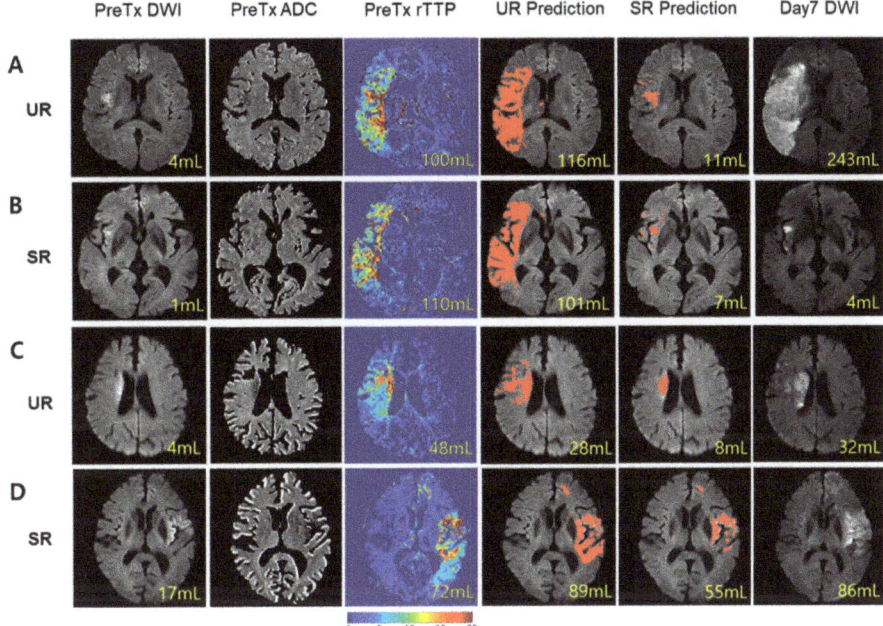

Figure 2. Sample external validation cases of SR- and UR-based infarct predictions. (**A**) A case of large infarct growth in a UR patient (intravenous thrombolysis, modified treatment in cerebral infarction (mTICI) = 0, and 90-day modified Rankin Scale (mRS) = 5). (**B**) A case of small infarct growth in an SR patient (endovascular therapy, mTICI = 2b, and 90-day mRS = 0). (**C**) A case of small infarct growth in a UR patient (endovascular therapy, mTICI = 1, and 90-day mRS = 2). (**D**) A case of large infarct growth in an SR patient (endovascular therapy, mTICI = 2b, and 90-day mRS = 5). Predicted infarct masks, shown in red, are overlaid on pre-treatment DWI images for UR and SR model predictions. All four patients had target mismatch presence but showed various degrees of infarct growth. The yellow numbers indicate the following volumes: (from left to right) baseline DWI lesion volume, baseline PWI lesion volume, UR-predicted infarct volume, SR-predicted infarct volume, and day-7 infarct volume.

In the UR model validation, the ICC between manual infarct volume and UR-predicted infarct volume was 0.73 (95% CI = 0.31–0.91, $p < 0.01$; Figure 3A). In the SR model validation, the ICC between manual infarct volume and SR-predicted infarct volume was 0.87 (95% CI = 0.73–0.94, $p < 0.001$; Figure 3B). The mean difference (95% LOA obtained from Bland–Altman analysis) was −32.5 mL (−126.9 mL, 61.9 mL) for the UR model validation and 3.5 mL (−48.2 mL, 55.2 mL) for the SR model validation.

In all the external validation subjects, the presented ML model had a median Dice similarity coefficient (DSC) of 0.49 (IQR, 0.37–0.59), which was comparable to the DSC of 0.53 (IQR, 0.31–0.68) in the study by Yu et al. [19]. The presented ML model had a median DSC of 0.43 (IQR, 0.20–0.52) in the SR external validation subjects and a median DSC of 0.58 (IQR, 0.55–0.67) in the UR external validation subjects.

In external validation SR patients ($n = 27$), there was a statistically significant difference in actual infarct growth volume between the mismatch and non-mismatch groups ($p = 0.02$; Figure 4A). It was also observed that there was a statistically significant difference in actual infarct growth volume between the low and high SR predicted infarct growth volume groups ($p = 0.01$; Figure 4B). *p*-values between the low and intermediate groups and between the intermediate and high groups were 0.08 and 0.15, respectively (Figure 4B).

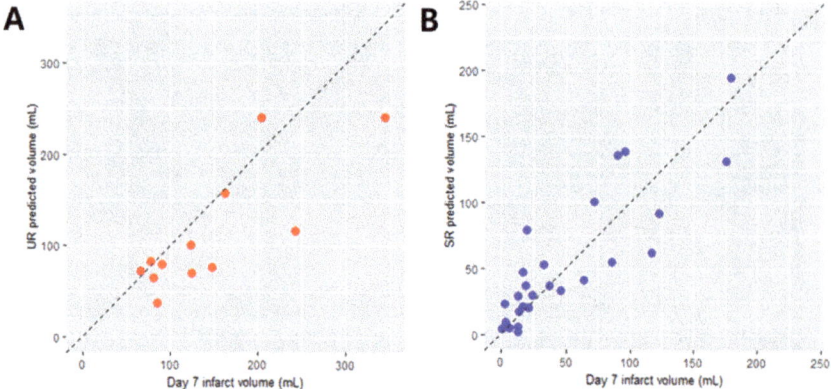

Figure 3. Correlation plots of (**A**) the UR-predicted infarct volume and (**B**) the SR-predicted infarct volume on the external validation UR and SR cohorts, respectively. The manual infarct volume measurement on day-7 DWI served as the reference.

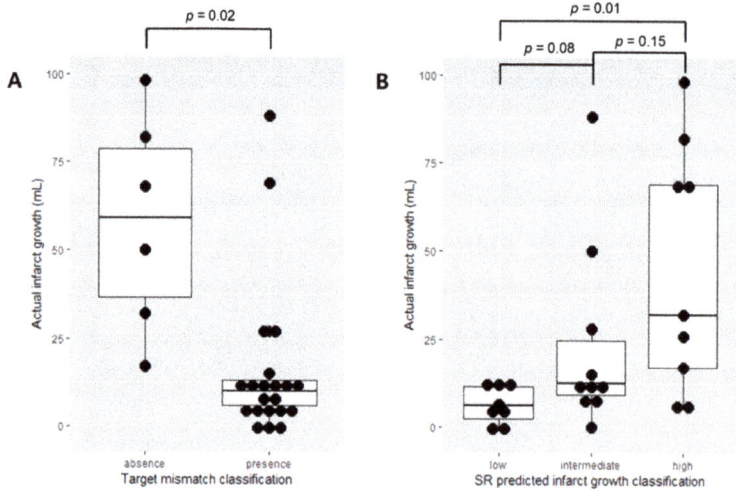

Figure 4. Infarct growth distribution in the external validation SR patients ($n = 27$). (**A**) Target mismatch classification. (**B**) SR-predicted infarct growth classification. In (**A**), the mismatch absence group shows a heterogeneous distribution of actual infarct growth. In (**B**), the high group (SR-predicted infarct growth ≥ 35 mL) shows a heterogeneous distribution of actual infarct growth, and the low group (SR-predicted infarct growth < 15 mL) shows the narrowest distribution of the actual infarct growth.

The percentage values of favorable clinical outcomes of the day-90 mRS score ≤ 1 for the mismatch presence and absence groups in overall SR patients were 50% and 36%, respectively (Figure 5A). The percentage values of favorable clinical outcomes were 61%, 56%, and 25%, respectively, for the low, intermediate, and high SR-predicted infarct growth groups (Figure 5A). In UR patients, the percentage values of favorable outcomes for the mismatch presence and absence groups were 14% and 0%, respectively, while they were 9%, 18%, and 7%, respectively, for the low, intermediate, and high UR-predicted infarct growth groups (Figure 5B).

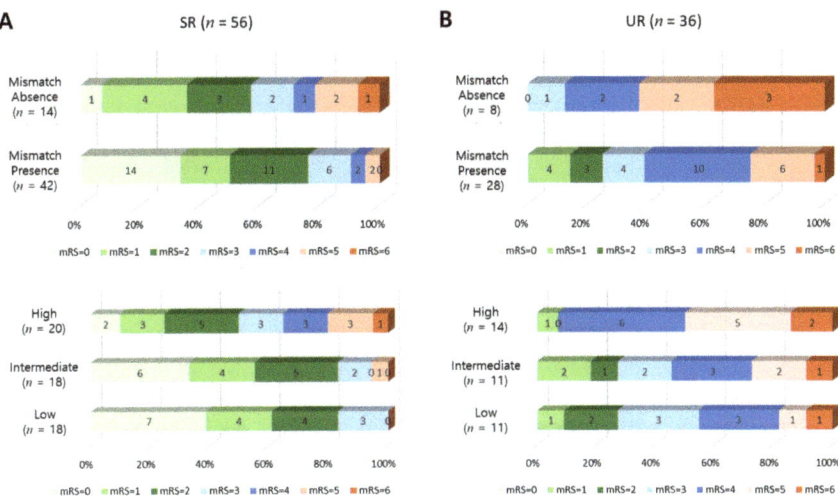

Figure 5. Distribution of modified Rankin Scale (mRS) scores at day-90 by target mismatch (top) and ML-predicted infarct growth (bottom). In both (**A**) SR and (**B**) UR patients, a lower ML-predicted infarct growth was related to a lower mRS score at day 90.

4. Discussion

This study suggests that the ML-predicted infarct growth volumes can offer a novel insight into selecting patients and predicting clinical outcome. The method may be a useful alternative to target mismatch, as it provides a direct way to measure infarct distribution and growth. Although the number of the mismatch absence group is small in this study, it indicates that the patient selection based on the ML-predicted infarct growth volume may have the infarct growth prediction performance comparable to target mismatch-based selection. In particular, the low infarct growth group showed a narrow distribution of the actual infarct growth, and this may indicate that once a patient was classified into the low group, a small infarct growth as well as a favorable clinical outcome would be highly likely. It is important to note that traditional PWI–DWI mismatch is evaluated only based on baseline DWI and PWI images without consideration of the final infarct images, while, in the presented approach, the SR and UR infarct volumes are estimated using ML models trained on baseline DWI and PWI images and the final infarct annotated images.

Ischemic penumbra is defined as a hypoperfused area that can regain function with rapid reperfusion [20]. This area is at a risk of infarction without rapid reperfusion, and infarct growth occurs in the absence of reperfusion. In the present study, mean infarct growth in the UR group was higher than that in the SR group, but the degree of infarct growth was highly variable in both UR and SR groups. The large variability of infarct growth within the SR (or UR) group may be attributed to the variable degrees of perfusion defect severities and ischemic damage in the penumbra zone or ischemic core.

Traditional threshold-based lesion volume estimation approaches have limitations, since the appropriate threshold values often depend on MRI sequence parameters, scanner vendors, and software analysis tools. ML takes a different perspective by learning a non-linear function from input/output relationships and has the potential to overcome the limitations of traditional threshold-based volume estimation approaches. Although the evaluation regarded traditional threshold-based methods used for target mismatch assessment as a reference, it is expected that the ML-based method could provide additional information in cases where threshold-based volume estimation is unsatisfactory. Until now, the Diffusion and perfusion imaging Evaluation For Understanding Stroke Evolution (DEFUSE) trial, Echo-Planar Imaging Thrombolytic Evaluation Trial (EPITHET), and other studies have attempted to find the optimal Tmax threshold and mismatch ratio [1,2,21,22]. Similarly, Olivot and colleagues showed that besides mismatch volume, lesion geography and structure also determine infarct growth [23]. Lastly, the rate of infarct growth during the few days after stroke onset varies substantially between patients, and certain patients have slow infarct growth while others have rapid infarct growth [24]. ML-based prediction has the potential to overcome the limitations of traditional approaches of estimating ischemic penumbra.

Current mismatch concepts provide information on the likelihood ratio and number needed to treat for a favorable outcome. In the Highly Effective Reperfusion evaluated in Multiple Endovascular Stroke trials (HERMES), a meta-analysis of individual patient data from five randomized trials of EVT, the odds ratio was 2.49 and the number needed to treat with EVT to reduce disability by at least one level of the mRS for one patient was 2.6 [25]. On the contrary, our ML-based prediction method can produce the visualization of the degree of DWI lesion growth, which can be shown to patients or their guardians, prior to revascularization therapy. ML predictions using our custom tool via post processing typically took approximately 8 min. Using the current strict recanalization criteria based on the mismatch concept, we can calculate treatment effect sizes, but at the cost of limiting the benefit to a small portion of our stroke patients [26]. With ML, treatment approaches may be more customized, rather than dichotomized into either withholding or offering treatment. In addition, Oppenheim and colleagues showed that in patients without SR, DWI volume > 145 mL within 14 h of onset reliably predicted a malignant MCA infarction [27]. ML-based prediction of infarct volume at the peak time of cytotoxic edema (at 3–4 days after the infarction) may guide early management, such as decompressive hemicraniectomy.

This study has several limitations. First, a larger mean difference of predicted infarct volume was observed for UR than for SR. The inaccuracy may be attributed to the large variability of infarct growth rate, which varies from person to person and is highly unpredictable [28]. It may be worth investigating the division of patient grouping based on the infarct growth rate and develop individual ML models. Second, a custom software tool was used to measure the pre-treatment PWI and DWI lesion volumes based on Tmax and ADC thresholds, for the target mismatch assessment. ML-based methods for lesion volume estimation may be alternative tools for mismatch evaluation [29,30]. Third, only ADC and rTTP were used for the ML model development in the present study. Consideration of other MRI sequences, such as fluid-attenuated inversion recovery (FLAIR), may improve the accuracy of infarct growth prediction [31]. Onset to imaging time can affect the volume of the ischemic penumbra zone, as well as the final infarct volume. Recently, the infarct growth rate estimated from the baseline DWI lesion volume and time of stroke onset was reported to be associated with penumbral salvage and clinical outcomes after EVT reperfusion [28]. In a similar fashion, we are currently investigating the feasibility of an improved prediction of infarct growth with the incorporation of relative FLAIR, which is indicative of a 'tissue clock', into the prediction model. Fourth, Lev and colleagues reported the importance of 'location-weighted' scoring over simple volumetric data of penumbra areas [32,33]. For instance, in patients with similar infarct volumes, different severities of neurologic deficits can be observed, depending on the clinical features and lesion site. Hence, location-weighted ML-based prediction of functional outcome is worthy of investigation. Fifth, clinical variables were not used in this study. Previous studies demonstrated the effectiveness of clinical variables in the prediction of infarct growth [34] and clinical outcome [35], while our study was solely based on image features. The inclusion of clinical variables may help improve the outcome prediction. Finally, this was a single-center study performed on a 3T scanner, with only a small number of patients available for analysis. A larger prospective study is necessary to evaluate the benefit of the ML-based method.

5. Conclusions

ML-based prediction of tissue fate was demonstrated using two ML models trained on data from patients with and without recanalization. The presented ML-based method provides the estimations of voxel-wise infarct distributions and final infarct volumes in cases of SR and UR. The classification of patients in terms of ML-predicted infarct growth offers novel and alternative ways to predict infarct growth and functional outcome, when compared with the traditional target mismatch classification. As ML is data-driven and allows sophisticated feature engineering, the ML prediction is expected to improve as more data are collected and careful ML modeling is made based on multi-modal MRI. The advancement of technology will implicate more accurate predictions of the final infarct distribution, potentially providing clinicians with precise information for the guidance of treatment selection and the prediction of clinical outcome.

Author Contributions: Conceptualization, O.Y.B. and Y.-C.K.; methodology, O.Y.B. and Y.-C.K.; software, Y.-C.K.; validation, O.Y.B., Y.-C.K., H.J.K., J.-W.C.; formal analysis, O.Y.B.; investigation, O.Y.B.; resources, O.Y.B., H.S.N., P.J., K.H.K., M.J.S.; data curation, O.Y.B., I.K.; writing—original draft preparation, O.Y.B., Y.-C.K.; writing—review and editing, O.Y.B., Y.-C.K., J.-W.C., H.K, W.-K.S., G.-M.K.; visualization, O.Y.B., Y.-C.K.; supervision, O.Y.B., G.-M.K.; project administration, O.Y.B., I.G.K.; funding acquisition, O.Y.B. All authors have read and agreed to the published version of the manuscript.

Funding: This research was supported by the National Research Foundation of Korea, grant numbers 2018R1A2B2003489 and 2018R1D1A1B07042692.

Conflicts of Interest: The authors declare no conflict of interest. The funding sources had no role in the design of the study; in the collection, analyses, or interpretation of data; in the writing of the manuscript, or in the decision to publish the results.

Appendix A

Comparison of Tmax > 6 s Volume and rTTP > 4.5 s Volume

A custom MATLAB (Mathworks, Natick, MA, USA) module was developed to calculate Tmax from PWI time series image data and compare it with rTTP. An axial slice with middle cerebral arteries was selected, and an arterial input function (AIF) was automatically calculated by the cluster analysis proposed by Mouridsen et al. [36]. Standard singular value decomposition (SVD) [37] was used to estimate Tmax, defined to be the delay of the peak of the residue function. Figure A1-A compares Tmax > 6 s volume with rTTP > 4.5 s volume. Pearson correlation coefficient between Tmax > 6 s and rTTP > 4.5 s volumes was 0.84 (95% CI = 0.75–0.89, *p*-value < 0.0001). The mean difference (95% limits of agreement from Bland-Altman analysis) was −2.4 mL (−66.3 mL, 61.5 mL). Figure A1-B compares Tmax > 10 s volume with rTTP > 9.5 s volume. Pearson correlation coefficient between Tmax > 10 s and rTTP > 9.5 s volumes was 0.81 (95% CI = 0.72–0.87, *p*-value < 0.0001). The mean difference (95% limits of agreement from Bland–Altman analysis) was 7.5 mL (−42.9 mL, 57.9 mL).

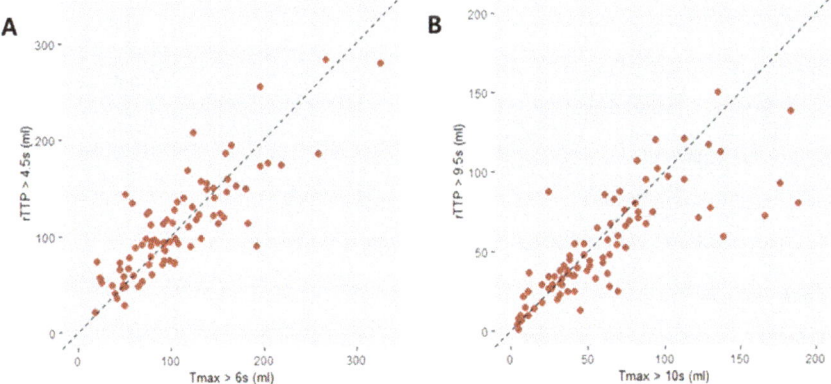

Figure A1. Comparison of time-to-maximum (Tmax) and relative time to peak (rTTP) lesion volumes. (**A**) Perfusion lesion volumes measured by Tmax and rTTP. (**B**) Severe ischemic lesion volumes measured by Tmax and rTTP.

References

1. Albers, G.W.; Thijs, V.N.; Wechsler, L.; Kemp, S.; Schlaug, G.; Skalabrin, E.; Bammer, R.; Kakuda, W.; Lansberg, M.G.; Shuaib, A.; et al. Magnetic resonance imaging profiles predict clinical response to early reperfusion: The diffusion and perfusion imaging evaluation for understanding stroke evolution (DEFUSE) study. *Ann. Neurol.* **2006**, *60*, 17–508. [CrossRef] [PubMed]
2. Albers, G.W.; Marks, M.P.; Kemp, S.; Christensen, S.; Tsai, J.P.; Ortega-Gutierrez, S.; McTaggart, R.A.; Torbey, M.T.; Kim-Tenser, M.; Leslie-Mazwi, T.; et al. Thrombectomy for Stroke at 6 to 16 Hours with Selection by Perfusion Imaging. *N. Engl. J. Med.* **2018**, *378*, 708–718. [CrossRef] [PubMed]
3. Bang, O.Y.; Chung, J.W.; Son, J.P.; Ryu, W.S.; Kim, D.E.; Seo, W.K.; Kim, G.M.; Kim, Y.C. Multimodal MRI-Based Triage for Acute Stroke Therapy: Challenges and Progress. *Front. Neurol.* **2018**, *9*, 586. [CrossRef] [PubMed]
4. Rosso, C.; Hevia-Montiel, N.; Deltour, S.; Bardinet, E.; Dormont, D.; Crozier, S.; Baillet, S.; Samson, Y. Prediction of infarct growth based on apparent diffusion coefficients: Penumbral assessment without intravenous contrast material. *Radiology* **2009**, *250*, 92–184. [CrossRef]
5. Kane, I.; Sandercock, P.; Wardlaw, J. Magnetic resonance perfusion diffusion mismatch and thrombolysis in acute ischaemic stroke: A systematic review of the evidence to date. *J. Neurol. Neurosurg. Psychiatry* **2007**, *78*, 485–491. [CrossRef]
6. Ma, H.K.; Zavala, J.A.; Churilov, L.; Ly, J.; Wright, P.M.; Phan, T.G.; Arakawa, S.; Davis, S.M.; Donnan, G.A. The hidden mismatch: An explanation for infarct growth without perfusion-weighted imaging/diffusion-weighted imaging mismatch in patients with acute ischemic stroke. *Stroke* **2011**, *42*, 662–668. [CrossRef]
7. Albers, G.W.; Goyal, M.; Jahan, R.; Bonafe, A.; Diener, H.C.; Levy, E.I.; Pereira, V.M.; Cognard, C.; Cohen, D.J.; Hacke, W.; et al. Ischemic core and hypoperfusion volumes predict infarct size in SWIFT PRIME. *Ann. Neurol.* **2016**, *79*, 76–89. [CrossRef]
8. Warach, S.; Pettigrew, L.C.; Dashe, J.F.; Pullicino, P.; Lefkowitz, D.M.; Sabounjian, L.; Harnett, K.; Schwiderski, U.; Gammans, R. Effect of citicoline on ischemic lesions as measured by diffusion-weighted magnetic resonance imaging. Citicoline 010 Investigators. *Ann. Neurol.* **2000**, *48*, 22–713. Available online: https://www.ncbi.nlm.nih.gov/pubmed/11079534 (accessed on 23 June 2020). [CrossRef]
9. Lucas, C.; Kemmling, A.; Bouteldja, N.; Aulmann, L.F.; Mamlouk, A.M.; Heinrich, M.P. Learning to Predict Ischemic Stroke Growth on Acute CT Perfusion Data by Interpolating Low-Dimensional Shape Representations. *Front. Neurol.* **2018**, *9*, 989. [CrossRef]
10. Nielsen, A.; Hansen, M.B.; Tietze, A.; Mouridsen, K. Prediction of Tissue Outcome and Assessment of Treatment Effect in Acute Ischemic Stroke Using Deep Learning. *Stroke* **2018**, *49*, 1394–1401. [CrossRef]
11. Pinto, A.; McKinley, R.; Alves, V.; Wiest, R.; Silva, C.A.; Reyes, M. Stroke Lesion Outcome Prediction Based on MRI Imaging Combined With Clinical Information. *Front. Neurol.* **2018**, *9*, 1060. [CrossRef] [PubMed]
12. Tang, T.Y.; Jiao, Y.; Cui, Y.; Zeng, C.H.; Zhao, Y.; Zhang, Y.; Peng, C.Y.; Yin, X.D.; Gao, P.Y.; Yang, Y.J.; et al. Development and validation of a penumbra-based predictive model for thrombolysis outcome in acute ischemic stroke patients. *EBioMedicine* **2018**, *35*, 251–259. [CrossRef] [PubMed]
13. McKinley, R.; Hani, L.; Gralla, J.; El-Koussy, M.; Bauer, S.; Arnold, M.; Fischer, U.; Jung, S.; Mattmann, K.; Reyes, M.; et al. Fully automated stroke tissue estimation using random forest classifiers (FASTER). *J. Cereb. Blood Flow Metab.* **2017**, *37*, 2728–2741. [CrossRef] [PubMed]
14. Wouters, A.; Christensen, S.; Straka, M.; Mlynash, M.; Liggins, J.; Bammer, R.; Thijs, V.; Lemmens, R.; Albers, G.W.; Lansberg, M.G. A Comparison of Relative Time to Peak and Tmax for Mismatch-Based Patient Selection. *Front. Neurol.* **2017**, *8*, 539. [CrossRef] [PubMed]
15. Calamante, F. Arterial input function in perfusion MRI: A comprehensive review. *Prog. Nucl. Magn. Reason. Spectrosc.* **2013**, *74*, 1–32. [CrossRef] [PubMed]
16. Ashburner, J. SPM: A history. *Neuroimage* **2012**, *62*, 791–800. [CrossRef]
17. Yushkevich, P.A.; Piven, J.; Hazlett, H.C.; Smith, R.G.; Ho, S.; Gee, J.C.; Gerig, G. User-guided 3D active contour segmentation of anatomical structures: Significantly improved efficiency and reliability. *Neuroimage* **2006**, *31*, 1116–1118. [CrossRef]
18. Pedregosa, F.; Varoquaux, G.; Gramfort, A.; Michel, V.; Thirion, B.; Grisel, O.; Blondel, M.; Prettenhofer, P.; Weiss, R.; Dubourg, V. Scikit-learn: Machine learning in Python. *J. Mach. Learn. Res.* **2011**, *12*, 2825–2830.

19. Yu, Y.; Xie, Y.; Thamm, T.; Gong, E.; Ouyang, J.; Huang, C.; Christensen, S.; Marks, M.P.; Lansberg, M.G.; Albers, G.W. Use of Deep Learning to Predict Final Ischemic Stroke Lesions from Initial Magnetic Resonance Imaging. *JAMA Netw. Open* **2020**, *3*, e200772. [CrossRef]
20. Astrup, J.; Siesjo, B.K.; Symon, L. Thresholds in cerebral ischemia—The ischemic penumbra. *Stroke* **1981**, *12*, 723–725. [CrossRef]
21. Zaro-Weber, O.; Fleischer, H.; Reiblich, L.; Schuster, A.; Moeller-Hartmann, W.; Heiss, W.D. Penumbra detection in acute stroke with perfusion magnetic resonance imaging: Validation with (15) O-positron emission tomography. *Ann. Neurol.* **2019**, *85*, 875–886. [CrossRef] [PubMed]
22. Kakuda, W.; Lansberg, M.G.; Thijs, V.N.; Kemp, S.M.; Bammer, R.; Wechsler, L.R.; Moseley, M.E.; Marks, M.P.; Albers, G.W. Optimal definition for PWI/DWI mismatch in acute ischemic stroke patients. *J. Cereb. Blood Flow Metab.* **2008**, *28*, 887–891. [CrossRef] [PubMed]
23. Olivot, J.M.; Mlynash, M.; Thijs, V.N.; Purushotham, A.; Kemp, S.; Lansberg, M.G.; Wechsler, L.; Gold, G.E.; Bammer, R.; Marks, M.P.; et al. Geography, structure, and evolution of diffusion and perfusion lesions in Diffusion and perfusion imaging Evaluation for Understanding Stroke Evolution (DEFUSE). *Stroke* **2009**, *40*, 3245–3251. [CrossRef]
24. Albers, G.W. Late Window Paradox. *Stroke* **2018**, *49*, 768–771. [CrossRef] [PubMed]
25. Goyal, M.; Menon, B.K.; van Zwam, W.H.; Dippel, D.W.; Mitchell, P.J.; Demchuck, A.M.; Davalos, A.; Majoie, C.B.; van der Lugt, A.; de Miquel, M.A.; et al. Endovascular thrombectomy after large-vessel ischaemic stroke: A meta-analysis of individual patient data from five randomised trials. *Lancet* **2016**, *387*, 1723–1731. [CrossRef]
26. Nogueira, R.G.; Ribo, M. Endovascular Treatment of Acute Stroke. *Stroke* **2019**, *50*, 2612–2618. [CrossRef]
27. Oppenheim, C.; Samson, Y.; Manai, R.; Lalam, T.; Vandamme, X.; Crozier, S.; Srour, A.; Cornu, P.; Dormont, D.; Rancurel, G.; et al. Prediction of malignant middle cerebral artery infarction by diffusion-weighted imaging. *Stroke* **2000**, *31*, 2175–2781. [CrossRef]
28. Wheeler, H.M.; Mlynash, M.; Inoue, M.; Tipirnini, A.; Liggins, J.; Bammer, R.; Lansberg, M.G.; Kemp, S.; Zaharchuck, G.; Straka, M.; et al. The growth rate of early DWI lesions is highly variable and associated with penumbral salvage and clinical outcomes following endovascular reperfusion. *Int. J. Stroke* **2015**, *10*, 723–729. [CrossRef]
29. Kim, Y.C.; Lee, J.E.; Yu, I.; Song, H.N.; Baek, I.Y.; Seong, J.K.; Jeong, H.G.; Kim, B.J.; Nam, H.S.; Chung, J.W.; et al. Evaluation of Diffusion Lesion Volume Measurements in Acute Ischemic Stroke Using Encoder-Decoder Convolutional Network. *Stroke* **2019**, *50*, 1444–1451. [CrossRef]
30. McKinley, R.; Hung, F.; Wiest, R.; Liebeskind, D.S.; Scalzo, F. A Machine Learning Approach to Perfusion Imaging with Dynamic Susceptibility Contrast MR. *Front. Neurol.* **2018**, *9*, 717. [CrossRef]
31. Livne, M.; Boldsen, J.K.; Mikkelsen, I.K.; Fiebach, J.B.; Sobesky, J.; Mouridsen, K. Boosted Tree Model Reforms Multimodal Magnetic Resonance Imaging Infarct Prediction in Acute Stroke. *Stroke* **2018**, *49*, 912–918. [CrossRef] [PubMed]
32. Lev, M.H. CT/NIHSS mismatch for detection of salvageable brain in acute stroke triage beyond the 3-h time window: Overrated or undervalued? *Stroke* **2007**, *38*, 2028–2029. [CrossRef] [PubMed]
33. Boers, A.M.M.; Jansen, I.G.H.; Brown, S.; Lingsma, H.F.; Beenen, L.F.M.; Devlin, T.G.; Roman, L.S.; Heo, J.H.; Ribo, M.; Almekhlafi, M.A.; et al. Mediation of the Relationship Between Endovascular Therapy and Functional Outcome by Follow-up Infarct Volume in Patients with Acute Ischemic Stroke. *JAMA Neurol.* **2019**, *76*, 194–202. [CrossRef] [PubMed]
34. Kamran, S.; Akhtar, N.; Alboudi, A.; Kamran, K.; Ahmad, A.; Inshasi, J.; Salam, A.; Shuaib, A.; Qidwai, U. Prediction of infarction volume and infarction growth rate in acute ischemic stroke. *Sci. Rep.* **2017**, *7*, 7565. [CrossRef] [PubMed]
35. Nishi, H.; Oishi, N.; Ishii, A.; Ono, I.; Ogura, T.; Sunohara, T.; Chihara, H.; Fukumitsu, R.; Okawa, M.; Yamana, N.; et al. Predicting Clinical Outcomes of Large Vessel Occlusion Before Mechanical Thrombectomy Using Machine Learning. *Stroke* **2019**, *50*, 2379–2388. [CrossRef]

36. Mouridsen, K.; Christensen, S.; Gyldensted, L.; Ostergaard, L. Automatic selection of arterial input function using cluster analysis. *Magn. Reason. Med.* **2006**, *55*, 524–531. [CrossRef]
37. Ostergaard, L.; Weisskoff, R.M.; Chesler, D.A.; Gyldensted, C.; Rosen, B.R. High resolution measurement of cerebral blood flow using intravascular tracer bolus passages. Part I: Mathematical approach and statistical analysis. *Magn. Reason. Med.* **1996**, *36*, 715–725. [CrossRef]

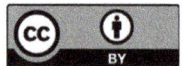

© 2020 by the authors. Licensee MDPI, Basel, Switzerland. This article is an open access article distributed under the terms and conditions of the Creative Commons Attribution (CC BY) license (http://creativecommons.org/licenses/by/4.0/).

Journal of
Clinical Medicine

Case Report

Acute Middle Cerebral Artery Occlusion Detection Using Mobile Non-Imaging Brain Perfusion Ultrasound—First Case

Mustafa Kilic [1], Christina Wendl [2], Sibylle Wilfling [1], David Olmes [1], Ralf Andreas Linker [1] and Felix Schlachetzki [1,*]

[1] Department of Neurology, Center for Vascular Neurology and Intensive Care, University of Regensburg, University Hospital Regensburg, Medbo Bezirksklinikum Regensburg, Universitaetsstr. 84, 93053 Regensburg, Germany; mustafa.kilic@medbo.de (M.K.); sibylle.wilfling@medbo.de (S.W.); david.olmes@medbo.de (D.O.); ralf.linker@medbo.de (R.A.L.)

[2] Center for Neuroradiology, University Hospital Regensburg, Medbo Bezirksklinikum Regensburg, Universitaetsstr. 84, 93053 Regensburg, Germany; christina.wendl@ukr.de

* Correspondence: felix.schlachetzki@klinik.uni-regensburg.de; Tel.: +49-941-941-3502; Fax: +49-941-941-3095

Abstract: Mobile brain perfusion ultrasound (BPU) is a novel non-imaging technique creating only hemispheric perfusion curves following ultrasound contrast injection and has been specifically designed for early prehospital large vessel occlusion (LVO) stroke identification. We report on the first patient investigated with the SONAS® system, a portable point-of-care ultrasound system for BPU. This patient was admitted into our stroke unit about 12 h following onset of a fluctuating motor aphasia, dysarthria and facial weakness resulting in an NIHSS of 3 to 8. Occlusion of the left middle cerebral artery occlusion was diagnosed by computed tomography angiography. BPU was performed in conjunction with injection of echo-contrast agent to generate hemispheric perfusion curves and in parallel, conventional color-coded sonography (TCCS) assessing MCAO. Both assessments confirmed the results of angiography. Emergency mechanical thrombectomy (MT) achieved complete recanalization (TICI 3) and post-interventional NIHSS of 2 the next day. Telephone follow-up after 2 years found the patient fully active in professional life. Point-of-care BPU is a non-invasive technique especially suitable for prehospital stroke diagnosis for LVO. BPU in conjunction with prehospital stroke scales may enable goal-directed stroke patient placement, i.e., directly to comprehensive stroke centers aiming for MT. Further results of the ongoing phase II study are needed to confirm this finding.

Keywords: prehospital stroke diagnosis; large vessel occlusion; ultrasound; thrombectomy; brain perfusion; SONAS®; prehospital stroke scales; point-of-care diagnostics

1. Introduction

Mechanical thrombectomy (MT) has evolved as the most efficient therapy in cerebral ischemic stroke due to large vessel occlusion (LVO) achieving a 20–27% absolute increase in patients regaining functional independence compared to patients without receiving MT mboxciteB1-jcm-1747802,B2-jcm-1747802. These impressive results, however, are being achieved by rigorous patient selection by cerebral perfusion imaging, achievement of successful recanalization and short symptom to recanalization times including transport to comprehensive stroke centers (CSC) [3,4]. In rural areas, stroke units (SU) and telestroke networks have been established only with intravenous thrombolysis (IVT) capabilities more than 20 years ago, and further transfer to CSC for MT is time-consuming, causing delay in the initiation of recanalization therapy.

Still, prehospital stroke detection algorithms employ clinical scales deemed imperfect for detecting LVO. Thus, transfer of severe stroke patient to either CSCs or the next regional SU remains a complex decision [5]. Ultrasound is currently the only mobile imaging modality widely available for brain vascular diagnostics. Our group demonstrated that transcranial color-coded sonography (TCCS) using mobile color-Duplex point-of care ultrasound (POCUS) can be performed in the prehospital phase with very high sensitivity and specificity for the detection of middle cerebral artery (MCA) occlusion [6,7]. Another highly efficient alternative, the mobile stroke units (mSU) with computed tomography (CT), including CT-angiography installed in an ambulance to perform at the patient's site, is of limited availability, costly and has a rather small range. The air-mobile SU version of the mSU is still in the concept phase [8,9]. However, the drawback of TCCS is the high neurological expertise requiring extensive practical and theoretical training programs for paramedics to employ the pathophysiological driven diagnostic concept for TCCS, i.e., focusing on the right middle cerebral artery in left-sided hemiparesis and neglect [10].

We recently published the results of a phase I study using a mobile battery driven brain perfusion ultrasound (BPU) device SONAS® (BURL Concepts, Inc., San Diego, CA, USA) in healthy volunteers with good correlation of measured hemispheric brain perfusion to perfusion weighted MRI [11]. This case report describes the BPU finding in a patient with acute MCA occlusion confirmed by CT-angiography and TCCS prior to MT.

2. Materials and Methods

During initiation of a phase I–II study at the University of Regensburg, Department of Neurology at the medbo Bezirksklinikum (approval by the local ethics committee, IRB protocol number 2018-001279-19, in accordance with the World Medical Association Declaration of Helsinki), an acute stroke patient was admitted and individual informed consent in the presence of his parents as well as post-hoc consent for publication 1 year later given. The phase I–II study SONAS enrolled acute stroke patients with perfusion CT and was registered at ClinicalTrials.gov (NCT03897153). In brief, patients with acute ischemic stroke within 24 h will be investigated using the SONAS® device after confirmation of an either proximal, middle or distal MCA main stem occlusion or distal internal carotid artery occlusion (including carotid-T occlusion). Confirmation of the LVO will be performed by cerebral magnetic resonance imaging (cMRI) or cerebral imaging computed tomography (cCT), including perfusion weighted (pw) imaging sequences. The study has now been completed and data analysis is in preparation.

2.1. Case Report

The 46-year-old male patient was transferred for suspected left hemispheric ischemia as on admission, he presented with moderate dysarthria, motor aphasia and mild facial paresis (NIHSS 3) starting early in the morning. He reported that about 4–5 weeks prior, one side of the face had felt strange for 10–15 min, suggestive of a transient ischemic attack. Admission was approximately 12 h after stroke onset. At this time, cCT was almost unremarkable (ASPECTS Score 9), while CT-angiography revealed proximal MCA occlusion (M1 segment) on the left side with good collateralization (collateral score 3–4, Figure 1). With fluctuating symptoms between progressive global aphasia and brachiocephalic hemiparesis (NIHSS 3 to 8), and an overall deficit relevant to daily living, the decision was made for MT, especially since no intravenous thrombolysis was initiated. Informed consent for additional ultrasonography was obtained from the patient and his parents and retrospectively. Both TCCS and BPU were performed in parallel to MT preparation in general anesthesia without causing a time delay.

Digital subtraction angiography demonstrated proximal MCA occlusion with good cortical collaterals via leptomeningeal anastomosis predominantly from the anterior cerebral artery (Figure 2). After successful MT (TICI 3), the patient was extubated and presented only mild word finding difficulties and minimal facial paresis (NIHSS 2). On telephone follow up two years later, he was back to work and neurologically unremarkable (modified Rankin Scale 0).

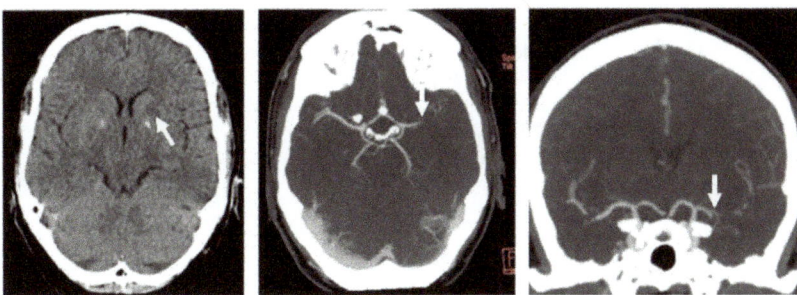

Figure 1. Left: unenhanced CT, putaminal hypodensity (arrow), ASPECTS score 9; **middle**: axial maximum intensity projection (MIP) reconstruction of CT-angiography showing left MCA occlusion (arrow); **right**: coronal MIP reconstruction of left MCA occlusion (arrow), good leptomeningeal collaterals can be seen.

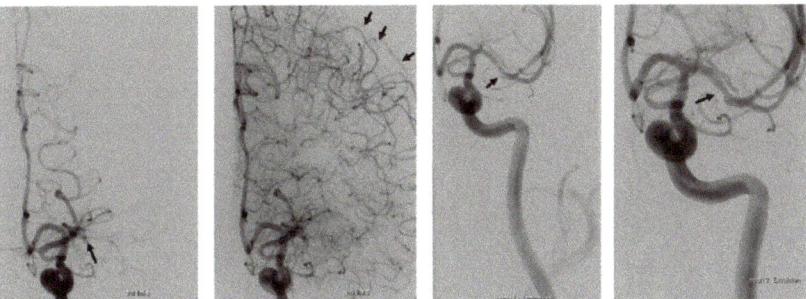

Figure 2. Digital subtraction angiography. **Left** to **right**: phase after contrast injection showing proximal MCA occlusion (arrow); demonstration of extensive leptomeningeal collaterals arising from the ACA (arrows); immediately after mechanical thrombectomy by first use of the stent retriever showing suspicious residual thrombus with mild lumen narrowing (arrow) and, right, complete recanalization with mild stenosis/vasospasm (TICI 3).

2.2. Transcranial Color-Coded Sonography (TCCS)

TCCS was performed using a standard color Duplex ultrasound system equipped with a low-frequency phased array transducer (Philips, Affiniti 70, S5-1 cardiac sector probe, Amsterdam, The Netherlands). Transtemporal insonation for detection of the basal cerebral arteries was performed as previously described [12]. In brief, after detection of a sufficient temporal bone window by identification of the mesencephalic peduncle and the contralateral skull in B-mode color Duplex mode helped to identify patent cerebral arteries with flow towards the transducer depicted in red, and flow away from the transducer in blue. Pulsed Doppler measurements were performed to quantify flow velocities. An occluded MCA can be assumed when the anterior cerebral artery can be depicted confirming a diagnostic useful temporal bone window.

2.3. Brain Perfusion Ultrasound (BPU) Using SONAS®

BPU was performed as previously described employing the CE-certified (Class IIa), non-imaging ultrasound device SONAS®, a portable, battery-powered device to generate hemispheric time intensity curves after injection of an ultrasound enhancing agent, which in this case was SonoVue® [11,13]. In brief, bilateral low-frequency transducer with low transmit frequencies and power (220 kHz, 2% alternating duty cycle from right to left, TIC and MI < 1.0) measure the 4th to 6th harmonic frequencies generated by intravenous 2.4 mL microbubble injection. Time to peak (TTP) curves are generated based on measurements contralateral, that is transmission and reception are on opposite sides of the head, and ipsilateral measurement, where transmission and receiving are ipsilateral (Figure 3). Using an automatic peak detection algorithm for both brain hemispheres separately, hemispheric TTP values are compared. The differential of peaks is computed and shown as a delta-TTP (dTTP) value.

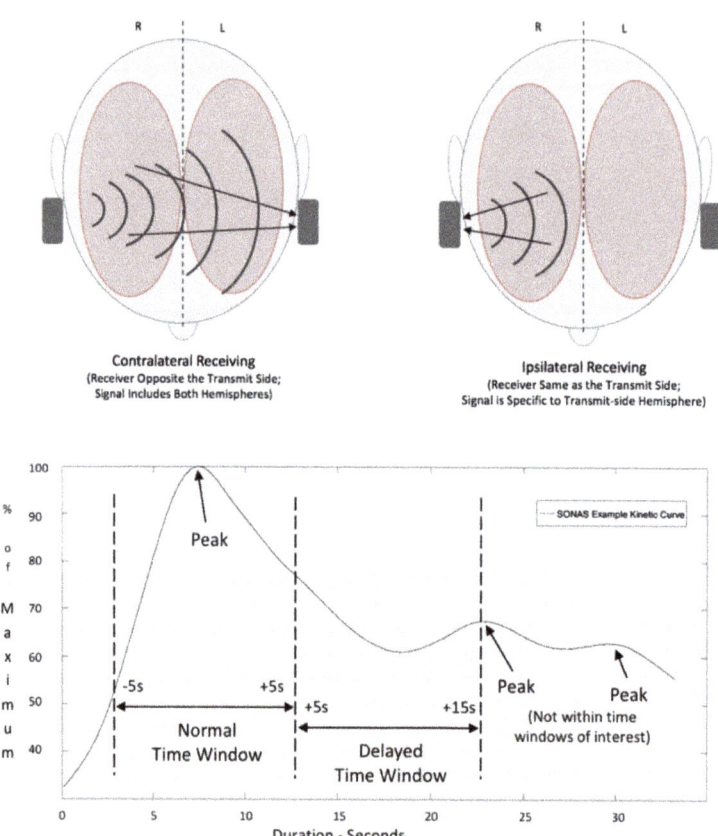

Figure 3. Upper figure: signal transmission and recording from both ultrasound transducers after injection of echo-enhancing agents demonstrating the mode of operation. R—right, L—left. Lower figure: time intensity curves after contrast agent injection with X-axis time after injection and Y-axis maximum signal backscatter analyzed automatically by BPU machine (SONAS®). The first peak is due to the first appearance of contrast agent while the second and third peaks are to due systemic reflow phenomenon.

3. Results

Prior to embolectomy and 30 min after neurological deterioration, both, BPU und TCCS were performed. BPU demonstrated significant delay in left hemispheric perfusion with a delay of 6.6 s (Figure 4).

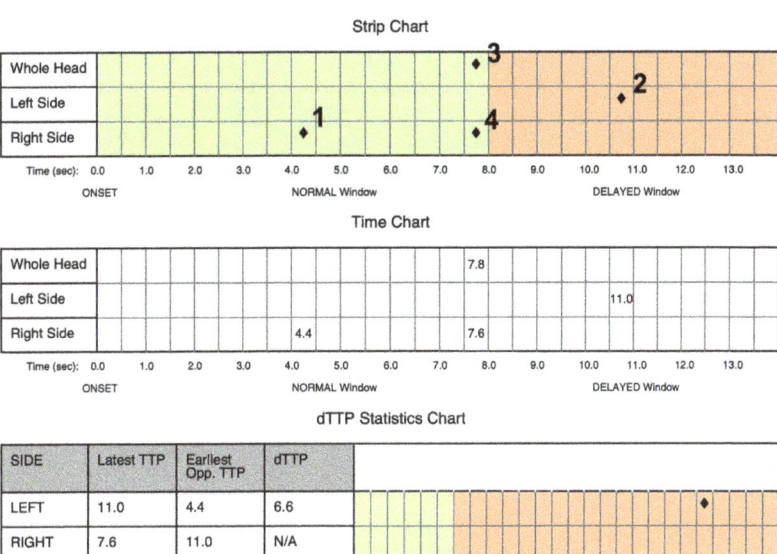

Figure 4. Analysis of time intensity curves representing brain perfusion ultrasound using SONAS®. Upper row: 1—first time-to-peak (TTP) in the "healthy" right hemisphere, 2—delayed left hemispheric peak, 3—peak of the whole brain, and 4—delayed second peak probably representing right anterior cerebral artery crossflow as the primary collateral pathway. Middle row: absolute time values of the peaks. Lower row: expression of the difference in time-to-peak values (delta-TTP) expressing the absolute perfusion deficit in the left hemisphere.

Conventional TCCS demonstrated only only slow proximal pseudo-venous flow in the proximal MCA (peak systolic flow less than 10 cm/s) consistent with MCA occlusion and relatively normal flow in the left ACA (Figure 5).

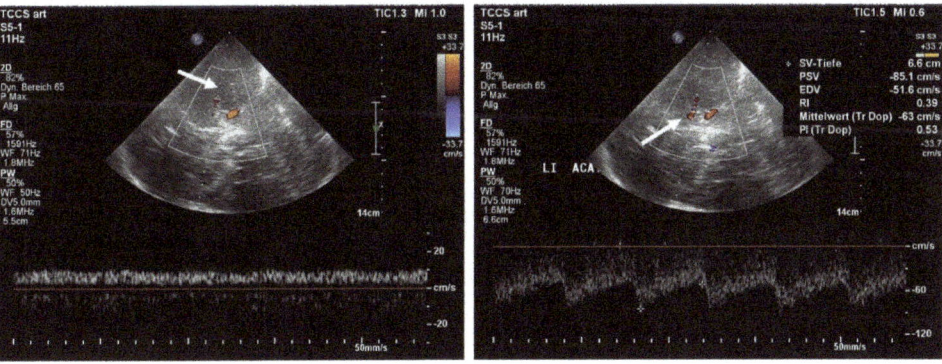

Figure 5. TCCS scan through the left temporal bone window with transcranial color-coded sonography in the upper and Doppler spectrum from the Doppler gate. **Left**: Doppler gate placed at the origin of the middle cerebral artery with absent color filling (arrow) in the M1 segment and pseudo-venous flow at the beginning of the M1-Segment (Doppler gate depth 55 mm). **Right**: anterior cerebral artery color-coded in red due to aliasing due to increased flow velocities with the Doppler gate placed at a depth of 66 mm in the A1-segment showing increased flow of 63 cm/s mean maximum flow and decreased resistance index of 0.39 all suggestive of collateral flow.

Case Report Continued

Decision for embolectomy under general anesthesia was made based on the persistent MCA occlusion and fluctuating course of neurological deficits (NIHSS 3 to 8). The first angiographic image was made at 20:45 h and complete TICI 3 recanalization was noted at 21:17 h. After extubation, NIHSS score was 3 and 2 in the following days. Neuropsychological testing showed mild cognitive impairment and indication for neurorehabilitation. At telephone follow-up 2 years later, the patient was again able to work and independent in daily life (mRS score of 0–1).

4. Discussion

This is the first report describing the application of BPU in a patient with acute MCA occlusion shown by CT-angiography and later digital subtraction angiography using a portable POCUS device for BPU (SONAS®) with comparison to standard TCCS as another mobile method for acute stroke diagnosis, while TCCS allowed MCA occlusion imaging with similar information as CT-angiography and DSA BPU depicts the subsequent brain perfusion changes. If replicated in the ongoing phase II study, BPU may be feasible in prehospital stroke diagnostics.

The progressive developments in the field of MT with high recanalization rates along with decreasing peri-interventional risk challenge the identification and allocation of acute stroke patients in the prehospital phase. In stroke patients in need for MT, direct transfer to an endovascular MT-capable center may be preferred as opposed to transport to the closest primary stroke center and secondary transport for MT [14]. To date, efforts have been made to identify LVO employing prehospital stroke scales as shown in the PRESTO study comparing eight scales employed by paramedics in the prehospital phase and identifying three scales with acceptable-to-good accuracy [15]. In another prospective study on patients with ischemic stroke entered in the Dyon stroke registry, Duloquin et al. applied 16 different prehospital stroke scales; however, a priori excluding patients with ICH severely reducing its value as a prehospital study [16]. Even with this drawback sensitivities of scales were still low (identification of LVO ranging between 0.64 to 0.79, sensitivity 59% to 93%, and specificity ranging from 34% to 89%, c-statistic) with 174 of 971 patients (17.9%) had LVO (defined as occlusion of M1 and M2-segment of the MCA and basilar artery occlusion). In a topical review from 2020, van Gaal and Demchuck listed common flaws of studies on the validity of prehospital stroke scales, among them, exclusion of ICH patients, lack of prospective studies in the field as opposed to application of stroke scales to pure ischemic stroke databases (exclusion, i.e., TIA, ICH, stroke mimics, amongst others), and whether or not these scales have indeed been tested by paramedics [17]. However, in a recent pilot study in the Baltimore metro area patients were re-routed CSCs for MT upon application of the Los Angeles Motor Scale. Consequently, significantly shorter procedural times from symptom to MT onset of 119 min were achieved [18]. While the faster initiation of MT showed a strong non-significant trend for better outcome, more than 50% of patients were allocated to the wrong clinic.

However, fast and goal-directed prehospital point-of-care diagnostics such as blood serum biomarkers and TCCS have been advocated to further accelerate the diagnostic and therapeutic stroke pathways in stroke patients [19–22]. Apart from mobile stroke units, only portable TCCS is a neuroimaging tool capable of visualizing LVO in the field, preferentially employing echo-enhancing agents [23,24]. In the patient described here, conventional TCCS identified left MCA occlusion in line with CT-angiography and digital subtraction angiography. BPU, which involves single-slice transcranial ultrasound using phased-array transducers and echo-enhancing agents to produce perfusion maps comparable to perfusion CT, is not currently mature enough to be used for routine practice, let alone prehospital use [25,26]. Yet, for conventional TCCS, detailed pathophysiological hypothesis of the stroke location and hands-on expertise in identifying an adequate temporal bone window is needed. However, many of these obstacles may be solved by employing telemetric and artificial intelligence support [27,28]. BPU using the SONAS® device differs significantly from TCCS and other transcranial ultrasound techniques as it lacks anatomical information and presents only perfusion curves [11]. However, the demonstrated delay in time-to-peak times of the left hemisphere together with the clinical information can be easily gathered with little expertise, ideal for application in the prehospital phase. Table 1 compares the basic findings, techniques, advantages and disadvantages of TCCS and non-imaging BPU using SONAS®.

Table 1. Comparison of TCCS and BPU.

	Brain Perfusion Ultrasound	**Transcranial Color-Coded Sonography**
Information	Hemispheric brain perfusion	Ipsilateral intracranial arteries
Operator qualification	Low due to automated analysis	High, requires anatomical knowledge for interpretation
Controls	Single button, sequential operation	Variable keyboard complexity, pro–grammable presets
Bone penetration	High	Low to high, can be increased using echo-enhancing agents
Echo-enhancing agents	Required	Optional
Presentation	Generation of time-intensity curves on-site	Real-time depiction of vessel occlusion
Potential additional information	Raised intracranial pressure	Intracerebral hemorrhage Brain parenchymal shift (i.e., midline displacement, intracerebral hemorrhage, hydrocephalus)

5. Conclusions

This is the first patient with MCA occlusion in whom both the BPU technique with the SONAS® device and standard TCCS were used to visualize MCA occlusion and the resulting perfusion deficit. The results of BPU using the SONAS® device were compared with conventional imaging (CT angiography, TCCS and DSA) and revealed a similar result. The user-friendly mode of operation of BPU requiring little additional skills indicate the potential of SONAS® to fasten stroke treatment when positively identifying LVO at the earliest time point possible after symptom onset. Goal-directed hospital admission for MT and fewer secondary transportations may enable faster symptom to recanalization times, and eventually better outcome. The results of the ongoing phase II study with the SONAS® device in acute ischemic stroke patients as well as further studies on lacunar infarction, intracerebral hemorrhage, minor strokes and stroke mimics are the prerequisite to define the full potential of BPU.

Author Contributions: M.K. and F.S. contributed equally to the patient investigation and data collection, analysis of the results, and writing of the manuscript. C.W., S.W., D.O. and R.A.L. contributed to the analytical methods and data analysis. The main draft was written by M.K. and F.S. All authors have read and agreed to the published version of the manuscript.

Funding: This research received no external funding.

Institutional Review Board Statement: Not applicable.

Informed Consent Statement: Consent to publish the results was given by all included participants especially the patient.

Data Availability Statement: The raw data underlying this article are intended for publication on a suitable platform and can be made available by the corresponding author on reasonable request.

Acknowledgments: The authors would like to thank the patient for approving the investigation and publication, and Burl Concepts, Inc. for technical support and data analysis of this extra patient.

Conflicts of Interest: The authors declare no conflict of interest.

References

1. Goyal, M.; Menon, B.K.; van Zwam, W.H.; Dippel, D.W.; Mitchell, P.J.; Demchuk, A.M.; Davalos, A.; Majoie, C.B.; van der Lugt, A.; de Miquel, M.A.; et al. Endovascular thrombectomy after large-vessel ischaemic stroke: A meta-analysis of individual patient data from five randomised trials. *Lancet* **2016**, *387*, 1723–1731. [CrossRef]
2. Jovin, T.G.; Nogueira, R.G.; Lansberg, M.G.; Demchuk, A.M.; Martins, S.O.; Mocco, J.; Ribo, M.; Jadhav, A.P.; Ortega-Gutierrez, S.; Hill, M.D.; et al. Thrombectomy for anterior circulation stroke beyond 6 h from time last known well (AURORA): A systematic review and individual patient data meta-analysis. *Lancet* **2022**, *399*, 249–258. [CrossRef]
3. Holodinsky, J.K.; Patel, A.B.; Thornton, J.; Kamal, N.; Jewett, L.R.; Kelly, P.J.; Murphy, S.; Collins, R.; Walsh, T.; Cronin, S.; et al. Drip and ship versus direct to endovascular thrombectomy: The impact of treatment times on transport decision-making. *Eur. Stroke J.* **2018**, *3*, 126–135. [CrossRef] [PubMed]
4. Weber, R.; Eyding, J.; Kitzrow, M.; Bartig, D.; Weimar, C.; Hacke, W.; Krogias, C. Distribution and evolution of acute interventional ischemic stroke treatment in Germany from 2010 to 2016. *Neurol. Res. Pract.* **2019**, *1*, 4. [CrossRef] [PubMed]
5. Jauch, E.C.; Schwamm, L.H.; Panagos, P.D.; Barbazzeni, J.; Dickson, R.; Dunne, R.; Foley, J.; Fraser, J.F.; Lassers, G.; Martin-Gill, C.; et al. Recommendations for Regional Stroke Destination Plans in Rural, Suburban, and Urban Communities from the Prehospital Stroke System of Care Consensus Conference: A Consensus Statement from the American Academy of Neurology, American Heart Association/American Stroke Association, American Society of Neuroradiology, National Association of EMS Physicians, National Association of State EMS Officials, Society of NeuroInterventional Surgery, and Society of Vascular and Interventional Neurology: Endorsed by the Neurocritical Care Society. *Stroke* **2021**, *52*, e133–e152.
6. Schlachetzki, F.; Herzberg, M.; Holscher, T.; Ertl, M.; Zimmermann, M.; Ittner, K.P.; Pels, H.; Bogdahn, U.; Boy, S. Transcranial ultrasound from diagnosis to early stroke treatment: Part 2: Prehospital neurosonography in patients with acute stroke: The Regensburg stroke mobile project. *Cerebrovasc. Dis.* **2012**, *33*, 262–271. [CrossRef] [PubMed]
7. Herzberg, M.; Boy, S.; Holscher, T.; Ertl, M.; Zimmermann, M.; Ittner, K.P.; Pemmerl, J.; Pels, H.; Bogdahn, U.; Schlachetzki, F. Prehospital stroke diagnostics based on neurological examination and transcranial ultrasound. *Crit. Ultrasound J.* **2014**, *6*, 3. [CrossRef]
8. Audebert, H.; Fassbender, K.; Hussain, M.S.; Ebinger, M.; Turc, G.; Uchino, K.; Davis, S.; Alexandrov, A.; Grotta, J.; Group, P. The PRE-hospital Stroke Treatment Organization. *Int. J. Stroke* **2017**, *12*, 932–940. [CrossRef]
9. Walter, S.; Zhao, H.; Easton, D.; Bil, C.; Sauer, J.; Liu, Y.; Lesmeister, M.; Grunwald, I.Q.; Donnan, G.A.; Davis, S.M.; et al. Air-Mobile Stroke Unit for access to stroke treatment in rural regions. *Int. J. Stroke* **2018**, *13*, 568–575. [CrossRef]
10. Kilic, M.; Pflug, K.; Theiss, S.; Webert, M.; Hirschmann, N.; Wagner, A.; Boy, S.; Ertl, M.; Linker, R.A.; Schlachetzki, F.; et al. Prehospital Identification of Middle Cerebral Artery Occlusion—A Stroke Education Program and Transcranial Ultrasound for Paramedics. *Austin. J. Clin. Neurol.* **2020**, *7*, 1142.
11. Kilic, M.; Scalzo, F.; Lyle, C.; Baldaranov, D.; Dirnbacher, M.; Honda, T.; Liebeskind, D.S.; Schlachetzki, F. A mobile battery-powered brain perfusion ultrasound (BPU) device designed for prehospital stroke diagnosis: Correlation to perfusion MRI in healthy volunteers. *Neurol. Res. Pract.* **2022**, *4*, 13. [CrossRef]
12. Gerriets, T.; Postert, T.; Goertler, M.; Stolz, E.; Schlachetzki, F.; Sliwka, U.; Seidel, G.; Weber, S.; Kaps, M. DIAS I: Duplex-sonographic assessment of the cerebrovascular status in acute stroke. A useful tool for future stroke trials. *Stroke* **2000**, *31*, 2342–2345. [CrossRef]
13. Bogdahn, U.; Holscher, T.; Rosin, L.; Gotz, B.; Schlachetzki, F. Contrast-Enhanced Transcranial and Extracranial Duplex Sonography: Preliminary Results of a Multicenter Phase II/III Study with SonoVuetrade mark. *Echocardiography* **1999**, *16 Pt 2*, 761–766. [CrossRef] [PubMed]
14. Goyal, M.; Marko, M. Optimising prehospital stroke triage in a changing landscape. *Lancet Neurol.* **2021**, *20*, 166–168. [CrossRef]
15. Duvekot, M.H.C.; Venema, E.; Rozeman, A.D.; Moudrous, W.; Vermeij, F.H.; Biekart, M.; Lingsma, H.F.; Maasland, L.; Wijnhoud, A.D.; Mulder, H.; et al. Comparison of eight prehospital stroke scales to detect intracranial large-vessel occlusion in suspected stroke (PRESTO): A prospective observational study. *Lancet Neurol.* **2021**, *20*, 213–221. [CrossRef]
16. Duloquin, G.; Graber, M.; Garnier, L.; Mohr, S.; Giroud, M.; Vergely, C.; Bejot, Y. Assessment of Clinical Scales for Detection of Large Vessel Occlusion in Ischemic Stroke Patients from the Dijon Stroke Registry. *J. Clin. Med.* **2021**, *10*, 5893. [CrossRef] [PubMed]
17. Van Gaal, S.; Demchuk, A. Clinical and Technological Approaches to the Prehospital Diagnosis of Large Vessel Occlusion. *Stroke* **2018**, *49*, 1036–1043. [CrossRef]
18. Haight, T.; Tabaac, B.; Patrice, K.A.; Phipps, M.S.; Butler, J.; Johnson, B.; Aycock, A.; Toral, L.; Yarbrough, K.L.; Schrier, C.; et al. The Maryland Acute Stroke Emergency Medical Services Routing Pilot: Expediting Access to Thrombectomy for Stroke. *Front. Neurol.* **2021**, *12*, 663472. [CrossRef]
19. Yperzeele, L.; Van Hooff, R.J.; De Smedt, A.; Valenzuela Espinoza, A.; Van de Casseye, R.; Hubloue, I.; De Keyser, J.; Brouns, R. Prehospital stroke care: Limitations of current interventions and focus on new developments. *Cerebrovasc. Dis.* **2014**, *38*, 1–9. [CrossRef]
20. Antipova, D.; Eadie, L.; Macaden, A.; Wilson, P. Diagnostic accuracy of clinical tools for assessment of acute stroke: A systematic review. *BMC Emerg. Med.* **2019**, *19*, 49. [CrossRef]

21. Ramos-Pachon, A.; Lopez-Cancio, E.; Bustamante, A.; de la Ossa, N.P.; Millan, M.; Hernandez-Perez, M.; Garcia-Berrocoso, T.; Cardona, P.; Rubiera, M.; Serena, J.; et al. D-Dimer as Predictor of Large Vessel Occlusion in Acute Ischemic Stroke. *Stroke* **2021**, *52*, 852–858. [CrossRef] [PubMed]
22. Luger, S.; Jaeger, H.S.; Dixon, J.; Bohmann, F.O.; Schaefer, J.; Richieri, S.P.; Larsen, K.; Hov, M.R.; Bache, K.G.; Foerch, C.; et al. Diagnostic Accuracy of Glial Fibrillary Acidic Protein and Ubiquitin Carboxy-Terminal Hydrolase-L1 Serum Concentrations for Differentiating Acute Intracerebral Hemorrhage from Ischemic Stroke. *Neurocrit. Care* **2020**, *33*, 39–48. [CrossRef] [PubMed]
23. Diaz-Gomez, J.L.; Mayo, P.H.; Koenig, S.J. Point-of-Care Ultrasonography. *N. Engl. J. Med.* **2021**, *385*, 1593–1602. [CrossRef] [PubMed]
24. Valaikiene, J.; Schlachetzki, F.; Azevedo, E.; Kaps, M.; Lochner, P.; Katsanos, A.H.; Walter, U.; Baracchini, C.; Bartels, E.; Skoloudik, D. Point-of-Care Ultrasound in Neurology—Report of the EAN SPN/ESNCH/ERcNsono Neuro-POCUS Working Group. *Ultraschall Med.* **2022**. [CrossRef] [PubMed]
25. Meairs, S. Contrast-enhanced ultrasound perfusion imaging in acute stroke patients. *Eur. Neurol.* **2008**, *59* (Suppl. S1), 17–26. [CrossRef]
26. Rim, S.J.; Leong-Poi, H.; Lindner, J.R.; Couture, D.; Ellegala, D.; Mason, H.; Durieux, M.; Kassel, N.F.; Kaul, S. Quantification of cerebral perfusion with "Real-Time" contrast-enhanced ultrasound. *Circulation* **2001**, *104*, 2582–2587. [CrossRef]
27. Antipova, D.; Eadie, L.; Makin, S.; Shannon, H.; Wilson, P.; Macaden, A. The use of transcranial ultrasound and clinical assessment to diagnose ischaemic stroke due to large vessel occlusion in remote and rural areas. *PLoS ONE* **2020**, *15*, e0239450. [CrossRef]
28. Mort, A.; Eadie, L.; Regan, L.; Macaden, A.; Heaney, D.; Bouamrane, M.M.; Rushworth, G.; Wilson, P. Combining transcranial ultrasound with intelligent communication methods to enhance the remote assessment and management of stroke patients: Framework for a technology demonstrator. *Health Inform. J.* **2016**, *22*, 691–701. [CrossRef]

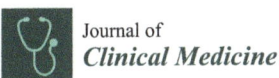

Article

Acute Management Should Be Optimized in Patients with Less Specific Stroke Symptoms: Findings from a Retrospective Observational Study

Simona Halúsková [1], Roman Herzig [1,*], Dagmar Krajíčková [1], Abduljabar Hamza [2], Antonín Krajina [3], Vendelín Chovanec [3], Miroslav Lojík [3], Jan Raupach [3], Ondřej Renc [3], Libor Šimůnek [1], Eva Vítková [1], Lukáš Sobíšek [1] and Martin Vališ [1]

1. Department of Neurology, Comprehensive Stroke Center, Charles University Faculty of Medicine and University Hospital, Sokolská 581, CZ-500 05 Hradec Králové, Czech Republic; sim.haluskova@gmail.com (S.H.); dagmar.krajickova@fnhk.cz (D.K.); libor.simunek@email.cz (L.Š.); eva@kinoaero.cz (E.V.); lukas.sobisek@yahoo.com (L.S.); valismar@seznam.cz (M.V.)
2. Department of Neurology, Charles University Faculty of Medicine, CZ-500 03 Hradec Králové, Czech Republic; hamzaabdulj@gmail.com
3. Department of Radiology, Comprehensive Stroke Center, Charles University Faculty of Medicine and University Hospital, CZ-500 05 Hradec Králové, Czech Republic; antonin.krajina@fnhk.cz (A.K.); chovanec.v@seznam.cz (V.C.); miroslav.lojik@fnhk.cz (M.L.); jan.raupach@fnhk.cz (J.R.); ondrej.renc@fnhk.cz (O.R.)
* Correspondence: herzig.roman@seznam.cz

Citation: Halúsková, S.; Herzig, R.; Krajíčková, D.; Hamza, A.; Krajina, A.; Chovanec, V.; Lojík, M.; Raupach, J.; Renc, O.; Šimůnek, L.; et al. Acute Management Should Be Optimized in Patients with Less Specific Stroke Symptoms: Findings from a Retrospective Observational Study. *J. Clin. Med.* **2021**, *10*, 1143. https://doi.org/10.3390/jcm10051143

Academic Editor: Hyo Suk Nam

Received: 25 January 2021
Accepted: 2 March 2021
Published: 9 March 2021

Publisher's Note: MDPI stays neutral with regard to jurisdictional claims in published maps and institutional affiliations.

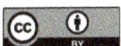

Copyright: © 2021 by the authors. Licensee MDPI, Basel, Switzerland. This article is an open access article distributed under the terms and conditions of the Creative Commons Attribution (CC BY) license (https://creativecommons.org/licenses/by/4.0/).

Abstract: Anterior circulation stroke (ACS) is associated with typical symptoms, while posterior circulation stroke (PCS) may cause a wide spectrum of less specific symptoms. We aim to assess the correlation between the initial presentation of acute ischemic stroke (AIS) symptoms and the treatment timeline. Using a retrospective, observational, single-center study, the set consists of 809 AIS patients treated with intravenous thrombolysis (IVT) and/or endovascular treatment (EVT). We investigate the impact of baseline clinical AIS symptoms and the affected vascular territory on recanalization times in patients treated with IVT only and EVT (±IVT). Regarding the IVT-only group, increasing the National Institutes of Health Stroke Scale (NIHSS) score on admission and speech difficulties are associated with shorter (by 1.59 ± 0.76 min per every one-point increase; $p = 0.036$, and by 24.56 ± 8.42 min; $p = 0.004$, respectively) and nausea/vomiting with longer (by 43.72 ± 13.13 min; $p = 0.001$) onset-to-needle times, and vertigo with longer (by 8.58 ± 3.84 min; $p = 0.026$) door-to-needle times (DNT). Regarding the EVT (±IVT) group, coma is associated with longer (by 22.68 ± 6.05 min; $p = 0.0002$) DNT, anterior circulation stroke with shorter (by 47.32 ± 16.89 min; $p = 0.005$) onset-to-groin time, and drooping of the mouth corner with shorter (by 20.79 ± 6.02 min; $p = 0.0006$) door-to-groin time. Our results demonstrate that treatment is initiated later in strokes with less specific symptoms than in strokes with typical symptoms.

Keywords: acute ischemic stroke; clinical symptoms; intravenous thrombolysis; endovascular therapy; recanalization times; clinical outcome

1. Introduction

Acute ischemic stroke (AIS) typically presents with the sudden onset of neurological deficit. Clinical manifestation depends mainly on the AIS localization and the volume of the affected brain tissue, which are associated with the involved vascular territory. Occlusion of the internal carotid arteries (ICA), middle cerebral arteries (MCA), and of the anterior cerebral arteries (ACA) or their branches results in anterior circulation stroke (ACS), accounting for approximately 70–80% of all AIS. Posterior circulation stroke (PCS) refers to any infarction localized in the regions supplied by the vertebrobasilar arterial system with reported prevalence ranging from 20 to 30% [1–4]. Symptoms of ACS include contralateral hemiparesis and/or hemianesthesia, central facial palsy, forced gaze deviation toward the lesion site, dysarthria, aphasia (dominant hemisphere), and neglect syndrome (non-dominant hemisphere). To contrast to ACS, PCS causes a wide spectrum of less specific symptoms, such as vertigo, headache, nausea and vomiting, diplopia, visual field disturbances, slurred speech, gait and limb ataxia, or alteration of consciousness [3,5].

Although the most common symptoms of ACS and PCS are well described, reliable differentiation between ACS and PCS can be challenging. How the stroke symptoms are described and how a patient presents at the emergency room affects the delay between stroke onset and the start of treatment. Several randomized controlled trials demonstrated that both intravenous thrombolysis (IVT) with the administration of recombinant tissue plasminogen activator (rtPA) and endovascular therapy (EVT) were highly time-sensitive treatments—the earlier they are commenced the better is the chance for achieving a favorable outcome [6,7]. Nevertheless, only a few studies assessed the impact of specific AIS symptoms on the recanalization times within the limited treatment window [8,9].

Our aim is to investigate the impact of initial presentation of AIS symptoms and the affected vascular territory on recanalization times in patients treated with IVT only and with EVT (±IVT).

2. Materials and Methods

2.1. Data Source and Study Population

All relevant data used for this retrospective analysis were manually extracted from hospital information systems and available individual patient medical charts, including documentation from the referring hospital (in the case of patients with secondary transport), emergency physician notes, neurology notes, and medication administration records.

During a retrospective, observational, single-center study, prospectively collected data of 809 consecutive AIS patients aged ≥18 years and treated with IVT only or EVT (±IVT) between 1 January 2013 and 31 December 2018 were analyzed. All EVT procedures were performed at the Comprehensive Stroke Center (CSC), Hradec Králové, Czech Republic. Ninety-eight patients from the EVT group received IVT in the primary stroke centers (PSC) according to the geographic area and then were subsequently transferred to our CSC. Patients experiencing in-hospital stroke (38) also were enrolled in this analysis. Each stroke was considered an independent event, regardless of whether it was the first hospital stay or a readmission. Patients were considered eligible for the analysis if data about the involvement of the particular territory (ACS or PCS) were available. Patients with an unclear stroke territory (e.g., thalamic infarcts or border zone infarcts in the posterior cerebral artery (PCA)/MCA watershed) or AIS involving both anterior and posterior circulation were excluded in the data collection phase already. ACS was classified as symptomatic ischemia involving the ICA, MCA, or ACA territories. PCS was defined as symptomatic ischemia occurring within the territory of the vertebral artery (VA), basilar artery (BA), or PCA. No additional exclusion criteria were applied. Initial routine investigation in the emergency room comprised neurological, physical, and laboratory examinations and assessment of the admission neurological deficit using the National Institutes of Health Stroke Scale (NIHSS) [10] performed by a certified neurologist.

2.2. Neuroimaging

All patients underwent the standardized stroke imaging protocol for the assessment of the eligibility for IVT and endovascular treatment EVT, as described in detail previously [11]. This protocol included non-enhanced computed tomography (CT) of the brain with the assessment of the Alberta Stroke Program Early CT Score (ASPECTS) and CT angiography (CTA) of the cervical and intracranial arteries. Patients treated beyond 6 h after the onset of the first symptoms, or with an unknown time of stroke onset, also underwent a perfusion CT scan [12]. Regarding patients needing secondary transport to the CSC and with preceding IVT administration in the PSC, a non-enhanced brain CT control was performed in the CSC prior to an intended EVT to exclude IVT-related hemorrhagic complications or the development of an extensive brain infarction only if the transport took more than one hour, and/or the patient's neurological status deteriorated significantly.

2.3. Recanalization Treatment

Recanalization treatment was performed in agreement with the valid national and international guidelines [13–17]. IVT with a standard dose of 0.9 mg/kg (maximum dose of 90 mg) of rtPA (Actilyse®; Boehringer Ingelheim, Ingelheim am Rhein, Germany) was administered within 4.5 h from the "last-known-well" condition, with 10% of the dose given as an intravenous initial bolus and the remaining 90% of the dose as a 60-min infusion in all patients fulfilling the inclusion and exclusion criteria.

A mechanical thrombectomy (MT) using stent-retrievers was started as soon as possible, without waiting for the effect of the IVT (if applied) and within a standard 6-h time window from AIS symptom onset in ACS patients with an ASPECTS ≥ 6 on a non-enhanced brain CT. Regarding ACS patients treated more than 6 h after AIS symptom onset, or with an unknown AIS onset time, a MT was indicated based on the perfusion CT results—it was performed in patients with a small ischemic core ($\leq$70 mL) [18] and with the presence of ischemic penumbra. Regarding patients with PCS due to BA occlusion, a MT was performed within a 24-h time window in the case of the absence of an extensive brain infarction. The choice of the particular stent-retriever used for clot extraction was at the discretion of the treating interventional neuroradiologist. Concerning most patients, a MT was performed under conscious sedation and general anesthesia was avoided whenever possible after evaluation by a dedicated anesthesiology team.

Concerning patients with concurrent ICA occlusion (so called "tandem occlusion"), carotid artery stenting was performed under local anesthesia using a standard catheterization approach from the femoral artery via an 8F or 9F sheath introduced into the common carotid artery. During most procedures a self-expandable carotid stent was implanted after predilatation using a low profile balloon as the first step, followed by a MT using a balloon-guiding catheter placed in the ICA above the level of the carotid stent.

2.4. Observed Parameters

The following parameters were observed in both the IVT only and EVT ($\pm$IVT) groups: patient age and sex, baseline neurological deficit (assessed using the NIHSS score), involved vascular territory (anterior/posterior), and the presence of nine selected clinical symptoms—limb weakness (mono- or hemiparesis/hemiplegia; HEMIPAR), facial palsy (drooping of the corner of the mouth; N VII), speech difficulties (dysarthria/phatic disorder; SPEECH), sensory impairment (hypoesthesia/anesthesia/paresthesias; SENSATION), visual disturbances (diplopia/visual field defects; VISION), vertigo (VERTIGO), headache (HEADACHE), nausea/vomiting (VOMIT), and loss of consciousness (COMA). Regarding patients with a previous stroke, only the occurrence of new symptoms or a clear progression of possible residual symptoms were included in the analysis. Concerning the EVT group, we additionally evaluated the use of IVT before the EVT and localization of the arterial occlusion—in the extracranial ICA (ICAe), intracranial ICA (ICAi), M1 segment of the MCA (MCA/M1), M2 segment of the MCA (MCA/M2), ACA, PCA, VA, or BA.

Regarding both groups, times of symptoms onset, times of arrival to the emergency department in our hospital, times of IVT bolus dose administration and, in the EVT ($\pm$IVT) group, arterial puncture times also were recorded. Based on these times, five time intervals were evaluated—onset-to-door time (ODT), onset-to-needle time (ONT) and door-to-needle time (DNT) in both groups and, onset-to-groin time (OGT) and door-to-groin puncture time (DGT) in the EVT ($\pm$IVT) group. Regarding patients with an unknown time of stroke onset, only the time intervals after their arrival to the hospital were analyzed.

2.5. Statistical Analysis

The IVT only and EVT ($\pm$IVT) groups were compared using a chi-square test of independence for categorical variables (sex, clinical symptoms occurrence, vascular territory). Group differences in medians were compared by a non-parametric Mann-Whitney U test with non-pooled SDs for numeric parameters like time intervals, the NIHSS, and age. The Benjamini-Hochberg procedure was used to minimize the false discovery rate. Regarding the IVT only group, we investigated whether there was a significant relationship between the key time intervals (ODT, ONT, DNT) and the independent variables (age, sex, admission NIHSS, involved vascular territory, and initial presenting symptoms of AIS). Regarding the EVT (±IVT) group, we determined five outcome time intervals (ODT, ONT, DNT, OGT, DGT) and we aimed to assess the relationship between those time points and specific independent variables (age, sex, admission NIHSS, involved vascular territory, initial clinical symptoms, use of IVT, and localization of the occlusion in particular arteries). The time-interval outcomes were log-transformed for regression modelling because they were positively skewed. The series of univariate linear regression models in both groups were fitted for logarithmized time intervals to identify the dependency on each parameter (explanatory variable). To find a combination of explanatory variables that were able to describe the dependent variable more precisely, we next used a multivariable linear model. The suitable combinations of explanatory variables were detected by two procedures—Stepwise selection (implemented in R package MASS) and by the "leapBackward" cross-validated (5-folds) method from package leaps. The best multivariable model was finally chosen according to three information criteria: adjusted R^2 (index of determination), PRESS (predicted residual error sum of squares) and RMSE (Residual Mean Square Error). All analyses were performed using the statistical software R (www.r-project.org/ (accessed on 9 March 2021).) version 3.5.3; the reported p values were two-tailed and a 5% significance level was chosen.

2.6. Ethics

The entire study was conducted in accordance with the Declaration of Helsinki of 1964 and its later amendments (including the last in 2013). All procedures were performed in accordance with institutional guidelines. The study was approved by the Ethics Committee of the University Hospital Hradec Králové (approval No. 202005 S05P). All conscious patients signed informed consent forms for the eligible and available diagnostics and treatment. Independent witnesses verified the signatures in cases in which there were technical problems.

3. Results

Out of 809 enrolled consecutive AIS patients, 398 (49.2%) patients were treated with IVT only and 411 (50.8%) with EVT (±IVT). The baseline characteristics of the study population are shown in Table 1. The majority (74.9%) of patients had isolated large vessel occlusion. Nevertheless, in some patients, occlusion of several arteries was present. The most common occlusion site was the MCA/M1 (found in 71.8% of patients), followed by the ICAi (15.1%), MCA/M2 (13.1%), ICAe (11.2%), BA (8.3%), PCA (2.9%), VA (2.7%) and ACA (1.9%). Tandem pathology (defined as ICA+MCA M1/M2 occlusion) was detected in 11.2% of patients. The symptoms of SENSATION, VISION, VERTIGO, HEADACHE, VOMIT, and COMA were significantly more frequent in the IVT only group, whereas symptoms HEMIPAR and N VII occurred significantly more often in the EVT (±IVT) group. Clinical symptoms HEMIPAR, N VII and SPEECH were significantly more frequent in patients with ACS, while symptoms VISION, VERTIGO, HEADACHE, VOMIT and COMA were detected more often in patients diagnosed with PCS (statistical evaluation was not possible in the case of the last three mentioned symptoms due to their minimal occurrence in the ACS group) (Table 2). Observed time intervals were available for the following numbers of patients in the particular groups: ODT in 314 (78.9%) and in 239 (58.2%), ONT in 331 (82.2%) and in 204 (49.6%), respectively, DNT in 375 (94.2%) and in 214 (52.1%). Regarding the EVT (±IVT) group, OGT values were available in 295 (71.8%) and DGT in 362 (88.1%) patients (Figure 1). ONT and DNT were significantly longer (approximately by 18 and 9 min, respectively) in the IVT only group.

Table 1. Baseline and outcome characteristics.

Characteristic	IVT Only Group	EVT (±IVT) Group	p
N	398 (49.2)	411 (50.8)	N/A
Age, (years) †	71.17 ± 12.75 (72.0)	71.99 ± 12.43 (74.0)	0.2354
Male sex	223 (56.0)	172 (41.8)	0.0001
NIHSS baseline †	7.68 ± 5.00 (6.0)	14.18 ± 6.04 (14.0)	<0.0001
Vascular territory			0.7798
Anterior	346 (86.9)	361 (87.8)	
Posterior	52 (13.1)	50 (12.2)	
Clinical symptoms			
Limb weakness (HEMIPAR)	314 (78.9)	388 (94.4)	<0.0001
Drooping of the mouth corner (N VII)	283 (71.1)	342 (83.2)	0.0001
Speech difficulties (SPEECH)	313 (78.6)	341 (83.0)	0.1582
Sensory impairment (SENSATION)	61 (15.3)	18 (4.4)	<0.0001
Visual problems (VISION)	28 (7.0)	14 (3.4)	0.0363
VERTIGO	37 (9.3)	9 (2.2)	0.0001
HEADACHE	16 (4.0)	2 (0.5)	0.0020
Nausea and/or vomiting (VOMIT)	29 (7.3)	9 (2.2)	0.0015
Loss of consciousness (COMA)	3 (7.5)	26 (6.3)	0.0001
IVT	398 (100.0)	253 (61.6)	<0.0001
Time intervals (min)			
Onset-to-door (ODT) †	97.14 ± 57.35 (80.5)	105.30 ± 70.82 (85.0)	0.4089
Onset-to-needle (ONT) †	143.57 ± 64.99 (135.0)	125.28 ± 45.51 (119.0)	0.0005
Door-to-needle (DNT) †	50.10 ± 21.70 (47.0)	41.17 ± 17.29 (40.0)	<0.0001
Onset-to-groin (OGT) †	N/A	207.13 ± 87.35 (185.0)	
Door-to-groin (DGT) †	N/A	75.17 ± 40.74 (73.0)	

Data are N (%) for categorical variables or mean ± SD (median) for numerical variables †. Regarding categorical variables, the groups are statistically compared by a chi-square test of independence; for numerical variables, differences in group medians are tested by a Mann-Whitney t-test. All p-values (two-sided alternative hypothesis) are reported after Benjamini-Hochberg correction; EVT, endovascular therapy; IVT, intravenous thrombolysis; N, number of patients; N/A, not applicable; NIHSS, National Institutes of Health Stroke Scale; SD, standard deviation.

Table 2. Occurrence of presenting clinical symptoms in anterior circulation stroke (ACS) and posterior circulation stroke (PCS) patients.

Clinical Symptom	Circulation		p
	ACS (N = 707)	PCS (N = 102)	
Limb weakness (HEMIPAR)	636 (89.96)	66 (64.71)	<0.0001
Drooping of the mouth corner (N VII)	588 (83.17)	37 (36.27)	<0.0001
Speech difficulties (SPEECH)	593 (83.88)	61 (59.8)	<0.0001
Sensory impairment (SENSATION)	64 (9.05)	15 (14.71)	0.105
Visual problems (VISION)	5 (0.71)	37 (36.27)	<0.0001
VERTIGO	2 (0.28)	44 (43.14)	<0.0001
HEADACHE	0 (0)	18 (17.65)	N/A
Nausea and/or vomiting (VOMIT)	1 (0.14)	37 (36.27)	N/A
Loss of consciousness (COMA)	9 (1.27)	20 (19.61)	N/A

Data are N (%). Symptoms with sufficient frequencies (occurrences) were statistically compared by a chi-square test of independence between ACS and PCS; all p-values (two-sided alternative hypothesis) are reported after Benjamini-Hochberg correction; ACS, anterior circulation stroke; N, number of patients; N/A, not applicable; PCS, posterior circulation stroke.

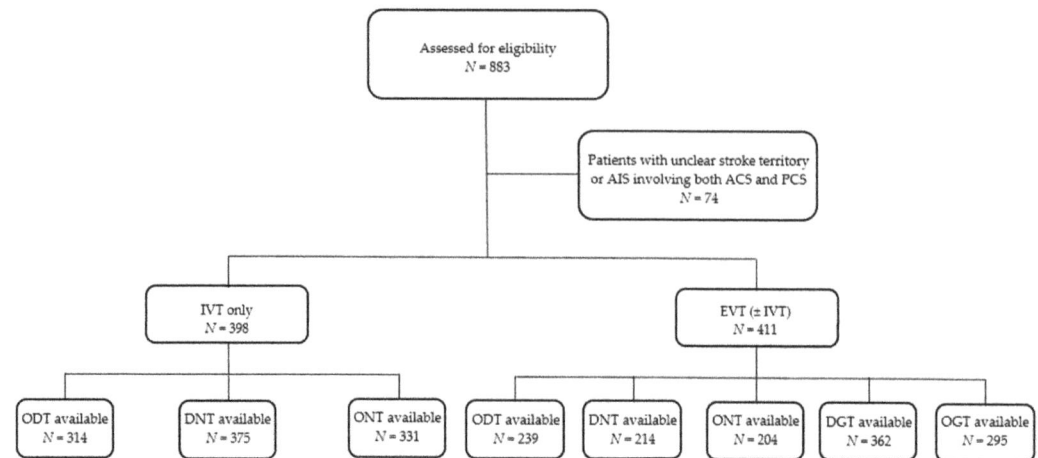

Figure 1. Flowchart of the study. ACS, anterior circulation stroke; AIS, acute ischemic stroke; DGT, door-to-groin puncture time; DNT, door-to-needle time; EVT, endovascular therapy; IVT, intravenous thrombolysis; N, Number; ODT, onset-to-door time; OGT, onset-to-groin time; ONT, onset-to-needle time; PCS, posterior circulation stroke.

Table 3 shows the results of the univariate regression analysis assessing the dependency of recanalization times on the observed parameters both in the IVT only and the EVT (±IVT) groups. The results of the multivariable linear model for recanalization times are presented in Table 4. Regarding the IVT only group, the ODT was best described by a combination of four variables—the baseline NIHSS score (every one-point increase in the NIHSS value is expected to shorten the ODT by 1.74 min) and the presence of clinical symptoms SPEECH (ODT shortening by 18.9 min), HEMIPAR (ODT shortening by 12.6 min) and VOMIT (ODT prolongation by 31.2 min). Similarly, the ONT was best characterized by a combination of four factors—admission NIHSS (every one-point increase in the NIHSS value is expected to shorten the ONT by 1.59 min) and the presence of clinical symptoms SPEECH (ONT shortening by 24.6 min), HEMIPAR (ONT shortening by 15.1 min) and VOMIT (ONT prolongation by 43.7 min). The clinical symptoms SPEECH and VERTIGO were defined as the best variables of DNT in IVT-treated patients, with DNT shortening by 5.2 min and prolongation by 8.6 min, respectively. Concerning the EVT (±IVT) group, no significant ODT predictor was identified. Affected anterior circulation and the presence of clinical symptom N VII had the highest predictive value for the ONT (with shortening by 24.8 and 15.8 min, respectively). Concerning the same group, only one explanatory variable was sufficient to accurately describe the remaining time intervals—presence of symptom COMA for the DNT (prolongation by 22.7 min), affected the anterior vascular territory for the OGT (shortening by 47.3 min) and presence of symptom N VII for the DGT (shortening by 20.8 min).

Table 3. Univariate regression analysis of the dependency of recanalization times.

Explanatory Variable (Predictor)	ODT		ONT			DNT		OGT	DGT
	IVT Only Group (N = 398)	EVT (±IVT) Group (N = 411)	IVT Only Group (N = 398)	EVT (±IVT) Group (N = 411)		IVT Only Group (N = 398)	EVT (±IVT) Group (N = 411)	EVT (±IVT) Group (N = 411)	EVT (±IVT) Group (N = 411)
Age, (years)	−0.0050 (0.0026); 0.076	−0.0021 (0.0030); 0.8174	−0.0034 (0.0022); 0.125	0.0025 (0.0019); 0.197		6.215×10^{-5} (1.558×10^{-3}); 0.968	0.0060 (0.0028); 0.0312	−0.0004 (0.0018); 0.798	0.0042 (0.0021); 0.0476
Male sex	−0.00007 (0.0661); 0.999	−0.2142 (0.0751); 0.0517	0.0207 (0.0573); 0.718	−0.0428 (0.0484); 0.377		−0.0134 (0.0395); 0.734	0.0314 (0.0676); 0.642	−0.1325 (0.0477); 0.0058	0.0275 (0.0553); 0.619
NIHSS baseline	−0.0270 (0.0065); 0.0006	−0.0111 (0.0068); 0.3363	−0.0174 (0.0057); 0.0027	−0.0033 (0.0049); 0.495		−0.0052 (0.0038); 0.178	0.0045 (0.0063); 0.474	−0.0047 (0.0041); 0.249	0.0026 (0.0047); 0.581
Posterior vascular territory	0.3190 (0.0927); 0.0021	0.2141 (0.1325); 0.3363	0.284 (0.0808); 0.0005	0.1889 (0.0866); 0.0304		0.1063 (0.0579); 0.0672	0.1701 (0.1277); 0.184	0.2232 (0.0791); 0.0051	0.1729 (0.0852); 0.0433
				Clinical symptoms					
Limb weakness (HEMIPAR)	−0.1927 (0.0785); 0.0271	−0.0868 (0.1662); 0.8278	−0.1673 (0.0681); 0.0146	−0.1384 (0.1328); 0.298		−0.0655 (0.0479); 0.173	0.0930 (0.1680); 0.58	−0.2052 (0.1081); 0.0585	−0.1231 (0.1217); 0.312
Drooping of the mouth corner (N VII)	−0.1554 (0.0712); 0.0486	−0.1816 (0.1060); 0.3363	−0.1619 (0.0619); 0.0093	−0.1678 (0.0694); 0.0165		−0.0669 (0.0431); 0.122	−0.1952 (0.0976); 0.0469	−0.0674 (0.0640); 0.293	−0.2539 (0.0763); 0.0009
Speech difficulties (SPEECH)	−0.2164 (0.0758); 0.0100	0.0069 (0.1155); 0.9530	−0.2275 (0.0662); 0.0006	−0.0366 (0.0714); 0.609		−0.1063 (0.0471); 0.0247	−0.0525 (0.1000); 0.6	−0.0752 (0.0675); 0.266	−0.099 (0.0767); 0.198
Sensory impairment (SENSATION)	0.0039 (0.0887); 0.9990	0.4925 (0.1955); 0.0909	0.0624 (0.0781); 0.424	−0.0707 (0.1121); 0.529		−0.0197 (0.0538); 0.715	0.0250 (0.2233); 0.911	0.2102 (0.1080); 0.0526	−0.1226 (0.1248); 0.327
Visual problems (VISION)	0.3724 (0.1180); 0.0046	0.2739 (0.2404); 0.5632	0.2694 (0.1039); 0.0099	0.1271 (0.1565); 0.418		0.0840 (0.0757); 0.268	−0.0596 (0.2491); 0.811	0.2008 (0.1466); 0.172	0.2197 (0.1513); 0.148
VERTIGO	0.37064 (0.1037); 0.0019	0.3421 (0.2625); 0.5335	0.3434 (0.0923); 0.0002	−0.0913 (0.1746); 0.602		0.1410 (0.0661); 0.0337	0.2770 (0.2484); 0.266	0.1908 (0.1688); 0.259	0.1165 (0.1744); 0.504
HEADACHE	0.2488 (0.1623); 0.1638	−0.1691 (0.5841); 0.8939	0.238 (0.1447); 0.101	−0.1183 (0.3468); 0.733		0.0359 (0.0970); 0.711	−0.2124 (0.4945); 0.668	−0.3638 (0.4105); 0.376	0.0696 (0.3666); 0.85
Nausea and/or vomiting (VOMIT)	0.4029 (0.1135); 0.0019	0.1496 (0.2408); 0.8278	0.357 (0.1012); 0.0004	0.3517 (0.1547); 0.0241		0.1181 (0.0731); 0.107	0.1613 (0.2041); 0.43	0.0456 (0.1692); 0.787	0.2319 (0.1844); 0.209
Loss of consciousness (COMA)	−0.2572 (0.4077); 0.6252	−0.0876 (0.1662); 0.8278	0.0447 (0.3643); 0.902	0.2309 (0.1237); 0.0636		0.3891 (0.2192); 0.0767	0.4960 (0.1745); 0.0049	0.1814 (0.0992); 0.0685	0.2670 (0.1181); 0.0244

Table 3. Cont.

Explanatory Variable (Predictor)	ODT		ONT		DNT		OGT	DGT
	IVT Only Group (N = 398)	EVT (±IVT) Group (N = 411)	IVT Only Group (N = 398)	EVT (±IVT) Group (N = 411)	IVT Only Group (N = 398)	EVT (±IVT) Group (N = 411)	EVT (±IVT) Group (N = 411)	EVT (±IVT) Group (N = 411)
Occlusion								
ICAe	N/A	−0.0803 (0.1091); 0.8174	N/A	−0.0622 (0.0692); 0.37	N/A	−0.0011 (0.0971); 0.991	−0.0035 (0.0713); 0.96	−0.1015 (0.0865); 0.242
ICAi	N/A	−0.0085 (0.0991); 0.9530	N/A	−0.0300 (0.0657); 0.648	N/A	0.0887 (0.0880); 0.315	−0.0481 (0.0657); 0.465	0.0743 (0.0740); 0.315
MCA/M1	N/A	−0.0175 (0.0860); 0.9229	N/A	−0.1082 (0.0554); 0.0524	N/A	−0.0994 (0.0789); 0.209	−0.1132 (0.0533); 0.0346	−0.1206 (0.0608); 0.0481
MCA/M2	N/A	−0.1073 (0.1091); 0.654	N/A	0.0470 (0.0703); 0.504	N/A	0.0536 (0.1000); 0.593	−0.0132 (0.0690); 0.848	0.0660 (0.0815); 0.418
ACA	N/A	−0.3067 (0.2627); 0.5632	N/A	−0.2934 (0.1736); 0.0925	N/A	0.1950 (0.2229); 0.383	−0.1851 (0.1689); 0.274	0.0331 (0.1848); 0.858
PCA	N/A	0.0849 (0.2410); 0.8861	N/A	0.3438 (0.1548); 0.0275	N/A	0.2230 (0.2228); 0.318	0.1866 (0.1565); 0.234	0.2837 (0.1576); 0.0727
VA	N/A	−0.1268 (0.2938); 0.8632	N/A	0.0970 (0.1565); 0.536	N/A	0.4025 (0.2476); 0.106	0.0744 (0.1691); 0.66	0.1508 (0.1656); 0.363
BA	N/A	0.3080 (0.1542); 0.2580	N/A	0.1902 (0.1114); 0.0894	N/A	0.0554 (0.1598); 0.729	0.2578 (0.0916); 0.0052	0.1518 (0.1049); 0.149
IVT	N/A	−0.4410 (0.0798); <0.0001	N/A	N/A	N/A	N/A	−0.0089 (0.0518); 0.863	−0.1019 (0.0572); 0.0757

Outputs from univariate regression models (OLS) for log transformed dependent variable (time intervals) are reported as follows: beta (SE); *p* value; ACA, anterior cerebral artery; BA, basilar artery; DGT, door-to-groin time; DNT, door-to-needle time; EVT, endovascular therapy; iCAe, extracranial internal carotid artery; ICAi, intracranial internal carotid artery; IVT, intravenous thrombolysis; MCA/ M1, M1 segment of the middle cerebral artery; MCA/M2, M2 segment of the middle cerebral artery; N, number of patients; N/A, not applicable; NIHSS, National Institutes of Health Stroke Scale; ODT, onset-to-door time; OGT, onset-to-groin time; ONT, onset-to-needle time; PCA, posterior cerebral artery; SE, standard error; VA, vertebral artery.

Table 4. Best multivariable models of observed time intervals.

Patient Group	Observed Time Interval (Outcome)	Explanatory Variable (Predictor)	Beta	Standard Error	p
IVT only	Onset-to-door time (ODT)	NIHSS	−1.741	0.687	0.0118
		Limb weakness (HEMIPAR)	−12.608	8.161	0.1233
		Speech difficulties (SPEECH)	−18.927	7.619	0.0135
		Nausea and/or vomiting (VOMIT)	31.159	11.748	0.0084
	Onset-to-needle time (ONT)	NIHSS	−1.5934	0.7575	0.036
		Limb weakness (HEMIPAR)	−15.0672	8.9026	0.092
		Speech difficulties (SPEECH)	−24.564	8.4185	0.004
		Nausea and/or vomiting (VOMIT)	43.7237	13.1284	0.001
	Door-to-needle time (DNT)	Speech difficulties (SPEECH)	−5.163	2.737	0.060
		VERTIGO	8.575	3.84	0.026
EVT (±IVT)	Onset-to-needle time (ONT)	Vascular territory—anterior	−24.76	12.99	0.058
		Drooping of the mouth corner (N VII)	−15.76	10.43	0.132
	Door-to-needle time (DNT)	Loss of consciousness (COMA)	22.675	6.046	0.0002
	Onset-to-groin time (OGT)	Vascular territory—anterior	−47.32	16.89	0.005
	Door-to-groin time (DGT)	Drooping of the mouth corner (N VII)	−20.794	6.015	0.0006

Beta is the estimated regression coefficient of the multivariable regression model (OLS) that can be interpreted as the population (point) estimate of the difference in the mean time from the reference group (no symptoms, posterior vascular territory). Beta for the NIHSS is the estimate of the marginal (unit) change, i.e., every one-point increase in the NIHSS value is expected to shorten the mean ONT in the IVT group by 1.59 min; EVT, endovascular therapy; IVT, intravenous thrombolysis; NIHSS, National Institutes of Health Stroke Scale.

4. Discussion

While there are many studies investigating the impact of the severity of the neurological deficit assessed by the NIHSS [19–23] or AIS localization (PCS versus ACS) [8,19,24] on specific treatment time intervals, studies focusing on individual stroke symptoms are rare [8,9]. According to our knowledge, our study is just the second original research manuscript dealing with this topic, as the study performed by Baraban et al. was published in the form of an abstract only [9].

During this study we identified several variables (the NIHSS value, anterior circulation, clinical symptoms HEMIPAR, N VII, SPEECH, VERTIGO, VOMIT, COMA) of five observed time intervals. Aligned with the previous literature, we observed that presenting symptoms did impact the treatment timeline [8,9,25]. Regarding AIS presenting with less specific symptoms (VERTIGO, VOMIT, COMA), the treatment was initiated later than in AIS with more defined clinical symptoms (HEMIPAR, N VII, SPEECH) related mainly to ACS. Since nonspecific symptoms such as VERTIGO and VOMIT, commonly occurring in PCS, overlap with more benign medical conditions like gastroenteritis, we assume that these patients will not have ONT, OGT, DNT, DGT only, but also ODT due to an inappropriate response (delay in calling 911 by patient/relative/friend). This hypothesis was confirmed by Baraban et al. who found that patients presenting with symptom SPEECH arrived at the hospital 14.2% faster ($p = 0.007$) and also had a 6.0% faster DNT ($p = 0.006$) than patients without these symptoms. Moreover, authors observed that those presenting with HEMIPAR had a 9.3% faster DNT ($p = 0.001$) and patients with other neurologic symptoms arrived 14.0% later than those without HEMIPAR ($p = 0.009$) [9]. According to Sarraj et al. [8], ONT was statistically different for the following clinical symptoms: N VII (153 versus 167 min in the case of its absence, $p = 0.044$), VOMIT (187 versus 156 min, $p = 0.009$), and COMA (153 versus 171 min, $p = 0.006$). DNT was significantly associated with HEMIPAR (74 versus 87 min in the case of its absence, $p = 0.014$) and VOMIT (96 versus 75 min, $p = 0.005$) [8]. Authors from Finland similarly demonstrated that AIS patients with a positive Face Arm Speech Time (FAST) test had a shorter DNT as well (48 versus 66 min, $p < 0.001$) [25]. Interestingly, in contrast to some previous reports in which HEMIPAR was associated with reduced DNT [8,9], in our study the presence of this symptom only insignificantly influenced ODT and ONT, even though it seems to be an easily recognizable stroke symptom. Conversely, the presence of the clinical symptom SPEECH was associated with a shorter ODT, ONT, and DNT in our IVT only group, and the presence of clinical symptom N VII was associated with a shorter ONT and DGT in our EVT (±IVT) group. The SPEECH symptom included not only dysarthria, but also phatic disorder, which represents a more remarkable neurological deficit. The symptom N VII, although representing a "minor stroke symptom", is easily recognizable by the public, similar to HEMIPAR. Even an isolated phatic disorder can justify the IVT procedure, as it might be associated with up to four points on the NIHSS, i.e., the cut-off point for rtPA administration) [13–17]. Although significant variables for the observed time intervals were slightly different in our and the above-mentioned studies, it was confirmed that patients with less specific symptoms experienced treatment delays. The symptom COMA represented the only exception—it was responsible for DNT prolongation in our EVT (±IVT) group by 22.7 min, but in the study by Sarraj et al., COMA significantly shortened ODT by approximately 12 min and ONT by approximately 18 min [8]. One possible interpretation could be the difference in the pre-hospital and intra-hospital management of comatose patients. Since COMA is a serious medical condition usually recognizable by the general public, the patient probably gets to the hospital quickly. However, the problem may be the intra-hospital delays due to the need for a systematic multidisciplinary approach to the unconscious patient, e.g., early physiological stabilization, activation of an anesthesia team, intubation for respiratory failure or airway protection [26]. Hassan et al. found that the mean time interval between the CT scan and the initiation of an endovascular procedure was significantly longer in patients who underwent preprocedural intubation (132 ± 102 versus 111 ± 47 min, $p < 0.0001$) [27]. Ultimately, our findings reflect a real clinical practice. There are several explanations of this phenomenon. Screening tools such as the FAST test developed for prehospital identification of AIS patients by checking for facial and/or arm weakness and speech disturbance are undoubtedly less sensitive for the identification of PCS compared to ACS [24,28,29]. Since symptoms of PCS can mimic other disorders, they can be misinterpreted easily and may lead to under-recognition considering initial nonfocal and nonspecific symptoms [24,30,31]. Both ONT and DNT were significantly longer in the PCS versus the ACS group (175 versus 155 min, $p = 0.0121$ and 90 versus 74 min, $p = 0.0026$, respectively) in the study published by Sarraj et al. [8]. Likewise, DNT was, on average, longer by 13 min in patients with PCS compared to ACS patients ($p < 0.001$) according to data reported by Sommer et al. [24]. During the Czech study which aimed to determine the predictors of calling 911 in reaction to stroke symptoms, responders identified SPEECH (37%) and HEMIPAR (34%) as the most typical symptoms of AIS [32]. A Swedish study reported that two-thirds of the population knew at least one stroke symptom, but only one-tenth knew three stroke symptoms [33]. Although public awareness of stroke has improved in recent years thanks to various mass media intervention campaigns advertising AIS symptoms, there is still a lack of recognition of mainly PCS symptoms, which implies a need for increased education not only of the general public, but also of paramedics and staff working in the emergency departments. It is obvious that the initial assessment phase is crucial, and better clinical recognition is urgently needed to optimize acute care. Even patients with less specific stroke symptoms must be promptly diagnosed and treated, although this still represents a challenge in emergency medicine. Last but not least, we found that every one-point increase in the admission NIHSS value was expected to shorten ONT by 1.59 min in the IVT only group. Most authors previously demonstrated that lower baseline NIHSS scores in AIS patients were associated with longer treatment times [20,23,34]. This fact is related to the above-discussed issue concerning an often difficult differential diagnosis of PCS. Since the NIHSS is weighted more toward ACS symptoms, it tends to underestimate the clinical severity in PCS, which is reflected by previous observations of overall lower NIHSS scores in patients with PCS compared to ACS [8,24,35,36]. During our study, "more defined" stroke symptoms, such as HEMIPAR, N VII and SPEECH were more frequent in the ACS, while in the PCS, "less defined" stroke symptoms, such as VISION, VERTIGO, HEADACHE, VOMIT and COMA were observed. However, ACS of low severity is also difficult to diagnose. Thus, this problem is not restricted to PCS.

Several limitations of the present study should be mentioned. First, it has a retrospective character with a sample extracted from a single stroke center database; therefore, the results may not be generalizable. Second, the data collection methods among databases may be the source of selection bias. Our study has the same limits as all non-randomized controlled trials. Third, reported data depend on the accuracy and the completeness of the medical records. Unfortunately, data missingness was present for some time outcomes, as mentioned above. We focused on five selected time intervals including onset-to-treatment, although the time of the stroke onset is often inaccurate. Actually, some strokes may have occurred during sleep and, in other cases, the witnesses were unable to recall the precise time of symptom onset. Conversely, the strength of this study is that it included a relatively large cohort of patients. We should note that, unlike other studies, we also evaluated the clinical profile behind the NIHSS values.

5. Conclusions

Our results demonstrated that initial presenting symptoms of AIS did influence the treatment timeline both in the pre-hospital and intra-hospital management phase. Patients with less specific stroke symptoms associated with posterior circulation experienced treatment delays. There is no doubt that the significant diagnostic ambiguity of PCS represents a serious issue in the field of emergency medicine. Therefore, an important research question for stroke specialists still remains regarding optimized logistics and acute phase management strategies. Analysis of a larger nationwide registry and of international registries would be beneficial to confirm our observations.

Author Contributions: Conceptualization, S.H. and R.H.; Data curation, S.H., R.H. and A.H.; Formal analysis, R.H. and L.S.; Funding acquisition, M.V.; Investigation, D.K., A.K., V.C., M.L., J.R., O.R., L.Š. and E.V.; Methodology, S.H. and R.H.; Project administration, S.H. and R.H.; Resources, R.H. and D.K.; Software, L.S.; Supervision, R.H.; Validation, R.H.; Visualization, S.H. and L.S.; Writing—original draft, S.H., R.H. and L.S.; Writing—review & editing, S.H., R.H., D.K., A.H., A.K., V.C., M.L., J.R., O.R., L.Š., E.V., L.S and M.V. All authors have read and agreed to the published version of the manuscript.

Funding: This work was supported in part by the Ministry of Health of the Czech Republic (grant number DRO—UHHK 00179906) and Charles University, Czech Republic (grant number PROGRES Q40).

Institutional Review Board Statement: The study was conducted according to the guidelines of the Declaration of Helsinki, and approved by the Ethics Committee of the University Hospital Hradec Králové, Czech Republic (approval No. 202005 S05P) on 21 April 2020.

Informed Consent Statement: Given the retrospective nature of the study, the individual consent to participate was not required after the approval from the local Ethics Committee.

Data Availability Statement: The datasets analyzed during the current study are available from the corresponding author on reasonable request.

Conflicts of Interest: The authors declare no conflict of interest. The funders had no role in the design of the study; in the collection, analyses, or interpretation of data; in the writing of the manuscript, or in the decision to publish the results.

References

1. De Marchis, G.M.; Kohler, A.; Renz, N.; Arnold, M.; Mono, M.L.; Jung, S.; Fischer, U.; Karameshev, A.I.; Brekenfeld, C.; Gralla, J.; et al. Posterior versus anterior circulation strokes: Comparison of clinical, radiological and outcome characteristics. *J. Neurol. Neurosurg. Psychiatry* **2011**, *82*, 33–37. [CrossRef] [PubMed]
2. Dorňák, T.; Herzig, R.; Kuliha, M.; Havlíček, R.; Školoudík, D.; Šaňák, D.; Köcher, M.; Procházka, V.; Lacman, J.; Charvát, F.; et al. Endovascular treatment of acute basilar artery occlusion: Time to treatment is crucial. *Clin. Radiol.* **2015**, *70*, e20–e27. [CrossRef]

3. Zürcher, E.; Richoz, B.; Faouzi, M.; Michel, P. Differences in ischemic anterior and posterior circulation strokes: A clinico-radiological and outcome analysis. *J. Stroke Cerebrovasc. Dis.* **2019**, *28*, 710–718. [CrossRef] [PubMed]
4. Frid, P.; Drake, M.; Giese, A.K.; Wasselius, J.; Schirmer, M.D.; Donahue, K.L.; Cloonan, L.; Irie, R.; Bouts, M.J.R.J.; McIntosh, E.C.; et al. Detailed phenotyping of posterior vs. anterior circulation ischemic stroke: A multi-center MRI study. *J. Neurol.* **2020**, *267*, 649–658. [CrossRef]
5. Tao, W.D.; Liu, M.; Fisher, M.; Wang, D.R.; Li, J.; Furie, K.L.; Hao, Z.L.; Lin, S.; Zhang, C.F.; Zeng, Q.T.; et al. Posterior versus anterior circulation infarction: How different are the neurological deficits? *Stroke* **2012**, *43*, 2060–2065. [CrossRef] [PubMed]
6. Emberson, J.; Lees, K.R.; Lyden, P.; Blackwell, L.; Albers, G.; Bluhmki, E.; Brott, T.; Cohen, G.; Davis, S.; Donnan, G.; et al. Effect of treatment delay, age, and stroke severity on the effects of intravenous thrombolysis with alteplase for acute ischaemic stroke: A meta-analysis of individual patient data from randomised trials. *Lancet* **2014**, *384*, 1929–1935. [CrossRef]
7. Saver, J.L.; Goyal, M.; van der Lugt, A.; Menon, B.K.; Majoie, C.B.; Dippel, D.W.; Campbell, B.C.; Nogueira, R.G.; Demchuk, A.M.; Tomasello, A.; et al. Time to treatment with endovascular thrombectomy and outcomes from ischemic stroke: A meta-analysis. *JAMA* **2016**, *316*, 1279–1288. [CrossRef]
8. Sarraj, A.; Medrek, S.; Albright, K.; Martin-Schild, S.; Bibars, W.; Vahidy, F.; Grotta, J.C.; Savitz, S.I. Posterior circulation stroke is associated with prolonged door-to-needle time. *Int. J. Stroke* **2015**, *10*, 672–678. [CrossRef]
9. Baraban, E.; Lucas, L.; Bhatt, A. Initial presenting stroke symptoms impact treatment timeline among ischemic stroke patients [abstract]. *Neurology* **2018**, *90* (Suppl. S15), P4.233.
10. Goldstein, L.B.; Samsa, G.P. Reliability of the National Institutes of Health Stroke Scale. Extension to non-neurologists in the context of a clinical trial. *Stroke* **1997**, *28*, 307–310. [CrossRef]
11. Krajíčková, D.; Krajina, A.; Herzig, R.; Lojík, M.; Chovanec, V.; Raupach, J.; Vítková, E.; Waishaupt, J.; Vyšata, O.; Vališ, M. Mechanical recanalization in ischemic anterior circulation stroke within an 8-hour time window. A real-world experience. *Diagn. Interv. Radiol.* **2017**, *23*, 465–471. [CrossRef]
12. Campbell, B.C.; Christensen, S.; Levi, C.R.; Desmond, P.M.; Donnan, G.A.; Davis, S.M.; Parsons, M.W. Cerebral blood flow is the optimal CT perfusion parameter for assessing infarct core. *Stroke* **2011**, *42*, 3435–3440. [CrossRef]
13. Jauch, E.C.; Saver, J.L.; Adams, H.P., Jr.; Bruno, A.; Connors, J.J.; Demaerschalk, B.M.; Khatri, P.; McMullan, P.W., Jr.; Qureshi, A.I.; Rosenfield, K.; et al. Guidelines for the early management of patients with acute ischemic stroke: A guideline for healthcare professionals from the American Heart Association/American Stroke Association. *Stroke* **2013**, *44*, 870–947. [CrossRef] [PubMed]
14. Neumann, J.; Tomek, A.; Školoudík, D.; Škoda, O.; Mikulík, R.; Herzig, R.; Václavík, D.; Bar, M.; Šaňák, D. Doporučený postup pro intravenózní trombolýzu v léčbě akutního mozkového infarktu—Verze 2014. *Cesk. Slov. Neurol. N.* **2014**, *77/110*, 381–385.
15. Powers, W.J.; Derdeyn, C.P.; Biller, J.; Coffey, C.S.; Hoh, B.L.; Jauch, E.C.; Johnston, K.C.; Johnston, S.C.; Khalessi, A.A.; Kidwell, C.S.; et al. 2015 American Heart Association/American Stroke Association focused update of the 2013 guidelines for the early management of patients with acute ischemic stroke regarding endovascular treatment: A guideline for healthcare professionals from the American Heart Association/American Stroke Association. *Stroke* **2015**, *46*, 3020–3035. [CrossRef]
16. Šaňák, D.; Neumann, J.; Tomek, A.; Školoudík, D.; Škoda, O.; Mikulík, R.; Herzig, R.; Václavík, D.; Bar, M.; Roček, M.; et al. Doporučení pro rekanalizační léčbu akutního mozkového infarktu—Verze 2016. *Cesk. Slov. Neurol. N.* **2016**, *79/112*, 231–234. [CrossRef]
17. Powers, W.J.; Rabinstein, A.A.; Ackerson, T.; Adeoye, O.M.; Bambakidis, N.C.; Becker, K.; Biller, J.; Brown, M.; Demaerschalk, B.M.; Hoh, B.; et al. 2018 guidelines for the early management of patients with acute ischemic stroke. A guideline for healthcare professionals from the American Heart Association/American Stroke Association. *Stroke* **2018**, *49*, e46–e110. [CrossRef] [PubMed]
18. Sanák, D.; Nosál', V.; Horák, D.; Bártková, A.; Zelenák, K.; Herzig, R.; Bucil, J.; Skoloudík, D.; Burval, S.; Cisariková, V.; et al. Impact of diffusion-weighted MRI-measured initial cerebral infarction volume on clinical outcome in acute stroke patients with middle cerebral artery occlusion treated by thrombolysis. *Neuroradiology* **2006**, *48*, 632–639. [CrossRef]
19. Ferrari, J.; Knoflach, M.; Seyfang, L.; Lang, W. Austrian Stroke Unit Registry Collaborators. Differences in process management and in-hospital delays in treatment with iv thrombolysis. *PLoS ONE* **2013**, *8*, e75378. [CrossRef]
20. Bhatt, A.; Lesko, A.; Lucas, L.; Kansara, A.; Baraban, E. Patients with low national institutes of health stroke scale scores have longer door-to-needle times: Analysis of a telestroke network. *J. Stroke Cerebrovasc. Dis.* **2016**, *25*, 2253–2258. [CrossRef]
21. Birnbaum, L.A.; Rodriguez, J.S.; Topel, C.H.; Behrouz, R.; Misra, V.; Palacio, S.; Patterson, M.G.; Motz, D.S.; Goros, M.W.; Cornell, J.E.; et al. Older stroke patients with high stroke scores have delayed door-to-needle times. *J. Stroke Cerebrovasc. Dis.* **2016**, *25*, 2668–2672. [CrossRef] [PubMed]
22. Kwei, K.T.; Liang, J.; Wilson, N.; Tuhrim, S.; Dhamoon, M. Stroke severity affects timing: Time from stroke code activation to initial imaging is longer in patients with milder strokes. *Neurologist* **2018**, *23*, 79–82. [CrossRef]
23. Jahan, R.; Saver, J.L.; Schwamm, L.H.; Fonarow, G.C.; Liang, L.; Matsouaka, R.A.; Xian, Y.; Holmes, D.N.; Peterson, E.D.; Yavagal, D.; et al. Association between time to treatment with endovascular reperfusion therapy and outcomes in patients with acute ischemic stroke treated in clinical practice. *JAMA* **2019**, *322*, 252–263. [CrossRef]
24. Sommer, P.; Seyfang, L.; Posekany, A.; Ferrari, J.; Lang, W.; Fertl, E.; Serles, W.; Töll, T.; Kiechl, S.; Greisenegger, S. Prehospital and intra-hospital time delays in posterior circulation stroke: Results from the Austrian Stroke Unit Registry. *J. Neurol.* **2017**, *264*, 131–138. [CrossRef]

25. Varjoranta, T.; Raatiniemi, L.; Majamaa, K.; Martikainen, M.; Liisanantti, J.H. Prehospital and hospital delays for stroke patients treated with thrombolysis: A retrospective study from mixed rural-urban area in Northern Finland. *Australas. Emerg. Care* **2019**, *22*, 76–80. [CrossRef]
26. Mowla, A.; Doyle, J.; Lail, N.S.; Rajabzadeh-Oghaz, H.; Deline, C.; Shirani, P.; Ching, M.; Crumlish, A.; Steck, D.A.; Janicke, D.; et al. Delays in door-to-needle time for acute ischemic stroke in the emergency department: A comprehensive stroke center experience. *J. Neurol. Sci.* **2017**, *376*, 102–105. [CrossRef]
27. Hassan, A.E.; Adil, M.M.; Zacharatos, H.; Rahim, B.; Chaudhry, S.A.; Tekle, W.G.; Qureshi, A.I. Should ischemic stroke patients with aphasia or high National Institutes of Health Stroke Scale score undergo preprocedural intubation and endovascular treatment? *J. Stroke Cerebrovasc. Dis.* **2014**, *23*, e299–e304. [CrossRef]
28. Gulli, G.; Markus, H.S. The use of FAST and ABCD2 scores in posterior circulation, compared with anterior circulation, stroke and transient ischemic attack. *J. Neurol. Neurosurg. Psychiatry* **2012**, *83*, 228–229. [CrossRef]
29. Berglund, A.; von Euler, M.; Schenck-Gustafsson, K.; Castrén, M.; Bohm, K. Identification of stroke during the emergency call: A descriptive study of callers' presentation of stroke. *BMJ Open* **2015**, *5*, e007661. [CrossRef]
30. Arch, A.E.; Weisman, D.C.; Coca, S.; Nystrom, K.V.; Wira, C.R., III; Schindler, J.L. Missed ischemic stroke diagnosis in the emergency department by emergency medicine and neurology services. *Stroke* **2016**, *47*, 668–673. [CrossRef]
31. Schneck, M.J. Current stroke scales may be partly responsible for worse outcomes in posterior circulation stroke. *Stroke* **2018**, *49*, 2565–2566. [CrossRef] [PubMed]
32. Mikulík, R.; Bunt, L.; Hrdlicka, D.; Dusek, L.; Václavík, D.; Kryza, J. Calling 911 in response to stroke: A nationwide study assessing definitive individual behavior. *Stroke* **2008**, *39*, 1844–1849. [CrossRef] [PubMed]
33. Nordanstig, A.; Jood, K.; Rosengren, L. Public stroke awareness and intent to call 112 in Sweden. *Acta Neurol. Scand.* **2014**, *130*, 400–404. [CrossRef] [PubMed]
34. Jung, S.; Rosini, J.M.; Nomura, J.T.; Caplan, R.J.; Raser-Schramm, J. Even faster door-to-alteplase times and associated outcomes in acute ischemic stroke. *J. Stroke Cerebrovasc. Dis.* **2019**, *28*, 104329. [CrossRef] [PubMed]
35. Förster, A.; Gass, A.; Kern, R.; Griebe, M.; Hennerici, M.G.; Szabo, K. Thrombolysis in posterior circulation stroke: Stroke subtypes and patterns, complications and outcome. *Cerebrovasc. Dis.* **2011**, *32*, 349–353. [CrossRef] [PubMed]
36. Inoa, V.; Aron, A.W.; Staff, I.; Fortunato, G.; Sansing, L.H. Lower NIH stroke scale scores are required to accurately predict a good prognosis in posterior circulation stroke. *Cerebrovasc. Dis.* **2014**, *37*, 251–255. [CrossRef]

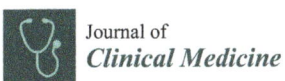

Article

Prediction of Infarct Growth and Neurological Deterioration in Patients with Vertebrobasilar Artery Occlusions

Seungyon Koh [1], Ji Hyun Park [2], Bumhee Park [2,3], Mun Hee Choi [1], Sung Eun Lee [1], Jin Soo Lee [1], Ji Man Hong [1] and Seong-Joon Lee [1,*]

[1] Department of Neurology, Ajou University School of Medicine, 164, World cup-ro, Yeongtong-gu, Suwon, Gyeonggi-do 16499, Korea; esin4498@gmail.com (S.K.); choimoonhee09@gmail.com (M.H.C.); plumpboy@hanmail.net (S.E.L.); jinsoo22@gmail.com (J.S.L.); dacda@hanmail.net (J.M.H.)
[2] Office of Biostatistics, Medical Research Collaborating Center, Ajou Research Institute for Innovative Medicine, Ajou University Medical Center, Suwon, Gyeonggi-do 16499, Korea; jhn1105@gmail.com (J.H.P.); bhpark@ajou.ac.kr (B.P.)
[3] Department of Biomedical Informatics, Ajou University School of Medicine, Suwon 16449, Korea
* Correspondence: editisan@gmail.com; Tel.: +82-31-219-5175; Fax: +82-31-219-5178

Received: 15 October 2020; Accepted: 21 November 2020; Published: 22 November 2020

Abstract: We aimed to identify predictors of infarct growth and neurological deterioration (ND) in vertebrobasilar occlusions (VBOs) with a focus on clinical-core mismatch. From 2010 to 2018, VBO patients were selected from a university hospital registry. In total, 138 VBO patients were included. In these patients, a posterior circulation Alberta Stroke Program Early CT score (PC-ASPECTS) less than 6 was associated with futile outcome. Within patients with feasible cores, a decrease in PC-ASPECTS score of 2 or more on follow-up imaging was classified as infarct growth and could be predicted by a National Institutes of Health Stroke Scale (NIHSS) mental status subset of 1 or higher (odds ratio (OR): 3.34, 95% confidence interval (CI) (1.19–9.38), $p = 0.022$). Among the 73 patients who did not undergo reperfusion therapy, 13 patients experienced ND (increase in discharge NIHSS score of 4 or more compared to the initial presentation). Incomplete occlusion (vs. complete occlusion, OR 6.17, 95% CI (1.11–34.25), $p = 0.037$), poorer collateral status (BATMAN score, OR: 1.91, 95% CI (1.17–3.48), $p = 0.009$), and larger infarct cores (PC-ASPECTS, OR: 1.96, 95% CI (1.11–3.48), $p = 0.021$) were predictive of ND. In patients with VBO, an initial PC-ASPECTS of 6 or more, but with a decrease in the mental status subset of 1 or more can predict infarct growth, and may be used as a criterion for clinical-core mismatch. ND in VBO patients presenting with milder symptoms can be predicted by incomplete occlusion, poor collaterals, and larger infarct cores.

Keywords: basilar artery; brain ischemia; intracranial atherosclerosis; embolism; infarction

1. Introduction

In anterior circulation stroke, endovascular treatment (EVT) for emergent large vessel occlusion is a well-established treatment. The indication is relatively clear, and its effectiveness has been proven through numerous randomized controlled trials (RCTs) [1]. While there have been no successful RCTs demonstrating the effectiveness of EVT in vertebrobasilar occlusion (VBO), it is strongly recommended that EVT be used for treating VBO [2]. In practice, however, decisions for EVT in VBO patients are complicated by diversity in clinical courses, such as prodromal symptoms, late progressions, and a wide range of clinical symptoms despite similar-looking vascular occlusions. Thus, there are some issues to be further resolved for EVT of VBO.

One major issue is generation of a clinical-core mismatch criterion in VBO. Time-based selection criteria for EVT in VBO may be complicated by heterogeneity in clinical presentation [3], and a clinical-core mismatch criterion can be supportive. The clinical-core mismatch criterion is used to identify patients with significant neurologic deficits but with limited infarct core that may benefit from EVT regardless of stroke onset-to-door time [4]. The clinical-core mismatch can predict infarct growth and maximize the treatment effect of EVT [5]. For example, the original reports have described an inclusion criteria of National Institutes of Health Stroke Scale (NIHSS) ≥10 with an infarct core of <31cc for anterior circulation large vessel occlusion patients [4]. In the anterior circulation, clinical-core mismatch is widely accepted as a predictor of infarct growth along with other methods such as diffusion-perfusion mismatch [6], or collateral status [7]. Theoretically, a clinical-core mismatch criteria can be superior to diffusion-perfusion mismatch or collateral status in VBO. Perfusion imaging of the posterior circulation is limited by its low spatial resolution, while leptomeningeal collateral assessment via noninvasive methods cannot be applied to the posterior circulation. However, whether to use the total NIHSS score, or to use special subsets of neurological deficits for the mismatch criteria to predict infarct growth, can be debatable. In the anterior circulation, cortical signs such as aphasia, extinction, and gaze deviation may be considered as a marker of hemispheric hypoperfusion [5]. It is not clear which neurological signs may represent this role in the posterior circulation.

A second major issue is neurological deterioration (ND). For VBO, even for patients that present with lower clinical severity, there is a high rate of neurological deterioration (ND). High rates of intracranial atherosclerotic occlusions are partly responsible. Owing to its longstanding diseased vessel status, patients with intracranial atherosclerotic occlusions may present with a wide variety of clinical severity, and experience a high rate of ND. While the pathomechanism underlying ND is diverse, late perfusion failure following ND are comparatively more common and often lead to devastating neurological outcomes. However, in VBO the actual frequency, the distributions of pathomechanism of the ND, and potential predictors are not well reported. Identification of such factors are needed to evaluate the feasibility of delayed or even preventive EVT.

The fact that there are high rates of intracranial atherosclerotic occlusions [7] in VBO is associated with both issues. However, such associations have not been appropriately addressed in previous studies; past literature describing clinical behaviors of VBO with regard to pathophysiology date back to the pre-EVT era [8], while reports of EVT in VBO seldom address the heterogeneity in clinical presentation. Further, the underlying occlusion etiology is difficult to verify in cases that do not undergo EVT, for identification of underlying stenosis can only be performed after recanalization is achieved [9]. However, recent studies focusing on pre-EVT identification of intracranial atherosclerotic occlusions have reported occlusion type analysis based on the idea that an embolus would likely become lodged at the site of an arterial bifurcation rather than being halted in the middle of the artery [10]. This etiologic classification was shown to be well-matched with post-procedural diagnosis especially in the VBO population [11], and used as a surrogate for intracranial atherosclerotic occlusions in both the anterior [12] and posterior [13] circulations.

Thus, in VBO patients, we aimed to describe the overall clinical picture that may benefit from reperfusion therapies, by addressing the issue of infarct growth and neurological deterioration. To achieve this goal, this study identified VBO patients based on presenting angiographic imaging and tissue imaging, rather than therapeutic modality or presenting time. In this population, we first aimed to generate a clinical-core mismatch criteria through identification of futile infarct cores and predictors of infarct growth, correcting for occlusion type. The total NIHSS score and its subsets were compared in this analysis. Second, in patients that did not undergo revascularization, the frequency, pathomechanism of ND, and its predictors were evaluated.

2. Materials and Methods

The data that support the findings of this study are available from the corresponding author, upon reasonable request.

2.1. Patient Selection

The flow chart for patient inclusion is summarized in Figure 1. From January 2010 to December 2018, all posterior circulation stroke patients were identified from Ajou Stroke Registry, a prospectively collected stroke registry from a university hospital stroke center. All patients admitted to the department of neurology for the treatment of acute ischemic stroke were registered regardless of the treatment or imaging. The basic demographics, the initial and follow-up NIHSS score at 2 h and 1, 3, 7, and 14 days, and the day of discharge, functional outcome as measured by modified Rankin scale (mRS) at discharge and at 3 months, laboratory tests, and the location of the infarction were collected from the registry. In all posterior circulation stroke patients included in the registry, patients with VBO was identified through medical record search for keywords "occlusion", or "stenosis" in baseline CTA or MRA reports, and further reviewed by two investigators (S.K., senior resident and S.-J.L., interventional neurologist) to identify an occlusion or near total occlusion in the basilar artery, bilateral vertebral artery, or dominant vertebral artery with no contralateral vertebral artery flow. Near total occlusions in which antegrade blood flow cannot be ascertained, or only minimal flow is suspected, was included because similar looking lesions present with a wide range of clinical severity, and in a large number of cases, antegrade blood flow cannot be ascertained without conventional angiography. Patients who had data regarding the initial and final infarct volumes available, which was assessed magnetic resonance imaging (MRI) or CT, were selected. Ethics approval was obtained from the local institutional review board, and the board waived the need for patient consent.

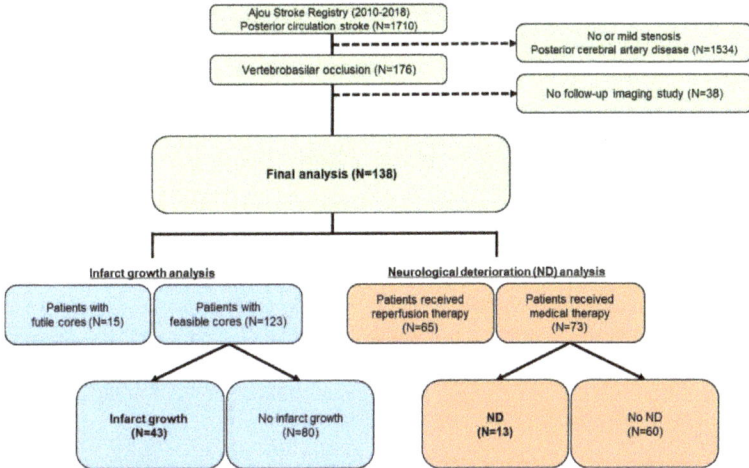

Figure 1. Flow chart of the patient selection process is provided in this flowchart. ND, neurological deterioration.

2.2. Variables and Image Analysis

Variables being investigated were obtained retrospectively by reviewing medical records. The NIHSS was divided into mental status, motor, and cranial and cerebellar subsets. The mental status subset included level of consciousness (LOC), LOC questions, and LOC commands; the motor subset included bilateral arm and leg scores; and the cranial and cerebellar subset included best gaze, facial palsy, dysarthria, language, and ataxia scores. This subset classification is summarized in

Figure 2. Prodrome was defined as a preceding fluctuation of neurological symptoms suggestive of a vertebrobasilar transient ischemic attack.

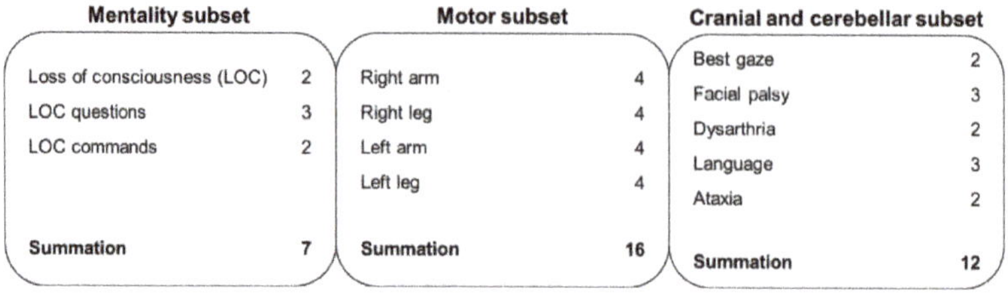

Mentality subset		Motor subset		Cranial and cerebellar subset	
Loss of consciousness (LOC)	2	Right arm	4	Best gaze	2
LOC questions	3	Right leg	4	Facial palsy	3
LOC commands	2	Left arm	4	Dysarthria	2
		Left leg	4	Language	3
				Ataxia	2
Summation	7	Summation	16	Summation	12

Figure 2. Classification of the NIHSS subsets for mental status, motor, and cranial and cerebellar scores.

The image analyses were performed using commercial image-viewing software (Picture Archiving and Communication System; Maroview 5.3 Infinitt Co., Seoul, Korea). It was performed by two investigators (S.K. and S.-J.L.) who were blinded of clinical information at the time of analyses. Disagreement was resolved by consensus. The location of the occlusion and the degree of occlusion were analyzed. For baseline infarct volume measurements, diffusion-weighted imaging (DWI) on MRI was used for all patients. For follow-up infarct volumes, DWI was utilized primarily, and non-contrast CT was used when follow-up MRI was not available. Follow-up imaging was performed within a week after the initial study. The infarct volume was semiquantitatively graded using a previously described scoring system: posterior circulation Alberta Stroke Program Early CT score (PC-ASPECTS) [14]. This scoring system is the posterior circulation-equivalent of Alberta Stroke Program Early CT Score used in the anterior circulation stroke, composed of 8 territories that are supplied by the vertebrobasilar vasculature. In comparison to the anterior circulation, higher points are given to the brainstem, and due to bone artifact or partial volume effect, it is commonly measured in MR DWI, where it has proven its predictive power [15]. PC-ASPECTS was scored as previously described, subtracting each assigned points when more than 20% involvement was found in the relevant territory [16]. Infarct growth was defined as a decrease in PC-ASPECTS of ≥2 points from the initial imaging study to the follow-up imaging study. Occlusion degree was classified into incomplete occlusion and complete occlusion based on CTA maximal intensity projection images or magnetic resonance angiography (MRA); it was classified as a complete occlusion when anterograde luminal flow was definitely missing and as an incomplete occlusion when the presence of anterograde luminal flow was uncertain or minimal flow was suspected. Occlusion types were classified into truncal type occlusion (TTO) suggestive of intracranial atherosclerotic occlusions and branching site occlusion (BSO) suggestive of embolic occlusions [7,17]: Non-visualization of the basilar artery bifurcation site due to thrombus indicates BSO, and sparing of the bifurcation site indicates TTO [11]. Baseline collateral status and thrombus burden were also evaluated based on CTA or MRA using the Basilar Artery on Computed Tomography Angiography (BATMAN) score [18]. An example of determining the PC-ASPECTS and BATMAN score in a patient is presented in Figures 3 and 4.

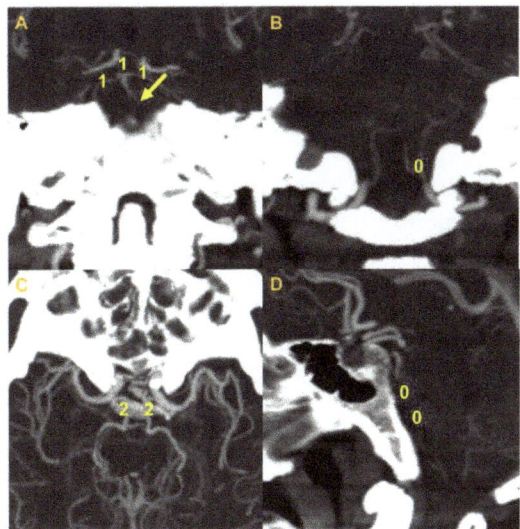

Figure 3. An example of a BATMAN score from a truncal-type occlusion from the cohort. (**A**) Coronal reconstruction of the MIP image of the basilar artery. Occlusion at the vertebrobasilar artery with visualization of the distal part and the basilar top is seen. Both PCAs are visualized. For the BATMAN score, each 1 point is given for the distal BA, and both PCAs. (**B**) Coronal MIP image of bilateral VAs. Note that both VAs are occluded. Zero point was given. (**C**) Axial MIP image showing both posterior communicating arteries. Two points for each communicating artery was given. (**D**) Sagittal MIP image showing occluded proximal and mid-BA. Zero points were given for each part of the BA, constituting a total BATMAN score of 7. BATMAN, Basilar Artery on Computed Tomography Angiography; BA, basilar artery; MIP, maximal intensity projection; PCA, posterior cerebral artery; VA, vertebral artery.

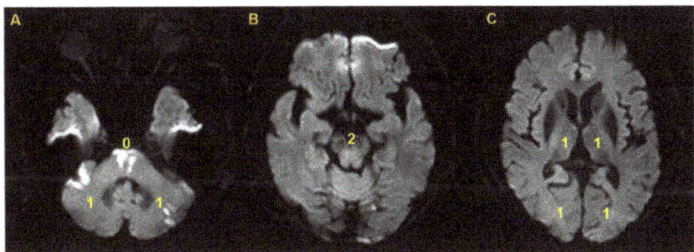

Figure 4. An example of a calculation of PC-ASPECTS from diffusion-weighted image. (**A**) Diffusion restriction is seen at the pontine level. Two points were subtracted at this level. Even though scattered infarction was noted in the bilateral cerebellum, lesions did not exceed 20% of the territories. (**B**) No acute infarction was noted at the midbrain level. (**C**) No acute infarction was noted in the bilateral thalami and PCA territories. This constitutes a total score of 8. PC-ASPECTS, Posterior Circulation-Alberta Stroke Program Early Computed Tomography Score; PCA, posterior cerebral artery.

2.3. Identification of the Clinical-Core Mismatch Criteria That Predicts Infarct Growth

For the generation of the clinical-core mismatch, the core criterion and clinical criterion was sequentially generated. For the core criterion, the futile core was calculated with PC-ASPECTS, by generating an initial PC-ASPECTS score that is highly specific to result in futile outcomes (3 months mRS 5-6) irrespective of treatment. Infarct volumes that do not meet the futile core criterion were considered feasible cores, and clinical mismatch criterion was evaluated within these patients. Significant cut-off values of NIHSS scores and subset scores were generated, which was predictive of infarct growth. For this, area under the receiver operating characteristic curve (AUC) analysis was performed along with expert opinion. Among the clinical scores, the best parameter predictive of infarct growth with other potentially significant variables included in multiple logistic regression analysis was identified as an optimal clinical-core mismatch criterion. The occlusion type was included in the logistic regression analysis to account for occlusion etiology.

2.4. Identification of Factors Predictive of Neurological Deterioration

In patients that did not perform EVT, the presence of ND was assessed. ND was defined as an increase in the NIHSS score by 4 or more points between the point of admission and discharge [19]. ND was classified according to its pathomechanism. Clinical profile and imaging findings were compared between patients who experienced ND and those who did not. Multiple logistic regression analysis was performed, including clinically important variables, to identify the independent predictors of ND.

2.5. Statistical Analysis

Variables are expressed as numbers (percentage), and median (interquartile range) value. Continuous variables were compared using Student's t-test or the Mann-Whitney U test. Categorized variables were compared using the chi-square test or Fisher's exact test. Normality of the distribution was assessed using the Kolmogorov-Smirnov test. Multiple logistic regression was performed for identification of best clinical-core mismatch criteria predictive of infarct growth and for identification of predictors of ND. Multiple logistic regression analysis included clinically important variables. For the multivariate analysis, predictive power was calculated for statistically significant variables. We calculated the power at the 0.05 significance level with a two-sided test for a multiple logistic regression model by using formulae given by Hsieh (1998) [20]. For this analysis, a power of 80% is generally considered acceptable in terms of sample size. Data are presented as the mean ± standard deviation, number (%), or median [interquartile range (IQR)] as appropriate for data type and distribution. All statistical analyses were performed using IBM SPSS Statistics version 25 (IBM Corp., Armonk, NY, USA) and R version 3.6.3. A p-value < 0.05 was considered statistically significant.

3. Results

From January 2010 to December 2018, 1710 posterior circulation stroke patients were identified. Patients that did not fulfill the criteria for CT-based VBO were excluded, leaving 176 VBO patients. All patients underwent MRI at admission. Among them, 138 patients who had follow-up imaging study using MRI (77/138, 55.8%) or CT (61/138, 44.2%), were selected and included in the analysis. Median follow-up imaging interval was 4 (IQR, 2–5) days.

3.1. Infarct Growth and Generation of Clinical-Core Mismatch Criteria

3.1.1. Generation of Core Criterion

In the 138 patients, infarct core was analyzed with PC-ASPECTS. Decreases in PC-ASPECTS could significantly predict futile outcomes with an AUC of 0.761 (0.680–0.842), and the dichotomized PC-ASPECTS score of less than 6 showed a sensitivity of 25.4% and specificity of 100% for futile outcomes irrespective of treatment. Fifteen patients presented with a PC-ASPECTS score of less than 6. The rest 123 patients were considered to present with feasible cores for reperfusion therapy, and were included in the clinical criterion analysis.

3.1.2. Generation of Clinical Criterion That Can Predict Infarct Growth

In the 123 patients (mean age: 67 ± 13; male: 85/123, 69.1%), 43 (35.0%) patients met the infarct growth definition. When patients with infarct growth and those without were compared, infarct growth group had lower rates of male sex, (53.5% vs. 77.5%, p = 0.006) and higher NIHSS scores at presentation (18 (8–22) vs. 7 (3–16), $p = 0.007$). Patients presenting with a NIHSS score 11 or more were significantly more frequent in the infarct growth group (67.4% vs. 40.0%, $p = 0.004$), as was mental status subset score of 1 or higher (83.7% vs. 51.2%, $p < 0.001$), motor subset score of 5 or higher (58.1% vs. 27.5%, $p = 0.001$), and cranial and cerebellar subset score of 4 or higher (74.4% vs. 48.8%, $p = 0.006$). Location of occlusion of the distal or proximal basilar artery (BA) was more frequently observed in the infarct growth group, in contrast to the higher number of vertebral artery (VA) occlusions in the non-infarct growth population ($p = 0.014$). In patients that experienced infarct growth, EVT was more frequently performed (60.5% vs. 36.3%, $p = 0.010$), representing patient selection in clinical practice. A good outcome was much less frequently observed in the infarct growth group (14.0% vs. 65.0%, $p < 0.001$). The two groups did not differ in terms of occlusion types (for TTO, 55.8% vs. 72.5%, $p = 0.061$), PC-ASPECTS (9 (8–10) vs. 9 (8–10), $p = 0.928$), or BATMAN scores (5 (3–7) vs. 6 (5–8), $p = 0.090$) (Table 1).

Table 1. Comparison of patients who experienced infarct growth and who did not.

Variables	Infarct Growth (N = 43)	No Infarct Growth (N = 80)	p Value
Age	72 (59–80)	66 (55–75)	0.114
Sex, male	23 (53.5%)	62 (77.5%)	0.006
HTN	21 (48.8%)	47 (58.8%)	0.292
DM	13 (30.2%)	22 (27.5%)	0.749
Atrial fibrillation	12 (27.9%)	17 (21.3%)	0.407
Presence of prodrome	8 (18.6%)	11 (13.8%)	0.477
Onset-to-door time (h)	3 (1–7)	3 (2–11.75)	0.857
NIHSS at presentation	18 (8–22)	7 (3–16)	0.007
NIHSS ≥11	29 (67.4%)	32 (40.0%)	0.004
Subset mental status scores	4 (1–6)	1 (0–4)	0.065
Mental status ≥1	36 (83.7%)	41 (51.2%)	<0.001
Subset motor scores	6 (2–8)	2 (0–5.75)	0.003
Motor ≥5	25 (58.1%)	22 (27.5%)	0.001
Subset cranial and cerebellar scores	5 (3–7)	3 (2–6)	0.048
Cranial and cerebellar ≥4	32 (74.4%)	39 (48.8%)	0.006
Occlusion degree			0.518
Complete occlusion	34 (79.1%)	67 (83.8%)	
Incomplete occlusion	9 (20.9%)	13 (16.3%)	
Occlusion location			0.014
distal BA	11 (25.6%)	10 (12.5%)	
proximal BA	23 (53.5%)	33 (41.3%)	
VA	9 (20.9%)	37 (46.3%)	
Occlusion type			0.061
Truncal-type occlusion	24 (55.8%)	58 (72.5%)	
Branching-site occlusion	19 (44.2%)	22 (27.5%)	
PC-ASPECTS	9 (8–10)	9 (8–10)	0.928
BATMAN	5 (3–7)	6 (5–8)	0.090
Reperfusion (EVT ± IV thrombo-lysis)	26 (60.5%)	29 (36.3%)	0.010
Final PC-ASPECTS	5 (3–7)	9 (8–10)	<0.001
Good outcomes (mRS 0–2)	6 (14.0%)	52 (65.0%)	<0.001

Numbers are represented by numbers (percentage), median value [interquartile range]; HTN, hypertension; DM, diabetes mellitus; NIHSS, National Institutes of Health Stroke Scale; BA, basilar artery; VA, vertebral artery; PC-ASPECTS, Posterior Circulation-Alberta Stroke Program Early Computed Tomography Score; BATMAN, Basilar Artery on Computed Tomography Angiography score; EVT ± IV thrombolysis, endovascular treatment with or without intravenous thrombolysis; mRS, modified Rankin scale.

When adjusted for age, sex, occlusion type, reperfusion therapy, BATMAN, and PC-ASPECTS, only mental status subset score of 1 or higher significantly predicted infarct growth (OR: 3.34, 95% CI (1.19–9.38), $p = 0.022$, predictive power: 93.65%), while total NIHSS, motor subset, and cranial and cerebellar subset cut-off values did not (Table 2).

Table 2. Comparison of logistic regression models for predicting infarct growth using cut-off values generated by NIHSS and its subset scores.

	Variables	OR	95% CI	p Value
Model 1	NIHSS at presentation≥11	2.16	0.83–5.65	0.116
	Age	1.01	0.98–1.05	0.570
	Sex	2.39	0.96–5.91	0.060
	TTO (vs. BSO)	0.93	0.35–2.43	0.876
	EVT ± IV thrombolysis	1.58	0.66–3.79	0.309
	PC-ASPECTS (per 1 point decrease)	0.93	0.65–1.33	0.682
	BATMAN (per 1 point decrease)	1.16	0.92–1.46	0.220
Model 2	Subset mental status ≥ 1	3.34	1.19–9.38	0.022
	Age	1.01	0.98–1.05	0.586
	Sex	2.19	0.88–5.43	0.092
	TTO (vs. BSO)	1.00	0.38–2.65	0.996
	EVT ± IV thrombolysis	1.48	0.61–3.55	0.383
	PC-ASPECTS (per 1 point decrease)	0.95	0.67–1.34	0.760
	BATMAN (per 1 point decrease)	1.17	0.92–1.47	0.200
Model 3	Subset motor ≥ 5	2.44	0.96–6.25	0.062
	Age	1.01	0.97–1.04	0.673
	Sex	2.13	0.86–5.30	0.104
	TTO (vs. BSO)	0.95	0.36–2.50	0.909
	EVT ± IV thrombolysis	1.50	0.61–3.65	0.376
	PC-ASPECTS (per 1 point decrease)	0.93	0.65–1.33	0.695
	BATMAN (per 1 point decrease)	1.19	0.94–1.49	0.150
Model 4	Subset cranial and cerebellar ≥ 4	1.73	0.64–4.69	0.285
	Age	1.01	0.98–1.05	0.542
	Sex	0.44	0.18–1.07	0.069
	TTO (vs. BSO)	0.85	0.33–2.18	0.729
	EVT ± IV thrombolysis	1.57	0.63–3.94	0.333
	PC-ASPECTS (per 1 point decrease)	0.99	0.71–1.39	0.963
	BATMAN (per 1 point decrease)	1.15	0.92–1.45	0.229

OR, odds ratio; CI, confidence interval; NIHSS, National Institutes of Health Stroke Scale; TTO, truncal-type occlusion; BSO, branching-site occlusion; EVT ± IV thrombolysis, endovascular treatment with or without intravenous thrombolysis; PC-ASPECTS, Posterior Circulation-Alberta Stroke Program Early Computed Tomography Score; BATMAN, Basilar Artery on Computed Tomography Angiography score.

3.2. Neurological Deterioration and Its Predictors

Among the 138 total population, 73 VBO patients (age: 68 ± 14; male: 54/73, 74.0%) did not receive reperfusion therapy. The patients presented with a median NIHSS score of 5 (2–15), and a median time interval of 7 (3–26) hours. The majority of the population presented with a TTO (54/73, 74.0%) suggestive of intracranial atherosclerosis. Predictors of neurological deterioration were evaluated in them. In the 73 patients, ND occurred in 13 (17.8%) patients. Causes of ND was infarct growth in 8 (61.5%), lacunar progression in 4 (30.8%), and brainstem compression in 1 (7.7%). Table 3 summarizes the differences in clinical and imaging characteristics between the ND group and those without ND. When patients with ND and no-ND were compared, there were no differences in baseline demographics, except for a higher rate of prodrome (46.2% vs. 11.7%, p = 0.003). There were no differences in NIHSS total or subset scores or onset-to-door time. Only 2/13 (15.4%) of the patients that experienced ND could achieve good outcomes, compared to 38/60 (63.3%) in the no-ND group (p = 0.002).

Table 3. Comparison of patients who experienced neurological deterioration and who did not, in those that did not undergo endovascular treatment.

Variables	ND (N = 13)	No-ND (N = 60)	p Value
Age	73 (48–77)	69.5 (56–77.75)	0.375
Sex, male	11 (84.6%)	43 (71.7%)	0.335
HTN	9 (69.2%)	35 (58.3%)	0.467
DM	7 (53.8%)	19 (31.7%)	0.130
Atrial fibrillation	1 (7.7%)	18 (30.0%)	0.097
Presence of prodrome	6 (46.2%)	7 (11.7%)	0.003
Onset-to-door time (h)	5 (2–28.5)]	7 (3–24)	0.870
NIHSS at presentation	7 (2.5–13.5)	4.5 (1.25–16.75)	0.438
Subset mental status scores	0 (0–2)	1 (0–3.75)	0.577
Subsetmotorscores	2 (0–5)	0 (0–4.75)	0.318
Subset cranial and cerebellar scores	3 (2–5)	2.5 (1–5.75)	0.934
Occlusion degree			0.020
Complete occlusion	7 (53.8%)	50 (83.3%)	
Incomplete occlusion	6 (46.2%)	10 (16.7%)	
Occlusion location			0.250
distal BA	0 (0.0%)	8 (13.3%)	
proximal BA	5 (38.5%)	27 (45.0%)	
VA	8 (61.5%)	25 (41.7%)	
Occlusion type			0.018
Truncal-type occlusion	13 (100.0%)	41 (68.3%)	
Branching-site occlusion	0 (0.0%)	19 (31.7%)	
PC-ASPECTS	8 (7–9.5)	9.5 (8–10)	0.144
BATMAN	5 (3.5–6)	6 (5–8)	0.077
Final PC-ASPECTS	8 (6–9.5)	9 (7–10)	0.935
Good outcomes (mRS 0–2)	2 (15.4%)	38 (63.3%)	0.002

Numbers are represented by numbers (percentage), median value [interquartile range]; HTN, hypertension; DM, diabetes mellitus; NIHSS, National Institutes of Health Stroke Scale; BA, basilar artery; VA, vertebral artery; PC-ASPECTS, Posterior Circulation-Alberta Stroke Program Early Computed Tomography Score; BATMAN, Basilar Artery on Computed Tomography Angiography score; mRS, modified Rankin scale.

Incomplete occlusion compared to complete occlusion was more frequently observed in the ND group (46.2% vs. 16.7%, $p = 0.020$). The initial infarct volume represented by PC-ASPECTS and collateral status represented by the BATMAN score did not differ in the univariate analysis. In the multivariate analysis for prediction of ND, an incomplete occlusion (OR: 6.17, 95% CI (1.11–34.25), $p = 0.037$, predictive power: 54.31%), decreases in collaterals as measured by BATMAN scores (per 1 point decrease, OR: 1.91, 95% CI (1.17–3.11), $p = 0.009$, predictive power: 45.43%), and larger infarct cores measured by decreases in PC-ASPECTS (OR: 1.96, 95% CI (1.11–3.48), $p = 0.021$, predictive power: 12.86%) could predict neurological deterioration with age, onset-to-door time, and NIHSS score at presentation as covariables (Table 4).

Table 4. Logistic regression model for prediction of neurological deterioration in vertebrobasilar occlusion patients that did not undergo endovascular treatment.

Variables	OR	95% CI	p Value
Incomplete occlusion (vs. complete occlusion)	6.17	1.11–34.25	0.037
BATMAN (per 1 point decrease)	1.91	1.17–3.11	0.009
PC-ASPECTS (per 1 point decrease)	1.96	1.11–3.48	0.021
Age	0.96	0.91–1.02	0.208
Onset-to-door time (h)	0.97	0.94–1.00	0.087
NIHSS at presentation (per 1 point increase)	0.88	0.77–1.01	0.072

OR, odds ratio; CI, confidence interval; BATMAN, Basilar Artery on Computed Tomography Angiography score; PC-ASPECTS, Posterior Circulation-Alberta Stroke Program Early Computed Tomography Score; NIHSS, National Institutes of Health Stroke Scale.

4. Discussion

In this retrospective study, we found that in VBO patients, an initial PC-ASPECTS of 6 or more, but with a decrease in the mental status subset of 1 or more can predict infarct growth, and may be used as a criterion for clinical-core mismatch. In patients who did not receive reperfusion therapy, an incomplete occlusion rather than complete occlusion based on CT angiography, a poorer collateral circulation status, and larger initial infarct cores were predictive of ND.

The current study has some clinical implications. It is to our knowledge, the first study to generate a clinical-core mismatch criterion in VBO. It is highly likely that EVT for VBO will significantly improve patient outcomes even in the late time window [21], and this criteria may be able to guide patient selection. This criteria may also guide patient selection in the early time window, especially when the NIHSS score is lower. In contrast to the anterior circulation, trials even with contemporary EVT for VBO have shown negative results [22,23]; however, in the recent BASICS trial, subgroup analysis showed that there was a significant difference in outcome favoring EVT in patients with moderate to severe stroke, or NIHSS score ≥ 10 [23], which emphasizes the value of patient selection for clinical trial success. An NIHSS score ≥ 11 was used as a potential cut-off point in our study but did not reach statistical significance. In contrast, a decrease in mental status could significantly predict infarct growth. Often, the NIHSS cut off for performing thrombolysis and EVT is arbitrary, even in the anterior circulation. The presence of cortical signs may guide decision in the anterior circulation, for it can be considered a marker of hemispheric hypoperfusion [5]. Our results suggest that decreases in mental status may be considered as such a marker in the posterior circulation, and can be a more intuitive approach for reperfusion decisions.

The causes of ND, and its predictors also suggest potential clinical implications. In patients that did not undergo immediate reperfusion therapies, the majority of patients were TTO. Therefore, intracranial atherosclerotic pathology would have been responsible for ND in a large number of cases. When we take a look at the causes of ND, the major cause of ND was growth in infarct size. This may occur from arterial embolism, in situ thrombosis, or hemodynamic insufficiency [24]. The second most common cause, lacunar progression, would also be due to branch occlusion within the atherosclerotic plaque. ND could be predicted by incomplete occlusions and poor collaterals. Such patients may benefit from delayed EVT if the patient progresses, or can be potential candidates for preventive intra-arterial tirofiban injection [25], for it can stabilize the irritable plaque surface safely [11].

This study failed to show an association between collateral scores and future infarct growth. Collaterals [26] in the anterior circulation is a major parameter that determines the extent and speed of infarct growth. The BATMAN score measures the collateral status along with the thrombus burden [18]. However, the abundance of atherosclerotic VBO in this study may have diluted the significance of collaterals since atherosclerotic occlusions result in higher collaterals [27] while presenting with a wide range of clinical severity. BATMAN scores, however, predicted ND in a more homogenous set of VBO patients, who were largely atherosclerotic and presented with milder symptoms. Furthermore, the Western literatures, which are most likely comprised of a more homogenous population of embolic VBO, continuously reported the prognostic value of collaterals [18] and the use of collaterals as a marker for response to EVT in extended time windows [21]. Such findings show that the interpretation of collaterals should be performed in a homogenous set of occlusion etiologies.

Interestingly, an incomplete occlusion was not predictive of a less likelihood of infarct growth, but was associated with later neurological deterioration. An incomplete occlusion was classified as possible or uncertain minimal antegrade flow based on CT angiography maximal intensity projection images because similar-looking incomplete atherosclerotic VBO lesions may present with a wide range of clinical symptoms. Indeed, differences in complete or incomplete occlusion did not predict infarct growth. It was, however, predictive of ND, suggesting that patients with critically reduced antegrade flow may be hemodynamically and neurologically unstable compared to patients with chronic complete occlusions, in which collaterals have already been developed.

The present study has some limitations. First, the initial patient selection was based solely on imaging criteria without consideration of clinical severity or time metrics. Thus, the VBO group included in this study differs from literatures that include more homogenous population of VBO that received EVT. This selection criteria for VBO was used to generate a clinical criteria predictive of infarct growth. However, this may result in heterogeneity in disease etiology and treatment course, and over-representation of atherosclerotic VBO. Accordingly, the results of this study needs to be interpreted with care. Second, while only MR DWI was used for the initial PC-APSECTS scores, both MRI and CT was used for the follow-up PC-ASPECTS grading. As CT evaluation of the brainstem can be limited by bone artifact or partial volume effect [28], this must be mentioned as a limitation of this study. However, we believe that this factor would not have significantly influenced the results of the study for two reasons. At the time of follow-up imaging, ischemic lesions change to frank hypodensity, which is more easily visualized in the brainstem then early ischemic changes. Further, PC-ASPECTS is evaluated only in the pons and midbrain of the brainstem and does not include the medulla, where the brainstem ischemia is most difficult to visualize by CT. Third, for the analysis of clinical-core mismatch, futile infarct cores should ideally be evaluated in patients with timely successful reperfusion. However, due to the limited number of VBO patients, a futile infarct core was generated using the total population, and a PC-ASPECTS cutoff which was highly specific for futile outcomes were used instead. This is apparently a limitation of the study. Last, due to the small number of patients included, the statistical power of the multivariable analysis in identification of neurological deterioration is lower than generally accepted. In this regard, the values generated in this study need to be validated in further studies.

5. Conclusions

Infarct growth in VBO can be predicted by clinical-core mismatch, especially any decreases in mental status in patients with feasible PC-ASPECTS scores. Neurological deterioration is encountered in VBO patients who present with minor symptoms and can be predicted by incomplete occlusion rather than complete occlusion along with poorer collateral status and larger initial infarct core. These results need to be externally validated in larger cohorts. The value of the clinical-core mismatch criteria in maximizing VBO EVT efficacy needs to be validated in a prospective trial.

Author Contributions: Conceptualization, S.K. and S.-J.L.; methodology, S.K., and S.-J.L.; formal analysis, S.K., J.H.P., B.P., and S.-J.L.; investigation, S.K., M.H.C., S.E.L., J.S.L., J.M.H., and S.-J.L.; resources, J.S.L., J.M.H., and S.-J.L.; data curation, S.K. and S.-J.L.; writing—original draft preparation, S.K. and S.-J.L.; writing—review and editing, S.K., M.H.C., S.E.L., J.S.L., J.M.H., and S.-J.L.; supervision, S.-J.L. All authors have read and agreed to the published version of the manuscript.

Funding: This research received no external funding.

Conflicts of Interest: The authors declare no conflict of interest.

References

1. Goyal, M.; Menon, B.K.; van Zwam, W.H.; Dippel, D.W.; Mitchell, P.J.; Demchuk, A.M.; Dávalos, A.; Majoie, C.B.; van der Lugt, A.; de Miquel, M.A.; et al. Endovascular thrombectomy after large-vessel ischaemic stroke: A meta-analysis of individual patient data from five randomised trials. *Lancet* **2016**, *387*, 1723–1731. [CrossRef]
2. Kayan, Y.; Meyers, P.M.; Prestigiacomo, C.J.; Kan, P.; Fraser, J.F.; Society of NeuroInterventional Surgery. Current endovascular strategies for posterior circulation large vessel occlusion stroke: Report of the Society of NeuroInterventional Surgery Standards and Guidelines Committee. *J. Neurointerv. Surg.* **2019**, *11*, 1055–1062. [CrossRef]
3. Mattle, H.P.; Arnold, M.; Lindsberg, P.J.; Schonewille, W.J.; Schroth, G. Basilar artery occlusion. *Lancet Neurol.* **2011**, *10*, 1002–1014. [CrossRef]

4. Nogueira, R.G.; Jadhav, A.P.; Haussen, D.C.; Bonafe, A.; Budzik, R.F.; Bhuva, P.; Yavagal, D.R.; Ribo, M.; Cognard, C.; Hanel, R.A.; et al. Thrombectomy 6 to 24 hours after stroke with a mismatch between deficit and infarct. *N. Engl. J. Med.* **2018**, *378*, 11–21. [CrossRef]
5. Nogueira, R.G.; Kemmling, A.; Souza, L.M.; Payabvash, S.; Hirsch, J.A.; Yoo, A.J.; Lev, M.H. Clinical diffusion mismatch better discriminates infarct growth than mean transit time-diffusion weighted imaging mismatch in patients with middle cerebral artery-M1 occlusion and limited infarct core. *J. Neurointerv. Surg.* **2017**, *9*, 127–130. [CrossRef]
6. Albers, G.W.; Marks, M.P.; Kemp, S.; Christensen, S.; Tsai, J.P.; Ortega-Gutierrez, S.; McTaggart, R.A.; Torbey, M.T.; Kim-Tenser, M.; Leslie-Mazwi, T.; et al. Thrombectomy for stroke at 6 to 16 hours with selection by perfusion imaging. *N. Engl. J. Med.* **2018**, *378*, 708–718. [CrossRef] [PubMed]
7. Baek, J.H.; Kim, B.M.; Kim, D.J.; Heo, J.H.; Nam, H.S.; Song, D.; Bang, O.Y. Importance of truncal-type occlusion in stentriever-based thrombectomy for acute stroke. *Neurology* **2016**, *87*, 1542–1550. [CrossRef] [PubMed]
8. Ferbert, A.; Bruckmann, H.; Drummen, R. Clinical features of proven basilar artery occlusion. *Stroke* **1990**, *21*, 1135–1142. [CrossRef] [PubMed]
9. Lee, J.S.; Hong, J.M.; Lee, K.S.; Suh, H.I.; Demchuk, A.M.; Hwang, Y.H.; Kim, B.M.; Kim, J.S. Endovascular Therapy of Cerebral Arterial Occlusions: Intracranial Atherosclerosis versus Embolism. *J. Stroke Cerebrovasc. Dis.* **2015**, *24*, 2074–2080. [CrossRef] [PubMed]
10. Baek, J.H.; Kim, B.M. Angiographical Identification of Intracranial, Atherosclerosis-Related, Large Vessel Occlusion in Endovascular Treatment. *Front. Neurol.* **2019**, *10*, 298. [CrossRef] [PubMed]
11. Lee, J.S.; Hong, J.M.; Kim, J.S. Diagnostic and Therapeutic Strategies for Acute Intracranial Atherosclerosis-related Occlusions. *J. Stroke* **2017**, *19*, 143–151. [CrossRef] [PubMed]
12. Baek, J.H.; Kim, B.M.; Heo, J.H.; Kim, D.J.; Nam, H.S.; Kim, Y.D. Outcomes of Endovascular Treatment for Acute Intracranial Atherosclerosis-Related Large Vessel Occlusion. *Stroke* **2018**, *49*, 2699–2705. [CrossRef] [PubMed]
13. Lee, S.J.; Hong, J.M.; Choi, J.W.; Park, J.H.; Park, B.; Kang, D.H.; Kim, Y.W.; Kim, Y.S.; Hong, J.H.; Yoo, J.; et al. Predicting Endovascular Treatment Outcomes in Acute Vertebrobasilar Artery Occlusion: A Model to Aid Patient Selection from the ASIAN KR Registry. *Radiology* **2020**, *294*, 628–637. [CrossRef] [PubMed]
14. Puetz, V.; Khomenko, A.; Hill, M.D.; Dzialowski, I.; Michel, P.; Weimar, C.; Wijman, C.A.; Mattle, H.P.; Engelter, S.T.; Muir, K.W.; et al. Extent of hypoattenuation on CT angiography source images in basilar artery occlusion: Prognostic value in the Basilar Artery International Cooperation Study. *Stroke* **2011**, *42*, 3454–3459. [CrossRef] [PubMed]
15. Nagel, S.; Herweh, C.; Kohrmann, M.; Huttner, H.B.; Poli, S.; Hartmann, M.; Hahnel, S.; Steiner, T.; Ringleb, P.; Hacke, W. MRI in patients with acute basilar artery occlusion—DWI lesion scoring is an independent predictor of outcome. *Int. J. Stroke* **2012**, *7*, 282–288. [CrossRef] [PubMed]
16. Khatibi, K.; Nour, M.; Tateshima, S.; Jahan, R.; Duckwiler, G.; Saver, J.; Szeder, V. Posterior Circulation Thrombectomy-pc-ASPECT Score Applied to Preintervention Magnetic Resonance Imaging Can Accurately Predict Functional Outcome. *World Neurosurg.* **2019**, *129*, e566–e571. [CrossRef] [PubMed]
17. Baek, J.H.; Kim, B.M.; Yoo, J.; Nam, H.S.; Kim, Y.D.; Kim, D.J.; Heo, J.H.; Bang, O.Y. Predictive Value of Computed Tomography Angiography-Determined Occlusion Type in Stent Retriever Thrombectomy. *Stroke* **2017**, *48*, 2746–2752. [CrossRef]
18. Alemseged, F.; Shah, D.G.; Diomedi, M.; Sallustio, F.; Bivard, A.; Sharma, G.; Mitchell, P.J.; Dowling, R.J.; Bush, S.; Yan, B.; et al. The Basilar Artery on Computed Tomography Angiography Prognostic Score for Basilar Artery Occlusion. *Stroke* **2017**, *48*, 631–637. [CrossRef]
19. Lin, L.C.; Lee, T.H.; Chang, C.H.; Chang, Y.J.; Liou, C.W.; Chang, K.C.; Lee, J.D.; Peng, T.Y.; Chung, J.; Chen, S.C.; et al. Predictors of clinical deterioration during hospitalization following acute ischemic stroke. *Eur. Neurol.* **2012**, *67*, 186–192. [CrossRef]
20. Hsieh, F.Y.; Bloch, D.A.; Larsen, M.D. A simple method of sample size calculation for linear and logistic regression. *Stat. Med.* **1998**, *17*, 1623–1634. [CrossRef]
21. Alemseged, F.; Van der Hoeven, E.; Di Giuliano, F.; Shah, D.; Sallustio, F.; Arba, F.; Kleinig, T.J.; Bush, S.; Dowling, R.J.; Yan, B.; et al. Response to Late-Window Endovascular Revascularization Is Associated With Collateral Status in Basilar Artery Occlusion. *Stroke* **2019**, *50*, 1415–1422. [CrossRef] [PubMed]

22. Liu, X.; Dai, Q.; Ye, R.; Zi, W.; Liu, Y.; Wang, H.; Zhu, W.; Ma, M.; Yin, Q.; Li, M.; et al. Endovascular treatment versus standard medical treatment for vertebrobasilar artery occlusion (BEST): An open-label, randomised controlled trial. *Lancet Neurol.* **2020**, *19*, 115–122. [CrossRef]
23. Schonewille, W.J. A Randomized Acute Stroke Trial of Endovascular Therapy in Acute Basilar Artery Occlusion. Presented at the ESO-WSO 2020 Major Clinical Trials Webinar, ESOC European Stroke Organisation, 13 May 2020; Available online: https://eso-wso-conference.org/eso-wso-may-webinar/ (accessed on 12 October 2020).
24. Bang, O.Y. Intracranial atherosclerosis: Current understanding and perspectives. *J. Stroke* **2014**, *16*, 27–35. [CrossRef] [PubMed]
25. Kim, Y.W.; Sohn, S.I.; Yoo, J.; Hong, J.H.; Kim, C.H.; Kang, D.H.; Kim, Y.S.; Lee, S.J.; Hong, J.M.; Choi, J.W.; et al. Local tirofiban infusion for remnant stenosis in large vessel occlusion: Tirofiban ASSIST study. *BMC Neurol.* **2020**, *20*, 284. [CrossRef]
26. Hwang, Y.H.; Kang, D.H.; Kim, Y.W.; Kim, Y.S.; Park, S.P.; Liebeskind, D.S. Impact of time-to-reperfusion on outcome in patients with poor collaterals. *AJNR Am. J. Neuroradiol.* **2015**, *36*, 495–500. [CrossRef]
27. Chang, F.C.; Luo, C.B.; Chung, C.P.; Kuo, K.H.; Chen, T.Y.; Lee, H.J.; Lin, C.J.; Lirng, J.F.; Guo, W.Y. Influence of Vertebrobasilar Stenotic Lesion Rigidity on the Outcome of Angioplasty and Stenting. *Sci. Rep.* **2020**, *10*, 3923. [CrossRef]
28. Monnin, P.; Sfameni, N.; Gianoli, A.; Ding, S. Optimal slice thickness for object detection with longitudinal partial volume effects in computed tomography. *J. Appl. Clin. Med. Phys.* **2017**, *18*, 251–259.

Publisher's Note: MDPI stays neutral with regard to jurisdictional claims in published maps and institutional affiliations.

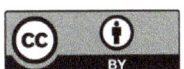

© 2020 by the authors. Licensee MDPI, Basel, Switzerland. This article is an open access article distributed under the terms and conditions of the Creative Commons Attribution (CC BY) license (http://creativecommons.org/licenses/by/4.0/).

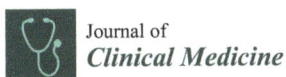

Article

Temporal Trends and Risk Factors for Delayed Hospital Admission in Suspected Stroke Patients

Moritz Kielkopf [1], Thomas Meinel [1], Johannes Kaesmacher [2], Urs Fischer [1], Marcel Arnold [1], Mirjam Heldner [1], David Seiffge [1], Pasquale Mordasini [3], Tomas Dobrocky [3], Eike Piechowiak [3], Jan Gralla [3] and Simon Jung [1],*

1. Department of Neurology, Inselspital, Bern University Hospital, University of Bern, 3010 Bern, Switzerland; moritz.kielkopf@insel.ch (M.K.); thomas.meinel@insel.ch (T.M.); urs.fischer@insel.ch (U.F.); marcel.arnold@insel.ch (M.A.); mirjam.heldner@insel.ch (M.H.); david.seiffge@insel.ch (D.S.)
2. Institute of Diagnostic and Interventional Neuroradiology, Institute of Diagnostic, Interventional and Pediatric, Radiology and Department of Neurology, University Hospital Bern, Inselspital, University of Bern, 3010 Bern, Switzerland; johannes.kaesmacher@insel.ch
3. University Institute of Diagnostic and Interventional Neuroradiology, Inselspital, Bern University Hospital, University of Bern, 3010 Bern, Switzerland; Pasquale.Mordasini@insel.ch (P.M.); Tomas.dobrocky@insel.ch (T.D.); eike.piechowiak@insel.ch (E.P.); Jan.gralla@insel.ch (J.G.)
* Correspondence: simon.jung@insel.ch; Tel.: +41-32-632-21-11

Received: 20 June 2020; Accepted: 22 July 2020; Published: 25 July 2020

Abstract: (1) Background: The benefit of acute ischemic stroke (AIS) treatment declines with any time delay until treatment. Hence, factors influencing the time from symptom onset to admission (TTA) are of utmost importance. This study aimed to assess temporal trends and risk factors for delays in TTA. (2) Methods: We included 1244 consecutive patients from 2015 to 2018 with suspected stroke presenting within 24 h after symptom onset registered in our prospective, pre-specified hospital database. Temporal trends were assessed by comparing with a cohort of a previous study in 2006. Factors associated with TTA were assessed by univariable and multivariable regression analysis. (3) Results: In 1244 patients (median [IQR] age 73 [60–82] years; 44% women), the median TTA was 96 min (IQR 66–164). The prehospital time delay reduced by 27% in the last 12 years and the rate of patients referred by Emergency medical services (EMS) increased from 17% to 51% and the TTA for admissions by General Practitioner (GP) declined from 244 to 207 min. Factors associated with a delay in TTA were stroke severity (beta−1.9; 95% CI−3.6 to −0.2 min per point NIHSS score), referral by General Practitioner (GP, beta +140 min, 95% CI 100–179), self-admission (+92 min, 95% CI 57–128) as compared to admission by emergency medical services (EMS) and symptom onset during nighttime (+57 min, 95% CI 30–85). Conclusions: Although TTA improved markedly since 2006, our data indicates that continuous efforts are mandatory to raise public awareness on the importance of fast hospital referral in patients with suspected stroke by directly informing EMS, avoiding contact of a GP, and maintaining high effort for fast transportation also in patients with milder symptoms.

Keywords: time to admission; prehospital delay; stroke; prior stroke

1. Introduction

The benefit of acute ischemic stroke (AIS) management is strongly time dependent. Using advanced imaging techniques, the time window for recanalization therapies has extended over the last decades. Thrombolysis has shown to improve outcome in selected patients up to 9 h after symptom onset [1], while endovascular thrombectomy lowered disability in selected patients with a large vessel occlusion up to 16–24 h after onset [2,3]. However, for endovascular treatment and thrombolysis [4–6] as well as conservative medical management [7] the time from symptom onset to initiation of therapy remains a decisive factor for functional outcome [6]. While efforts to reduce the door-to-treatment time have led to significant improvements [8], the development of prehospital delays in AIS remains controversial. Various global reviews reported divergent results with regard to the prehospital time improvement and the factors leading to delay [9–11]. For example, the impact of a previous cerebrovascular event (pCVE), i.e., previous stroke or transient ischemic attack (TIA) in the patient medical history on the time to hospital admission (TTA) remains uncertain. Additionally, there is a lack of data on the impact of optimized prehospital workflows.

Therefore, the aim of the study was to assess factors associated with TTA delays of suspected stroke patients referred to the Stroke Center Bern. In addition, we aimed to analyze temporal trends of TTA delay in comparison with a previous study cohort in 2006 [12].

2. Experimental Section

2.1. Material and Methods

Consecutive patients with a final diagnosis of AIS, TIA, amaurosis fugax, cerebral venous thrombosis or stroke mimics were analyzed. These events may typically present with symptoms compatible with AIS and demand the same diagnostic procedure as well as the ignition of the so called, stroke chain of survival [8]. Patients treated at emergency department from 01 February 2015 to 26 December 2018 were included. Demographic data and baseline variables were collected prospectively in our Bernese Stroke Database. The primary outcome variable (TTA) was defined as the time from onset of neurological symptoms to the time of hospital arrival. In the database, hospital arrival is declared as the time when patients were registered at the triage of the Emergency Department. We included patients presenting between 5 min and 24 h after symptom onset. Exclusion criteria were in-hospital strokes, wake-up strokes, as well as inter-hospital referrals. All inclusion and exclusion criteria and inclusion chart are presented in Figure 1.

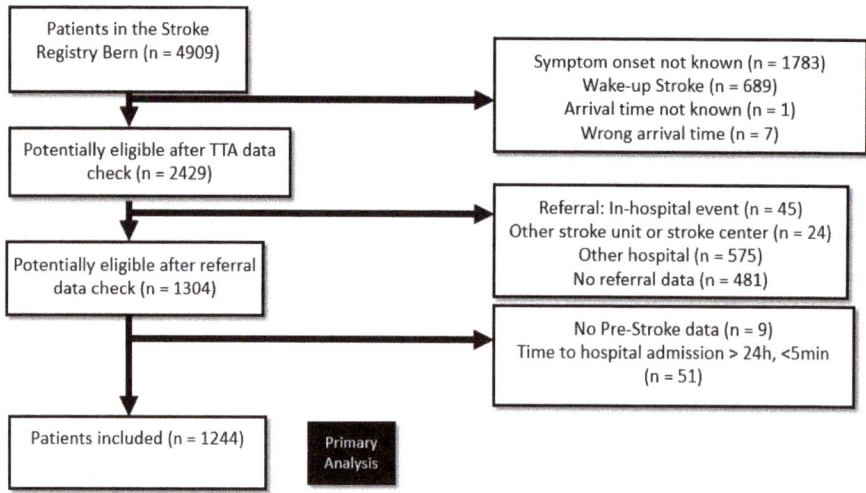

Figure 1. Inclusion Criteria in the main analysis.

To asses temporal trends in TTA delay we compared our data with a previous study in 2006. To ensure comparability we applied the same inclusion criteria to our dataset as in 2006 in a sub analysis. Therefore we included inter-hospital referrals (n = 652) and wake up strokes in the sub analysis. In patients with wake up stroke and patients who were found unconscious or aphasic, the wake up time or time of finding the patients was considered as the start of TTA. Furthermore, in subgroup analysis, the time span was restricted to a maximum of 48 h after symptom onset and only ischemic strokes and TIAs were included.

2.2. Statistical Analysis

To assess which factors were associated with prehospital delays, we compared patients with a fast (<96 min) and a long (>96 min) TTA using the median TTA as the cut-off point. To determine significant differences, we used appropriate statistical measures (χ^2 test for categorical variables, Fisher's exact test for categorical variables, Mann-Whitney-U-Test for non-normally continuous or ordinally scaled variables, and Welch's t-test for independent normally distributed data). To document the variance of continuous variables, we present results as median and interquartile range (IQR). We included variables with a *p*-value of <0.2 (statistical criterion), analyzed (multi)collinearity between variables and hence selected pathophysiologically plausible variables for the final multivariate model.

For the primary analysis the association of factors with TTA was assessed using linear regression adjusting for the following confounders: sex (categorical), age (continuous), diabetes mellitus (categorical), referral by GP as compared to EMS (categorical), self-referral GP as compared to EMS (categorical), presentation during daytime (categorical), stroke severity (NIHSS on admission [13], ordinal), systolic blood pressure on admission (mmHG, ordinal) and pCVE (categorical). We calculated (adjusted) beta regression coefficients (β) and corresponding 95% confidence intervals. All statistical analyses were performed using SPSS (IBM Corp. Released 2017. IBM SPSS Statistics for Windows, Version 25.0. Armonk, NY, USA: IBM Corp.). All *p* values are 2-sided, with $p < 0.05$ considered statistically significant. No adjustments for multiple testing were applied and patients with missing data items were excluded from the multivariate analysis.

3. Results

Of 4909 patients in the registry, 1244 patients complied with the inclusion criteria and were included in this analysis (see Figure 1 for reasons of exclusion). Median age was 73 years (60–82), 44% were female, median NIHSS score 4 (1–11). In total, 62.6% of patients presented within 0–2 h after symptom onset, 21.3% of patients within 2–4 h, 7.1% within 4–6 h, 2.4% within 6–8 h and only 6.5% of patients beyond 8 h after symptom onset (Figure 2). 81% of patients had an AIS as final diagnosis, whereas 19% suffered from other vascular emergencies (TIA, amaurosis fugax, cerebral venous thrombosis or stroke mimics). The median TTA was 96 min (IQR 66–164).

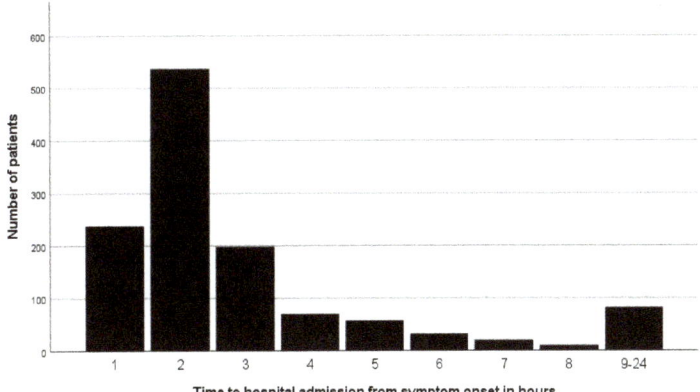

Figure 2. Prehospital delay time of patients with acute cerebrovascular event in hours.

Of 4909 patients in the registry, 2088 patients complied with the inclusion criteria from 2006 as mentioned above. The median TTA was 132 min (IQR 79–244) in comparison to 180 min in 2006 and

86% patients arrived within 6 h (75% in 2006). In 2018 51% of this patient group were referred by EMS compared to 17% in 2006. The exact comparison to the study conducted in 2006 is shown in Table 1.

Table 1. Comparison of adj. TTA and adj. referral pathways in acute stroke 2018 with 2006.

	2018	2006
EMS referral	51% (1063/2088)	17% (105/615)
GP referral *	7% (151/2088)	38% (233/615)
Self-referral	11% (222/2088)	12% (46/615)
Inter-hospital referral	31% (651/2088)	38% (231/615)
Median TTA	132 min	180 min
EMS referral Ambulance (Median TTA)	88 min	80 min
Helicopter (Median TTA)	99 min	93 min
GP ** (Median TTA)	207 min	224 min
SR (Median TTA)	140 min	174 min
Inter-hospital (Median TTA)	209 Min	195 min

The data from 2006 are the results of a previous study analyzing the time to admission in AIS, conducted within the same stroke network. * The data of 2006 include 64/233 patients referred by so-called Emergency doctors (ED), a system of familiar physicians who take regular terms in an emergency service outside the hospital. ** In 2006 only patients with direct GP-referral (n = 169) are considered for exact delay comparison (ED referrals excluded). SR, self-referral; GP, general practitioner; EMS, emergency medical services; TTA, time to hospital admission.

Factors Associated with TTA Delay

In univariable analysis the following factors were significantly associated with shorter TTA: referral by EMS, ischemic stroke event type, more severe stroke according to the NIHSS score, and higher systolic blood pressure on admission. Additionally the number of patients with a medical history of diabetes or with at least three vascular risk factors was significantly lower in the fast arrival group. Baseline characteristics of patients according to time from symptom onset to hospital admission are shown in the Appendix A, Table A1.

Variables associated with TTA in multivariable analysis were stroke severity (beta −1.9; 95% CI −3.6 to −0.2 min per point NIHSS score), referral by General Practitioner (GP) as compared to admission by EMS (beta + 140 min, 95% CI 100–179), self-admission as compared to admission by EMS (+92 min, 95% CI 57–128) and symptom onset during nighttime (+57 min, 95% CI−85 to−30, Table 2). There was no significant association of age, sex, blood pressure, and diabetes in the multivariable linear regression model. (Table 2).

In total, 319 patients (26%) were not referred by EMS of whom 134 were referred by GP (11%) and 185 by self-referral (15%). Patients not primarily admitted by EMS had less severe stroke (median NIHSS score 1, IQR 0–3 vs. 5, 2–11, $p < 0.001$), and were younger (67 years, 50–78 vs. 74, 62–83, $p < 0.001$). 302/1244 (24.3%) of the included patients have already suffered a pCVE. As compared to patients without pCVE, these patients were older, had a different referral pattern, more often a pre-existing disability, a worse vascular risk profile, and more often preceding antithrombotic therapy.

Table 2. Factors associated with time to admission (linear regression analysis).

Variable	Beta	95% CI	p-Value
Sex	16.5	−7.0–40.0	0.169
Age	−0.2	−1.0–0.6	0.589
Diabetes Mellitus	12.5	−19.4–44.5	0.442
General Practitioner	139.7	100.3–179.2	0.000 †
Self-Referral	92.1	56.6–127.5	0.000 †
Daytime	−57.5	−85.0–(−29.9)	0.000 †
PCVE	1.4	−26.0–28.7	0.921
NIHSS score to admission	−1.9	−3.6–(−0.2)	0.028 †
Blood pressure systolic (mmHg)	0.17	−0.3–0.6	0.434

† Statistically significant. Beta, Regression coefficient in its influence in mins. on TTA; Daytime, Daytime from 7 a.m.–7 p.m. ; PCVE, Previous cerebrovascular event ; NIHSS score, National Institute of Health Stroke Scale.

There was no difference in TTA between patients with a pCVE (94 min, IQR 64–160) as compared to patients without a pCVE (100 min, IQR 70–183, $p = 0.078$) in univariate analysis. After adjustments for confounders, pCVE was not associated with TTA (beta +1 min, 95% CI −26–+29 min).

4. Discussion

The main findings of our registry-based study of 1244 patients with acute vascular events presenting between 2015 and 2018 are:

(1) The median TTA was 96 min (IQR 66–164). (2) The prehospital time delay reduced by 27% in the last 14 years. (3) Self-referral or referral by a GP, lower NIHSS score and nighttime symptom onset were associated with a delay in TTA in both univariable and multivariable analysis. (4) Referral by EMS was the only modifiable variable associated with shorter TTA in both univariable and multivariable analysis. (5) A pCVE had no influence on TTA neither in univariable nor multivariable analysis.

Our results demonstrate that prehospital delay in patients with symptoms compatible with an acute vascular emergency are still considerable. The median TTA was around 1.5 h in our study, which is among the shortest reported prehospital times in different stroke networks, but is still too long [9,14]: Whereas 63% of patients arrived within 2 h, one of five patients (22%) arrived later than 3 h after symptom onset.

Previous studies on temporal trends of TTA revealed conflicting results. Whereas some studies indicated an improvement in TTA over the years [10,15], a meta-analysis on global cross-sectional studies could not find an improvement in TTA [9]. In this context the adj. TTA analyzation was carried out to carefully investigate time trends based on the same geographic, infrastructural and social characteristics. In the adjusted subgroup analysis, the median TTA was 132 min, corresponding to an absolute reduction of 48 min (27%) compared to 14 years ago. The median TTA for patients referred by GP dropped from 224 min in 2006 to 207 min in 2018 and for self-referral patients from 174 min in 2006 to 140 min in 2018 [12]. The fastened referral times are probably at least the the result of the efforts made in stroke information campaigns in the Bernese region. The key messages of the information campaigns were to avoid GP contact when stroke symptoms occur and to refer severe affected patients direct to a Stroke-Unit center. Indeed, the referral rate by EMS increased from 17% in 2006 to 51% in 2018 whereas GP referrals decreased from 38% to 7% and inter-hospital referrals from 38% to 31%.

The EMS referral times itself did not change over time. This might indicate that this referral pathway might already be close to its optimal speed. Our data indicates that continuous efforts are mandatory to raise public awareness on the importance of fast hospital referral in patients with suspected stroke by directly informing EMS, avoiding presentation at a GP, and maintaining high effort for fast transportation also in patients with milder symptoms.

The analysis of factors that contribute to TTA delays revealed referral by GP, self-referral, nighttime event and low NIHSS score. Referral by GP was associated with an approximated time delay of 2 h, self-referral with a time delay of 1.5 h and wake up stroke with 1 h delay. Our findings are in line with multiple studies investigating the impact of EMS over the last 10 years [16–18]. Age, sex and vascular risk factors had no significant influence in our multivariate analysis.

In concordance with the results from 2006, patients with pCVE showed a non-significant trend to longer TTA. At first glance, this seems surprising as these patients presumably have been informed about cerebrovascular diseases and the time is brain concept. Nevertheless, this is in line with previous studies suggesting that better stroke knowledge does not necessarily increase EMS use [14,16,19,20].

Limitations and Strengths

The strengths of our study are the size of the cohort, and the longitudinal comparison within the same network/population after several years. A limitation is a potential bias due to the exclusion of patients with unknown symptom onset, who potentially tend to show a TTA above average (n = 1783). In addition, the overall GP referrals in 2006 included 64/233 patients from so called Emergency doctors (ED), a system of familiar physicians who take regular terms in an emergency service outside the hospital, which restricts in some way the comparability of the two cohorts.

5. Conclusions

Referral by EMS, high NIHSS scores and symptom onset during daytime are independently associated with shorter TTA. The median TTA was 96 min, resulting in considerable improvement compared to our previous study roughly 10 years ago, mainly due to an increase of the referrals by EMS (17% to 51%). Continuous efforts are mandatory instructing stroke patients with vascular risk factors and their relatives, as well as GPs, to immediately request EMS assistance in case of suspected stroke.

Author Contributions: Conceptualization, U.F., M.A., J.G. and S.J.; Data curation, M.K.; Formal analysis, M.K.; Methodology, T.M.; Project administration, S.J.; Supervision, S.J.; Validation, T.M. and S.J.; Writing—original draft, M.K. and T.M.; Writing—review & editing, J.K., M.H., D.S., P.M., T.D., E.P. and S.J. All authors have read and agreed to the published version of the manuscript.

Funding: This research received no external funding.

Conflicts of Interest: The authors declare no conflict of interest.

Appendix A

Table A1. Baseline characteristics of patients according to time from symptom onset to hospital admission.

	n	Hospital Arrival within 96 min	Hospital Arrival after 96 min	*p*-Value
Age (IQR/median)	1244	62.27–82/73.45	57.58–82.1/73.15	0.113
Men (number, %)	1244	352/622 (56.6%)	351/622 (56.4%)	0.954
Referral (number, %) Self Referral Emergency service (144) General Practitioner	1244	73/622 (11.7%) 521/622 (83.8%) 28/622 (4.5%)	112/622 (18%) 404/622 (65%) 106/622 (17%)	0.000 †
Type of event (number, %) Ischemic Stroke Transient ischemic attack Others	1244	524/622 (84.2%) 89/622 (14.3%) 9/622 (1.4%)	483/622 (70.4%) 104/622 (16.7%) 35/622 (5.6%)	0.002 †

Table A1. Cont.

	n	Hospital Arrival within 96 min	Hospital Arrival after 96 min	p-Value
Daytime (number, %)	1244	488/622 (78.5%)	463/622 (74.4%)	0.109
PS-Disability mRS (number, %)	946			0.975
0		324/490 (66.1%)	300/456 (65.6%)	
1		96/490 (19.6%)	87/456 (19%)	
2		28/490 (5.7%)	30/456 (6.6%)	
3		31/490 (6.3%)	31/456 (6.8%)	
4		11/490 (2.2%)	9/456 (2%)	
Medical History (number, %)		141/622 (22.7%)	161/621 (25.9%)	0.181
PCVE		82/621 (13.2%)	115/621 (18.5%)	0.010 †
Diabetes		396/619 (64%)	408/616 (66.2%)	0.405
Hyperlipidemia		435/621 (70%)	429/620 (69.2%)	0.743
Hypertension		191/620 (30.8%)	191/620 (30.8%)	1.0
Atrial fibrillationAny		547/618 (88.5%)	547/610 (89.7%)	0.514
of this conditions >3 RF		202/618 (32.7%)	236/610 (38.7%)	0.028 †
Living situation–at home (number, %)	1240	589/620 (95%)	581/620 (93.7%)	0.325
NIHSS (IQR/median)	1186	2–13/5, n = 609	1–8/3, n = 577	0.000 †
Blood pressure systolic (mmHg) (IQR/median)	1231	140–177/160, n = 615	135–175/155, n = 616	0.032

Others, retinal infarct, amaurosis fugax, sinus vein thrombosis and stroke mimics; mRS, modified Rankin Scale; PS, Pre stroke; PCVE, Previous cerebrovascular event; RF, risk factor; NIHSS score, National Institute of Health Stroke Scale; Daytime, Daytime from 7 a.m.–7 p.m.

References

1. Campbell, B.C.V.; De Silva, D.A.; MacLeod, M.R.; Coutts, S.B.; Schwamm, L.H.; Davis, S.M.; Donnan, G.A. Ischaemic stroke. *Nat. Rev. Dis. Prim.* **2019**, *5*, 70. [CrossRef] [PubMed]
2. Nogueira, R.G.; Jadhav, A.P.; Haussen, D.C.; Bonafé, A.; Budzik, R.F.; Bhuva, P.; Yavagal, D.R.; Ribo, M.; Cognard, C.; Hanel, R.A.; et al. Thrombectomy 6 to 24 hours after stroke with a mismatch between deficit and infarct. *N. Engl. J. Med.* **2018**, *378*, 11–21. [CrossRef] [PubMed]
3. Albers, G.W.; Marks, M.P.; Kemp, S.; Christensen, S.; Tsai, J.P.; Ortega-Gutierrez, S.; McTaggart, R.A.; Torbey, M.T.; Kim-Tenser, M.; Leslie-Mazwi, T.; et al. Thrombectomy for stroke at 6 to 16 hours with selection by perfusion imaging. *N. Engl. J. Med.* **2018**, *378*, 708–718. [CrossRef] [PubMed]
4. Meinel, T.R.; Kaesmacher, J.; Mordasini, P.; Mosimann, P.J.; Jung, S.; Arnold, M.; Heldner, M.R.; Michel, P.; Hajdu, S.D.; Ribo, M.; et al. Outcome, efficacy and safety of endovascular thrombectomy in ischaemic stroke according to time to reperfusion: Data from a multicentre registry. *Ther. Adv. Neurol. Disord.* **2019**, *12*, 1756286419835708. [CrossRef] [PubMed]
5. Saver, J.L.; E Smith, E.; Fonarow, G.C.; Reeves, M.J.; Zhao, X.; Olson, D.M.; Schwamm, L.H. GWTG-stroke steering committee and investigators The "Golden Hour" and acute brain ischemia. *Stroke* **2010**, *41*, 1431–1439. [CrossRef] [PubMed]
6. Saver, J.L.; Goyal, M.; Van Der Lugt, A.; Menon, B.K.; Majoie, C.B.L.M.; Dippel, D.W.J.; Campbell, B.C.; Nogueira, R.G.; Demchuk, A.M.; Tomasello, A.; et al. Time to treatment with endovascular thrombectomy and outcomes from ischemic stroke: A meta-analysis. *JAMA* **2016**, *316*, 1279–1288. [CrossRef] [PubMed]
7. Rothwell, P.M.; Algra, A.; Chen, Z.; Diener, H.-C.; Norrving, B.; Mehta, Z. Effects of aspirin on risk and severity of early recurrent stroke after transient ischaemic attack and ischaemic stroke: Time-course analysis of randomised trials. *Lancet* **2016**, *388*, 365–375. [CrossRef]
8. Meretoja, A.; Strbian, D.; Mustanoja, S.; Tatlisumak, T.; Lindsberg, P.J.; Kaste, M. Reducing in-hospital delay to 20 minutes in stroke thrombolysis. *Neurology* **2012**, *79*, 306–313. [CrossRef] [PubMed]
9. Pulvers, J.N.; Watson, J.D.G. If time is brain where is the improvement in prehospital time after stroke? *Front. Neurol.* **2017**, *8*, 617. [CrossRef] [PubMed]

10. Evenson, K.R.; Foraker, R.E.; Morris, D.L.; Rosamond, W.D. A comprehensive review of prehospital and in-hospital delay times in acute stroke care. *Int. J. Stroke* **2009**, *4*, 187–199. [CrossRef] [PubMed]
11. Furlan, A.J. Endovascular therapy for stroke—It is about Time. *N. Engl. J. Med.* **2015**, *372*, 2347–2349. [CrossRef] [PubMed]
12. Agyeman, O.; Nedeltchev, K.; Arnold, M.; Fischer, U.; Remonda, L.; Isenegger, J.; Schroth, G.; Mattle, H.P. Time to admission in acute ischemic stroke and transient ischemic attack. *Stroke* **2006**, *37*, 963–966. [CrossRef] [PubMed]
13. Brott, T.; Adams, H.P.; Olinger, C.P.; Marler, J.R.; Barsan, W.G.; Biller, J.; Spilker, J.; Holleran, R.; Eberle, R.; Hertzberg, V. Measurements of acute cerebral infarction: A clinical examination scale. *Stroke* **1989**, *20*, 864–870. [CrossRef] [PubMed]
14. Teuschl, Y.; Brainin, M. Stroke education: Discrepancies among factors influencing prehospital delay and stroke knowledge. *Int. J. Stroke* **2010**, *5*, 187–208. [CrossRef] [PubMed]
15. Papapanagiotou, P.; Iacovidou, N.; Spengos, K.; Xanthos, T.; Zaganas, I.; Aggelina, A.; Alegakis, A.; Vemmos, K. Temporal Trends and associated factors for pre-hospital and in-hospital delays of stroke patients over a 16-year period: The Athens study. *Cerebrovasc. Dis.* **2011**, *31*, 199–206. [CrossRef] [PubMed]
16. Fladt, J.; Meier, N.; Thilemann, S.; Polymeris, A.; Traenka, C.; Seiffge, D.J.; Sutter, R.; Peters, N.; Gensicke, H.; Flückiger, B.; et al. Reasons for Prehospital Delay in Acute Ischemic Stroke. *J. Am. Heart Assoc.* **2019**, *8*, e013101. [CrossRef] [PubMed]
17. Salisbury, H.R.; Banks, B.J.; Footitt, D.R.; Winner, S.J.; Reynolds, D.J. Delay in presentation of patients with acute stroke to hospital in Oxford. *QJM Mon. J. Assoc. Physician* **1998**, *91*, 635–640. [CrossRef] [PubMed]
18. Morris, D.L.; Rosamond, W.; Madden, K.; Schultz, C.; Hamilton, S. Prehospital and emergency department delays after acute stroke. *Stroke* **2000**, *31*, 2585–2590. [CrossRef] [PubMed]
19. Derex, L.; Adeleine, P.; Nighoghossian, N.; Honnorat, J.; Trouillas, P. Factors influencing early admission in a French stroke unit. *Stroke* **2002**, *33*, 153–159. [CrossRef] [PubMed]
20. Lecouturier, J.; Murtagh, M.J.; Thomson, R.; Ford, G.; White, M.; Eccles, M.P.; Rodgers, H. Response to symptoms of stroke in the UK: A systematic review. *BMC Health Serv. Res.* **2010**, *10*, 157. [CrossRef] [PubMed]

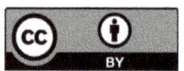

© 2020 by the authors. Licensee MDPI, Basel, Switzerland. This article is an open access article distributed under the terms and conditions of the Creative Commons Attribution (CC BY) license (http://creativecommons.org/licenses/by/4.0/).

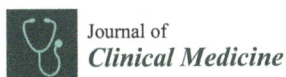

Article

Dynamic Hyperglycemic Patterns Predict Adverse Outcomes in Patients with Acute Ischemic Stroke Undergoing Mechanical Thrombectomy

Giovanni Merlino [1,2,*,†], Carmelo Smeralda [2,3,†], Massimo Sponza [4], Gian Luigi Gigli [2,5], Simone Lorenzut [1], Alessandro Marini [2,3], Andrea Surcinelli [2,3], Sara Pez [2,3], Alessandro Vit [4], Vladimir Gavrilovic [4] and Mariarosaria Valente [2,3]

1. Stroke Unit, Department of Neuroscience, Udine University Hospital, 33100 Udine, Italy; simone.lorenzut@asufc.sanita.fvg.it
2. Clinical Neurology, Udine University Hospital, 33100 Udine, Italy; carmelosmeralda@gmail.com (C.S.); gigli@uniud.it (G.L.G.); alemarini00@gmail.com (A.M.); andsurcinelli@gmail.com (A.S.); sarapez91@gmail.com (S.P.); mariarosaria.valente@uniud.it (M.V.)
3. DAME, University of Udine, 33100 Udine, Italy
4. Division of Vascular and Interventional Radiology, Udine University Hospital, 33100 Udine, Italy; massimo.sponza@asufc.sanita.fvg.it (M.S.); alessandro.vit@asufc.sanita.fvg.it (A.V.); vladimir.gavrilovic@asufc.sanita.fvg.it (V.G.)
5. DMIF, University of Udine, 33100 Udine, Italy
* Correspondence: giovanni.merlino@asufc.sanita.fvg.it; Tel.: +39-043-255-2720
† These authors contributed equally to this study.

Received: 5 May 2020; Accepted: 18 June 2020; Published: 20 June 2020

Abstract: Background: Admission hyperglycemia impairs outcome in acute ischemic stroke (AIS) patients undergoing mechanical thrombectomy (MT). Since hyperglycemia in AIS represents a dynamic condition, we tested whether the dynamic patterns of hyperglycemia, defined as blood glucose levels > 140 mg/dl, affect outcomes in these patients. Methods: We retrospectively analyzed data of 200 consecutive patients with prospective follow-up. Based on blood glucose level, patients were distinguished into 4 groups: (1) persistent normoglycemia; (2) hyperglycemia at baseline only; (3) hyperglycemia at 24-h only; and (4) persistent (at baseline plus at 24-h following MT) hyperglycemia. Results: AIS patients with persistent hyperglycemia have a significantly increased risk of poor functional outcome (OR 6.89, 95% CI 1.98–23.94, $p = 0.002$, for three-month poor outcome; OR 11.15, 95% CI 2.99–41.52, $p = 0.001$, for no major neurological improvement), mortality (OR 5.37, 95% CI 1.61–17.96, $p = 0.006$, for in-hospital mortality; OR 4.43, 95% CI 1.40–13.97, $p = 0.01$, for three-month mortality), and hemorrhagic transformation (OR 6.89, 95% CI 2.35–20.21, $p = 0.001$, for intracranial hemorrhage; OR 5.42, 95% CI 1.54–19.15, $p = 0.009$, for symptomatic intracranial hemorrhage) after endovascular treatment. These detrimental effects were partially confirmed after also excluding diabetic patients. The AUC-ROC showed a very good performance for predicting three-month poor outcome (0.76) in-hospital mortality (0.79) and three-month mortality (0.79). Conclusions: Our study suggests that it is useful to perform the prolonged monitoring of glucose levels lasting 24-h after MT.

Keywords: hyperglycemia; acute ischemic stroke; large vessel occlusion; mechanical thrombectomy

1. Background

Mechanical thrombectomy (MT) is the first-line treatment for acute ischemic stroke (AIS) due to large vessel occlusion (LVO) [1]. Several randomized, controlled trials reported that MT improves the outcome, in comparison with the best medical therapy [2–6]. In these studies, the prevalence of good outcome at three months was as high as 71% [2–6]. However, data coming from observational registries reported a significantly lower rate of patients with functional independence; this ranged between 34% and 39% [7–9]. In addition to blood pressure control and time to reperfusion, the glycemic status represents one of the most important modifiable predictors of adverse outcomes in patients undergoing MT [10–12].

Hyperglycemia impairs outcome in patients with AIS [13–15]. Among the several mechanisms implicated in this unfavorable association, it is important to remember that increased glucose levels in stroke patients alter the blood barrier permeability [16], exacerbate the thromboinflammatory cascade [17], induce acidosis [18], and increase oxidative stress response [19]. In AIS patients treated with alteplase, admission hyperglycemia has been associated with the increased risk of death, symptomatic intracranial hemorrhage (SICH), and poor functional status [20].

In recent years, the interest of the international scientific community shifted towards the role of altered glycemic status in affecting the outcome of AIS patients undergoing MT for LVO. Several studies observed that admission hyperglycemia reduced the likelihood of a good outcome in AIS patients treated with MT [21–24]. However, hyperglycemia may also occur during the post-operative period, both in diabetic and non-diabetic patients. A stress-response, characterized by excessive gluconeogenesis, glycogenolysis and insulin resistance with consequent hyperglycemia, is common after large strokes [25]. Recently, Li et al. investigated the role of post-operative hyperglycemia as a potential predictor of SICH in AIS patients treated with MT. The authors observed that, differently from glucose levels at admission, post-operative hyperglycemia increased the risk of the occurrence of SICH and parenchymal hematoma (PH) [26].

Since hyperglycemia in AIS represents a dynamic condition, we hypothesize that one isolated glucose test measure, performed at admission or within 24-h after MT, might be insufficient to understand the effects of the metabolic process on the ischemic brain. To date, only a few studies investigated the contribution of the dynamic patterns of hyperglycemia to stroke outcome [27–29]. These trials included only AIS patients treated and not treated with alteplase, whereas similar investigations in patients undergoing MT are lacking. We decided to perform this study with the aim of evaluating the impact of the dynamic patterns of hyperglycemia on stroke outcome, in AIS patients with LVO who were treated with MT.

2. Methods

2.1. Patients

This study is a retrospective analysis of consecutive patients with prospective follow-up admitted to the Udine University Hospital with AIS due to LVO, that were treated with MT from January 2015 to December 2019. Eligibility criteria for MT were the following: (1) presence of LVO in the anterior or posterior circulation, as revealed by CT angiography; (2) symptoms onset within 6 h for LVO in the anterior circulation and within 8 h for LVO in the posterior one; and (3) Alberta Stroke Program Early CT Score (ASPECTS) > 6 on direct CT scan. In our center, the following exclusion criteria for MT are in use: (1) life expectancy less than 12 months; (2) severe internal medicine diseases with signs of organ failure; and (3) platelet count less than 55,000 mmc. All patients treated with MT in our center were included in this study. No specific exclusion criteria were adopted. Patients showing symptoms onset within 4.5 h received alteplase in accordance with the international guidelines [1].

The study was approved by our local Ethics Committee (Ref. No. CEUR-2020-Os-173). Informed consent was obtained from the participants in this study, or their representatives.

2.2. Data Collection

The following variables were collected: age, sex, vascular risk factors, laboratory findings, including glycated hemoglobin (HbA1c), admission systolic blood pressure, and pharmacological treatment.

2.3. Vascular Risk Factors

Based on previous studies [30–32], we adopted the following definitions of vascular risk factors: (1) previous transient ischemic attack/stroke was defined if the patient had a history of ischemic (transient attack or stroke) or hemorrhagic cerebrovascular disease; (2) the presence of cardiovascular disease was based on the history of previous ischemic heart disease and/or revascularization treatment using percutaneous coronary intervention/coronary artery bypass grafting; (3) atrial fibrillation was defined if the patient had past medical history of atrial fibrillation that had been confirmed in medical records; (4) high blood pressure was defined as the history of hypertension and/or use of antihypertensive medication; (5) a history of diabetes mellitus that had been confirmed in medical records and/or use of insulin/oral hypoglycemic agents were considered for defining diabetes; (6) a presence of hypercholesterolemia was based on the use of lipid-lowering medications; (7) information on active tobacco use was used for defining patient as a current smoker.

2.4. Measurement of Blood Glucose

Blood glucose was measured at admission (baseline glucose level), before initiating any specific stroke treatment, and within 24 h after MT (post-operative glucose level). Based on previous studies on this topic, hyperglycemia was defined as a glucose level > 140 mg/dL [21–23]. Based on blood glucose level, patients were distinguished into 4 groups: (1) persistent normoglycemia, i.e., normoglycemia at baseline plus at 24-h; (2) hyperglycemia at baseline only; (3) hyperglycemia at 24-h only; and (4) persistent hyperglycemia, i.e., hyperglycemia at baseline plus at 24-h.

2.5. Clinical Assessment

2.5.1. Trial of ORG 10,172 in Acute Stroke Treatment classification

The trial of ORG 10,172 in acute stroke treatment (TOAST) classification was used to determine AIS subtypes based on their etiology. In particular, cerebrovascular events were distinguished as due to large artery atherosclerosis, cardioembolism, small-vessel occlusion, other determined etiology, and undetermined etiology [33].

2.5.2. National Institute of Health Stroke Scale Score

Stroke severity was determined with the National Institute of Health Stroke Scale (NIHSS) score, at admission and at discharge [34]. In accordance with many previous studies, we defined patients with major neurological improvement as those who had an improvement of ≥8 points on the NIHSS from baseline or a NIHSS score of 0 at discharge [35–37].

2.5.3. Modified Rankin Scale

Functional outcome was assessed by means of the modified Rankin scale (mRS) at admission based on pre-stroke disability and 3 months after stroke [38]. The mRS score after discharge was recorded at the patients' routine clinical visit or through telephone interviews with the patients or their immediate caregivers. The mRS score was dichotomized into: favorable outcome (0–2) and poor outcome (3–6).

2.5.4. Hemorrhagic Transformation

The presence of intracranial hemorrhage (ICH) was defined as any PH based on the European Cooperative Acute Stroke Study (ECASS) morphologic definitions (ECASS PH-1 or PH-2) [39], whereas the presence of SICH was based on the ECASS-III protocol [40].

2.6. Thrombectomy Procedure

We collected the following information: site of the cerebral artery occlusion, distinguished in middle cerebral artery (MCA), tandem (ICA + MCA), and vertebrobasilar; type of device used for MT procedure, classified as thromboaspiration, stent retriever, thromboaspiration plus stent retriever, and permanent stenting; presence or absence of secondary embolization; time from symptom onset to MT; procedure duration; recanalization rate, assessed at the end of MT, using the thrombolysis in cerebral infarction (TICI) classification and defined as successful recanalization when a TICI 2b-3 was achieved.

2.7. Outcome Measures

The following endpoints were analyzed: 3-month poor outcome, no major neurological improvement at discharge, in-hospital mortality, 3-month mortality, presence of ICH, and presence of SICH. All the outcome measures were collected as part of our routine clinical practice in patients affected by cerebrovascular events.

2.8. Statistical Analysis

Data are displayed in tables as median and interquartile range (IQR).

Differences between the 4 groups were assessed by means of the Chi square test or the Fisher's exact test, when appropriate, for categorial variables. One-way analysis of variance for normally distributed continuous variables, and the Kruskal–Wallis test for non-normally distributed continuous variables and for ordinal variables were used. Post-hoc analysis was performed by means of the Bonferroni test. The Kolmogorov–Smirnov test with Lilliefors significant correction was used to assess the normal distribution of data.

Multiple logistic regression analysis was performed to test the impact of hyperglycemia risk groups, with reference to the normoglycemia group. The potential confounding variables included in the model were: age, HbA1c values, use of antidiabetic drugs, intravenous thrombolysis before MT, baseline NIHSS score, pre-stroke mRS, time from symptom onset to MT, and successful recanalization. Systolic blood pressure > 180 mmHg was added to other confounders in the analysis, that evaluated the association between hyperglycemic patterns and hemorrhagic transformation (i.e., ICH, SICH) [1]. Multivariate analysis was performed for all the sample population and, later, only for patients without diabetes (subjects with a history of diabetes and/or with HbA1c values ≥ 6.5% were excluded from this analysis).

The utility of the hyperglycemic patterns in estimating unfavorable outcomes was tested with area under the receiver operating characteristic curve (AUC-ROC).

All probability values are two-tailed. A p value < 0.05 was considered statistically significant. Statistical analysis was carried out using the SPSS Statistics, Version 22.0 (Chicago, IL, USA).

3. Results

3.1. Baseline Characteristics

Among the 200 patients recruited during the study period, 116 (58%) had persistent normoglycemia, whereas 36 (18%) had elevated glucose only at baseline, 17 (8.5%) only at 24-h, and 31 (15.5%) persistent hyperglycemia. Oral antidiabetic agents were taken by 21 patients (10.5%), whereas only two patients were treated with insulin.

The general characteristics of the enrolled subjects are presented in Table 1. We did not observe any difference regarding age and sex between the 4 groups. The prevalence of diabetes mellitus and hypercholesterolemia was significantly higher in patients with persistent hyperglycemia than in the other three groups ($p = 0.001$). In addition, more than 80% of patients with persistent hyperglycemia was affected by hypertension. Compared to patients with persistent normoglycemia and baseline hyperglycemia, HbA1c values were significantly higher among subjects with persistent hyperglycemia

($p = 0.001$). Furthermore, these patients took slightly more antiplatelets. The use of alteplase before MT was similar among the groups. While admission NIHSS score was not different among the 4 groups, stroke severity at discharge was largely increased in patients with baseline and persistent hyperglycemia ($p = 0.04$).

Table 1. General characteristics of the subjects according to the hyperglycemic patterns.

	Persistent Normoglycemia ($n = 116$)	Baseline Hyperglycemia ($n = 36$)	24-h Hyperglycemia ($n = 17$)	Persistent Hyperglycemia ($n = 31$)	p
Demographic data					
Age, years	73 (67–80)	75 (68.2–82)	75 (66.5–78.5)	72 (69–79)	0.7
Males, n (%)	61 (52.6)	14 (38.9)	7 (41.2)	19 (61.3)	0.2
Vascular risk factors					
Previous transient ischemic attack/stroke, n (%)	11 (9.5)	2 (5.6)	3 (17.6)	3 (9.7)	0.6
Cardiovascular disease, n (%)	22 (19.0)	7 (19.4)	3 (17.6)	5 (16.1)	0.9
Atrial fibrillation, n (%)	31 (26.7)	13 (36.1)	3 (17.6)	6 (19.4)	0.4
Hypertension, n (%)	83 (72.2)	26 (72.2)	13 (76.5)	26 (83.9)	0.6
Diabetes mellitus, n (%)	7 (6.0)	6 (16.7)	3 (17.6)	13 (41.9)	0.001
Hypercholesterolemia, n (%)	25 (21.6)	9 (25.0)	1 (5.9)	13 (41.9)	0.03
Current smoking, n (%)	21 (18.1)	7 (19.4)	5 (29.4)	9 (29.0)	0.5
Laboratory findings					
HbA1c values, %	5.7 (5.4–6.0)	6.0 (5.7–6.4)	6.0 (5.9–6.4)	6.4 (5.8–7.1)	0.001
Total cholesterol, mg/dL	164 (145–195.5)	171 (145–194)	166 (122.2–206.7)	154 (135.2–170)	0.5
HDL cholesterol, mg/dL	51 (41–62)	50 (41–63.2)	47.5 (30.75–62.2)	46 (39–59)	0.7
LDL cholesterol, mg/dL	95 (77–121.2)	95.5 (80–121.2)	94.5 (67.2–124.5)	87 (68–101)	0.8
Triglycerides, mg/dL	92 (70–130.5)	85 (63–123)	73.5 (56.7–139)	95 (67.5–143.5)	0.4
Blood pressure					
Systolic blood pressure, mmHg	151 (130–170)	155 (143–163)	154 (145–168)	155 (138–180)	0.7
Antithrombotic treatment at admission					
Antiplatelets, n (%)	28 (24.1)	13 (36.1)	5 (29.4)	14 (45.2)	0.1
Anticoagulants, n (%)	16 (13.8)	6 (16.7)	2 (11.8)	3 (9.7)	0.9
Stroke subtypes based on TOAST classification					0.6
Large arterial atherosclerosis, n (%)	19 (16.4)	6 (16.7)	2 (11.8)	6 (19.4)	
Cardioembolism, n (%)	60 (51.7)	16 (44.4)	10 (58.8)	14 (45.2)	
Other determined etiology, n (%)	6 (5.2)	0 (0.0)	0 (0.0)	0 (0.0)	
Undetermined etiology, n (%)	31 (26.7)	14 (38.9)	5 (29.4)	11 (35.5)	
Baseline clinical characteristics					
Alteplase use before MT, n (%)	66 (56.9)	22 (61.1)	8 (47.1)	20 (64.5)	0.7
NIHSS score at admission	16.5 (13–20)	19 (15.2–22)	17 (14.5–19.5)	18 (15–22)	0.2
NIHSS score at discharge	3 (1–8.7)	9 (2–16.7)	7.5 (1.7–17.7)	12 (2.5–16.5)	0.04
Pre-stroke mRS 0–2, n (%)	103 (88.8)	34 (94.4)	17 (100)	28 (90.3)	0.4

HbA1c: glycated hemoglobin; MT: mechanical thrombectomy; NIHSS: National Institute of Health Stroke Scale; mRS: modified Rankin Scale.

Table 2 summarizes information on MT in the four groups. No significant difference was observed among the groups. As expected, MCA was the most common site of LVO in the four groups. The combined technique using thromboaspiration plus stent retriever was adopted in a large part of our sample (43.5%), whereas thrombectomy only with stent retriever was performed in only 6% of the patients. The median time between symptoms onset and MT was almost 220 min, while the procedure length was 70 min. The prevalence of successful recanalization was as high as 85%.

Table 2. Information on mechanical thrombectomy, according to the hyperglycemic patterns.

	Persistent Normoglycemia	Baseline Hyperglycemia	24-h Hyperglycemia	Persistent Hyperglycemia	p
	(n = 116)	(n = 36)	(n = 17)	(n = 31)	
Site of LVO					0.5
MCA, n (%)	80 (69.0)	22 (61.1)	13 (76.5)	24 (77.4)	
Tandem, n (%)	26 (22.4)	7 (19.4)	3 (17.6)	5 (16.1)	
Vertebrobasilar, n (%)	10 (8.6)	7 (19.4)	1 (5.9)	2 (6.5)	
Type of device use for MT					0.6
Thromboaspiration, n (%)	42 (36.2)	11 (30.6)	6 (35.3)	9 (29)	
Stent retriever, n (%)	5 (4.3)	2 (5.6)	2 (11.8)	3 (9.7)	
Thromboaspiration *plus* stent retriever, n (%)	49 (42.2)	17 (47.2)	9 (52.9)	12 (38.7)	
Permanent stenting, n (%)	20 (17.2)	6 (16.7)	0 (0.0)	7 (22.6)	
Other information on MT					
Secondary embolization, n (%)	6 (5.2)	4 (11.1)	3 (17.6)	3 (9.7)	0.3
Time from symptoms onset to MT, min	210 (170–260)	236 (205–270)	225 (195–310)	210 (155–255)	0.08
Procedure length, min	67.5 (50–98.7)	70 (50–85)	70 (42.5–95)	65 (40–120)	0.9
Successful recanalization rate, n (%)	102 (87.9)	29 (80.6)	13 (76.5)	26 (83.9)	0.5

MT: Mechanical thrombectomy; LVO: large vessel occlusion; MCA: middle cerebral artery.

3.2. Association of Hyperglycemic Patterns with Clinical Outcomes in Univariate Analysis

The rates of three-month poor outcome, three-month mortality, and SICH according to the hyperglycemic patterns are reported in Figures 1–3. The rates of three-month poor outcome, three-month mortality, and SICH prevalence of no major neurological improvement (24% for persistent normoglycemia, 55.9% for baseline hyperglycemia, 57.1% for 24-h hyperglycemia, and 66.7% for persistent hyperglycemia, $p = 0.001$), in-hospital mortality (10.3% for persistent normoglycemia, 5.6% for baseline hyperglycemia, 17.6% for 24-h hyperglycemia, and 32.3% for persistent hyperglycemia, $p = 0.006$), and ICH (19% for persistent normoglycemia, 22.2% for baseline hyperglycemia, 11.8% for 24-h hyperglycemia, and 54.8% for persistent hyperglycemia, $p = 0.001$) were statistically different among the four groups.

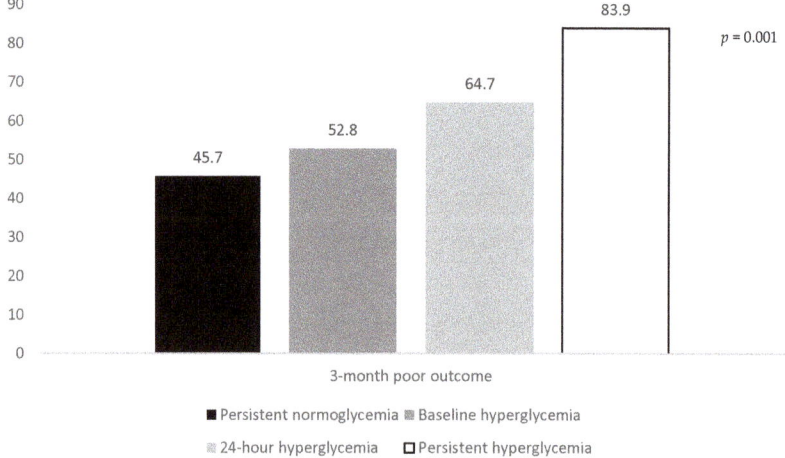

Figure 1. Rates of three-month poor outcome according to the hyperglycemic patterns.

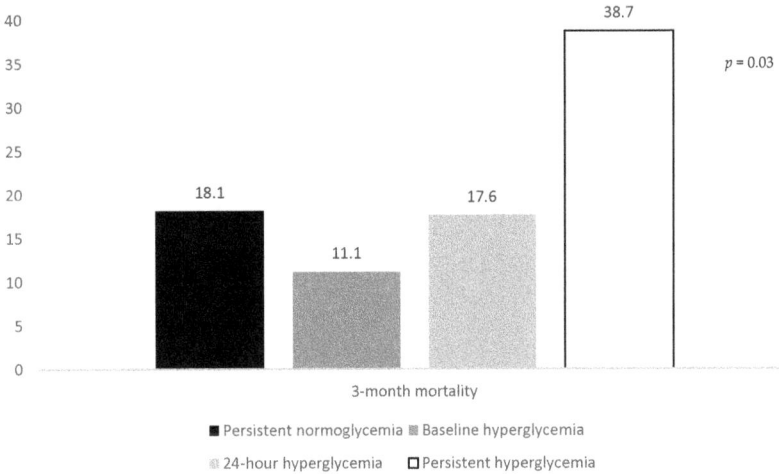

Figure 2. Rates of three-month mortality according to the hyperglycemic patterns.

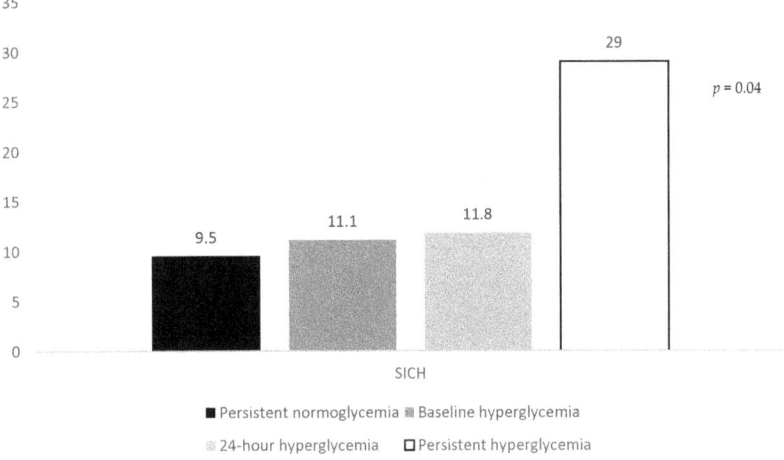

Figure 3. Rates of SICH according to the hyperglycemic patterns. SICH: symptomatic intracranial hemorrhage.

3.3. Association of Hyperglycemic Patterns with Clinical Outcomes in Multivariate Analysis

As reported in Table 3, all the outcomes were significantly associated with the presence of persistent hyperglycemia, even after controlling for confounders. Independent predictors, other than persistent hyperglycemia, were the following: (1) NIHSS score at admission (OR 1.11, 95% CI 1.04–1.18, $p = 0.002$) for three-month poor outcome; (2) baseline hyperglycemia (OR 3.37, 95% CI 1.39–8.19, $p = 0.007$), time from symptoms onset to MT (OR 1.01, 95% CI 1.00–1.01, $p = 0.02$), and successful recanalization (OR 0.22, 95% CI 0.07–0.66, $p = 0.007$) for no major neurological improvement; (3) age (OR 1.06, 95% CI 1.01–1.13, $p = 0.05$), NIHSS score at admission (OR 1.13, 95% CI 1.01–1.27, $p = 0.04$), and successful recanalization (OR 0.31, 95% CI 0.09–0.98, $p = 0.04$) for in-hospital mortality; (4) age (OR 1.08, 95% CI 1.02–1.13, $p = 0.008$), and pre-stroke mRS (OR 1.52, 95% CI 1.08–2.14, $p = 0.02$) for three-month mortality; systolic blood pressure > 180 mmHg for both (5) ICH (OR 3.33, 95% CI 1.43.31–7.79, $p = 0.005$), and (6) SICH (OR 9.69, 95% CI 3.55–26.47, $p = 0.001$).

Table 3. Logistic regression model: adjusted ORs (95% CIs) of hyperglycemic patterns, in relation to the respective outcomes.

	Persistent Normoglycemia	Baseline Hyperglycemia	24-h Hyperglycemia	Persistent Hyperglycemia
Three-month poor outcome [†]	1	0.99 (0.41–2.38)	1.75 (0.54–5.67)	6.89 (1.98–23.94) $p = 0.002$
No major neurological improvement at discharge [†]	1	3.37 (1.39–8.19) $p = 0.007$	3.41 (0.96–12.16)	11.15 (2.99–41.52) $p = 0.001$
In-hospital mortality [†]	1	0.39 (0.07–2.12)	2.67 (0.58–12.30)	5.37 (1.61–17.96) $p = 0.006$
Three-month mortality [†]	1	0.50 (0.14–1.82)	1.33 (0.31–5.66)	4.43 (1.40–13.97) $p = 0.01$
Presence of ICH [‡]	1	1.15 (0.43–3.08)	0.45 (0.08–2.44)	6.89 (2.35–20.21) $p = 0.001$
Presence of SICH [‡]	1	1.25 (0.33–4.71)	1.31 (0.21–8.31)	5.42 (1.54–19.15) $p = 0.009$

ICH: intracranial hemorrhage; SICH: symptomatic intracranial hemorrhage. [†] Adjusted for age, HbA1c values, use of antidiabetic drugs, intravenous thrombolysis, baseline NIHSS score, pre-stroke mRS, time from symptom onset to endovascular treatment, and successful recanalization. [‡] Adjusted for age, HbA1c values, use of antidiabetic drugs, intravenous thrombolysis, baseline NIHSS score, pre-stroke mRS, time from symptom onset to endovascular treatment, successful recanalization, and systolic blood pressure > 180 mmHg.

As summarized in Table 4, persistent hyperglycemia was independently associated with the outcome measures, with the exception of in-hospital mortality and three-month mortality, in non-diabetic patients. The independent predictors, other than persistent hyperglycemia, were the following: (1) age (OR 1.04, 95% CI 1.00–1.08, $p = 0.03$), and NIHSS score at admission (OR 1.12, 95% CI 1.04–1.20, $p = 0.002$) for three-month poor outcome; (2) baseline hyperglycemia (OR 4.43, 95% CI 1.57–12.53, $p = 0.005$), 24-h hyperglycemia (OR 4.29, 95% CI 1.01–12.53, $p = 0.05$), time from symptoms onset to MT (OR 1.01, 95% CI 1.00–1.01, $p = 0.04$), and successful recanalization (OR 0.23, 95% CI 0.06–0.84, $p = 0.03$) for no major neurological improvement; (3) NIHSS score at admission (OR 1.19, 95% CI 1.03–1.37, $p = 0.01$), and successful recanalization (OR 0.19, 95% CI 0.04–0.67, $p = 0.01$) for in-hospital mortality; (4) age (OR 1.08, 95% CI 1.02–1.15, $p = 0.009$), and pre-stroke mRS (OR 1.49, 95% CI 1.01–2.20, $p = 0.04$) for three-month mortality; and systolic blood pressure > 180 mmHg for both (5) ICH (OR 3.76, 95% CI 1.42–9.97, $p = 0.008$), and (6) SICH (OR 6.91, 95% CI 2.28–20.95, $p = 0.001$).

Table 4. Logistic regression model in non-diabetic patients: adjusted ORs (95% CIs) of hyperglycemic patterns in relation to the respective outcomes.

	Persistent Normoglycemia	Baseline Hyperglycemia	24-h Hyperglycemia	Persistent Hyperglycemia
three-month poor outcome [†]	1	1.20 (0.43–3.31)	3.01 (0.75–12.70)	4.91 (1.15–20.94) $p = 0.03$
No major neurological improvement at discharge [†]	1	4.43 (1.57–12.53) $p = 0.005$	4.29 (1.01–12.53) $p = 0.05$	8.62 (2.01–36.99) $p = 0.004$
In-hospital mortality [†]	1	0.25 (0.02–2.47)	3.27 (0.57–18.64)	2.80 (0.65–12.08)
three-month mortality [†]	1	0.49 (0.11–2.11)	1.24 (0.26–5.97)	1.81 (0.44–7.45)
Presence of ICH [‡]	1	0.93 (0.28–3.03)	0.16 (0.01–1.84)	7.15 (1.98–25.76) $p = 0.003$

Table 4. *Cont.*

	Persistent Normoglycemia	Baseline Hyperglycemia	24-h Hyperglycemia	Persistent Hyperglycemia
Presence of SICH [‡]	1	1.26 (0.29–5.52)	1.27 (0.18–9.07)	8.26 (1.95–35.01) $p = 0.004$

ICH: intracranial hemorrhage; SICH: symptomatic intracranial hemorrhage. [†] Adjusted for age, use of antidiabetic drugs, intravenous thrombolysis, baseline NIHSS score, pre-stroke mRS, time from symptom onset to treatment, and successful recanalization. [‡] Adjusted for age, use of antidiabetic drugs, intravenous thrombolysis, baseline NIHSS score, pre-stroke mRS, time from symptom onset to treatment, successful recanalization and systolic blood pressure > 180 mmHg.

3.4. Predictive Value of Hyperglycemic Patterns

In order to evaluate the diagnostic performance of the hyperglycemic patterns, as judged with AUC-ROC, we added them to the basic model that included the other independent predictors of each endpoint. After adding the hyperglycemic patterns to the basic model, the AUC-ROC value increased for predicting a three-month poor outcome from 0.70 (95% CI 0.63–0.77) to 0.76 (95% CI 0.69–0.82), for no major neurological improvement from 0.63 (95% CI 0.55–0.72) to 0.75 (95% CI 0.67–0.82), for in-hospital mortality from 0.69 (95% CI 0.59–0.78) to 0.79 (95% CI 0.71–0.87), for three-month mortality from 0.72 (95% CI 0.63–0.81) to 0.79 (95% CI 0.71–0.86), for ICH from 0.62 (95% CI 0.52–0.71) to 0.70 (95% CI 0.61–0.79), and for SICH from 0.71 (95% CI 0.59–0.83) to 0.77 (95% CI 0.66–0.88).

4. Discussions

In order to evaluate the impact of the dynamic patterns of hyperglycemia on stroke outcome in AIS patients with LVO treated with MT, we retrospectively analyzed the results observed in a series of consecutive patients with prospective follow-up. We demonstrated that AIS patients affected by LVO with persistent hyperglycemia, defined as blood glucose levels > 140 mg/dL at baseline plus at 24-h following MT, have a significantly increased risk of poor functional outcome, mortality, and hemorrhagic transformation after endovascular treatment. These detrimental effects were partially confirmed after also excluding diabetic patients.

Previous studies performed in AIS patients treated with MT used one isolated glucose test measurement at baseline for investigating the role of hyperglycemia as a predictor of unfavorable outcomes [21–24]. Taken together, results on admission hyperglycemia as a predictor of poor outcome in patients undergoing MT are contradictory, with some articles showing that hyperglycemia at admission was a predictor of a worse outcome [22,24], and others showing no effect of blood glucose levels [21,23]. To date, only one study investigated whether hyperglycemia after MT was associated with a worse outcome. Li et al. analyzed 156 patients and reported that post-operative hyperglycemia (1 mmol/L per increase, i.e., 18 mg/dl per increase) was an independent predictor of SICH (OR 1.20, 95% CI 1.06–1.36, $p = 0.008$) [26].

Differently from previous studies, we sought to investigate the clinical significance of the dynamic patterns of hyperglycemia in patients undergoing MT. Although no other study has been performed in this specific population, a post-hoc analysis of the ECASS-II trial lead the authors to conclude that, in addition to a single glucose measurement, the pattern of glycemic excursions should be considered in the prediction of stroke outcome [27]. A further study by Putaala et al. investigated 851 consecutive patients treated with alteplase. Differently from baseline normoglycemia, persistent and 48-h hyperglycemia predicted an unfavorable outcome, death, and SICH [28]. Similar results were reported by Yoo et al. [29]

Our findings show that the presence of glucose levels > 140 mg/dL at admission, plus at 24-h after MT, has harmful and detrimental effects, also in non-diabetic patients. It is very unlikely that this result may have been influenced by the use of alteplase prior to MT, since the use of alteplase was included in our multivariate analysis as confounder. A large number of patients with persistent hyperglycemia was functionally dependent at 3 months after stroke, their in-hospital and three-month mortality were as high as 32.3% and 38.7%, respectively, and finally, almost 30% of these patients experienced SICH. Apart from the endpoint called "no major neurological improvement at discharge", patients with isolated admission hyperglycemia did not show any increased risk of adverse outcomes. Similarly, isolated hyperglycemia at 24-h after MT was not associated with a worse functional outcome, as well as a higher likelihood of death and SICH. Persistent hyperglycemia also had detrimental effects in non-diabetic patients. In fact, patients with this abnormal glycemic pattern had a higher risk of functional dependence and hemorrhagic transformation than those with persistent normoglycemia. Differently, the presence of persistent hyperglycemia was not associated with in-hospital and three-month mortality among non-diabetics undergoing MT for AIS.

In our sample, persistent hyperglycemia might impair outcomes as a marker of diabetes mellitus. In fact, patients with persistent hyperglycemia were more frequently affected by the chronic metabolic disease and they showed values of HbA1c significantly higher than subjects with different glycemic profiles. Epidemiologic studies have shown that diabetes is a well-established independent, but modifiable risk factor for stroke; both ischemic and hemorrhagic stroke [41]. There are several possible mechanisms wherein diabetes leads to stroke, among them diabetic vasculopathy could be considered. This pathophysiological hypothesis would be in agreement with the observed association between persistent hyperglycemia and hypercholesterolemia, a known risk factor for atherosclerosis. Furthermore, AIS patients with persistent hyperglycemia took slightly more antiplatelets. Although several clues point to diabetes as the link between persistent hyperglycemia and adverse outcomes in patients undergoing MT, nevertheless, the metabolic disorder alone cannot explain the worse prognosis of hyperglycemic patients. In fact, HbA1c values did not represent an independent predictor of adverse outcomes in the multivariate analysis of our study.

Hyperglycemia occurs after an acute stress, such as stroke and myocardial infarction, by the activation of the hypothalamic-pituitary-adrenal axis [42,43]. Both human and animal studies showed that mortality rate, due to post-stress hyperglycemia, is high after both stroke and myocardial infarction [44]. Previous studies reported that post-stress hyperglycemia was strictly associated with stroke severity. Blood glucose increase was related to the severity of stroke in the study of Christensen et al. [45] Our results, regarding NIHSS score at discharge, are perfectly in line with these previous data. Moreover, we observed that persistent hyperglycemia was able to impair functional outcome and hemorrhagic transformation in non-diabetics. Thus, we postulate that post-stress hyperglycemia not only may occur, but also may cause severe consequences in AIS patients treated with MT.

The AUC-ROC analysis strongly supports the use of hyperglycemic patterns in order to predict outcomes in AIS patients with LVO undergoing MT.

Although our study would encourage to apply rigorous glycemic control for at least 24-h following MT to achieve better outcomes, to date, no evidence supports the concept that ensuring strict post-stroke normoglycemia improves outcome. A possible reason for this might have been the severe hypoglycemia occurred in the intravenous insulin treatment group [46]. In order to overcome the failing of insulin, a phase 2 trial (the TEXAIS trial) on exenatide is now enrolling AIS patients in Australia, New Zealand, and Finland [47].

There are several limitations in our study. This is an observational study performed in a single center with a limited simple size. Although the study was retrospective, we prospectively collected data in consecutive patients. Information on the use of lowering glucose drugs during hospitalization is lacking. In addition, even after controlling for known confounders, residual confounding from unobserved factors might have affected our results. Information on last food intake before admission blood sample was not collected and the lack of a common criterion might have changed values, depending on the length of previous fasting. Unfortunately, no information other than NIHSS score were collected on clinical conditions at discharge, thus limiting the possibility of excluding their influence on measures of follow up at three months. Finally, the sample size was too small for performing further statistical analysis, e.g., propensity matching analysis, able to confirm our preliminary results.

In conclusion, we demonstrated the utility of performing prolonged monitoring of glucose levels lasting 24-h after MT, instead of isolated blood glucose measurements. Further studies are needed to confirm these results in larger samples.

Author Contributions: Conceptualization, G.M. and C.S.; methodology, G.M. and C.S.; software, C.S. and S.L.; validation, S.L., G.L.G. and M.V.; formal analysis, G.M.; investigation, C.S., M.S., A.M., A.S., S.P., A.V., V.G.; data curation, G.M.; writing—original draft preparation, G.M.; writing—review and editing, G.M.; visualization, G.L.G.; supervision, M.V. All authors have read and agreed to the published version of the manuscript.

Conflicts of Interest: The authors declare that they have no competing interests.

References

1. Powers, W.J.; Rabinstein, A.A.; Ackerson, T.; Adeoye, O.M.; Bambakidis, N.C.; Becker, K.; Biller, J.; Brown, M.; Demaerschalk, B.M.; Hoh, B.; et al. American Heart Association Stroke Council. 2018 Guidelines for the early management of patients with acute ischemic stroke: A guideline for healthcare professionals from the American heart association/American stroke association. *Stroke* **2018**, *49*, e46–e110. [CrossRef]
2. Campbell, B.C.; Mitchell, P.J.; Kleinig, T.J.; Dewey, H.M.; Churilov, L.; Yassi, N.; Yan, B.; Dowling, R.J.; Parsons, M.W.; Oxley, T.J.; et al. EXTEND-IA Investigators. Endovascular therapy for ischemic stroke with perfusion-imaging selection. *N. Engl. J. Med.* **2015**, *372*, 1009–1018. [CrossRef] [PubMed]
3. Berkhemer, O.A.; Fransen, P.S.; Beumer, D.; van der Berg, L.A.; Lingsma, H.F.; Yoo, A.J.; Schonewille, W.J.; Vos, J.A.; Nederkoorn, P.J.; Wermer, M.J.; et al. MR CLEAN Investigators. A randomized trial of intraarterial treatment for acute ischemic stroke. *N. Engl. J. Med.* **2015**, *372*, 11–20. [CrossRef] [PubMed]
4. Goyal, M.; Demchuk, A.M.; Menon, B.K.; Eesa, M.; Rempel, J.L.; Thornton, J.; Roy, D.; Jovin, T.G.; Willinsky, R.A.; Sapkota, B.L.; et al. ESCAPE Trial Investigators. Randomized assessment of rapid endovascular treatment of ischemic stroke. *N. Engl. J. Med.* **2015**, *372*, 1019–1030. [CrossRef]
5. Saver, J.L.; Goyal, M.; Bonafe, A.; Diener, H.; Levy, E.I.; Pereira, V.M.; Albers, G.W.; Cognard, C.; Cohen, D.J.; Hacke, W.; et al. SWIFT PRIME Investigators. Stent-retriever thrombectomy after intravenous t-PA vs. t-PA alone in stroke. *N. Engl. J. Med.* **2015**, *372*, 2285–2295. [CrossRef] [PubMed]
6. Jovin, T.G.; Chamorro, A.; Cobo, E.; de Miquel, M.A.; Molina, C.A.; Rovira, A.; San Román, L.; Serena, J.; Abilleira, S.; Ribó, M.; et al. REVASCAT Trial Investigators. Thrombectomy within 8 h after symptom onset in ischemic stroke. *N. Engl. J. Med.* **2015**, *372*, 2296–2306. [CrossRef]
7. Merlino, G.; Sponza, M.; Petralia, B.; Vit, A.; Gavrilovic, V.; Pellegrin, A.; Rana, M.; Cancelli, I.; Naliato, S.; Lorenzut, S.; et al. Short and long-term outcomes after combined intravenous thrombolysis and mechanical thrombectomy versus direct mechanical thrombectomy: A prospective single-center study. *J. Thromb. Thrombolysis* **2017**, *44*, 203–209. [CrossRef]
8. Sallustio, F.; Koch, G.; Alemseged, F.; Konda, D.; Fabiano, S.; Pampana, E.; Morosetti, D.; Gandini, R.; Diomedi, M. Effect of mechanical thrombectomy alone or in combination with intravenous thrombolysis for acute ischemic stroke. *J. Neurol.* **2018**, *265*, 2875–2880. [CrossRef]
9. Minnerup, J.; Wersching, H.; Teuber, A.; Wellmann, J.; Eyding, J.; Weber, R.; Reimann, G.; Weber, W.; Krause, L.U.; Kurth, T.; et al. Outcome after thrombectomy and intravenous thrombolysis in patients with acute ischemic stroke: A prospective observational study. *Stroke* **2016**, *47*, 1584–1592. [CrossRef]
10. Cho, B.H.; Kim, J.T.; Lee, J.S.; Park, M.S.; Kang, K.W.; Choi, K.H.; Lee, S.H.; Choi, S.M.; Kim, B.C.; Kim, M.K.; et al. Associations of various blood pressure parameters with functional outcomes after endovascular thrombectomy in acute ischaemic stroke. *Eur. J. Neurol.* **2019**, *26*, 1019–1027. [CrossRef]
11. Maïer, B.; Dargazanli, C.; Bourcier, R.; Kyheng, M.; Labreuche, J.; Mosimann, P.J.; Puccinelli, F.; Taylor, G.; Le Guen, M.; Riem, R.; et al. Effect of steady and dynamic blood pressure parameters during thrombectomy according to the collateral status. *Stroke* **2020**, *51*, 1199–1206. [CrossRef] [PubMed]
12. Meinel, T.R.; Kaesmacher, J.; Mordasini, P.; Mosimann, P.J.; Jung, S.; Arnold, M.; Heldner, M.R.; Michel, P.; Hajdu, S.D.; Ribo, M.; et al. Outcome, efficacy and safety of endovascular thrombectomy in ischaemic stroke according to time to reperfusion: Data from a multicentre registry. *Ther. Adv. Neurol. Disord.* **2019**, *12*, 1756286419835708. [CrossRef] [PubMed]
13. Baird, T.A.; Parsons, M.W.; Phan, T.; Butcher, K.S.; Desmond, P.M.; Tress, B.M.; Colman, P.G.; Chambers, B.R.; Davis, S.M. Persistent poststroke hyperglycemia is independently associated with infarct expansion and worse clinical outcome. *Stroke* **2003**, *34*, 2208–2214. [CrossRef] [PubMed]

14. Fuentes, B.; Castillo, J.; San José, B.; Leira, R.; Serena, J.; Vivancos, J.; Dávalos, A.; Nuñez, A.G.; Egido, J.; Díez-Tejedor, E. Stroke Project of the Cerebrovascular Diseases Study Group, Spanish Society of Neurology The prognostic value of capillary glucose levels in acute stroke: The GLycemia in Acute Stroke (GLIAS) study. *Stroke* **2009**, *40*, 562–568. [CrossRef] [PubMed]
15. Capes, S.E.; Hunt, D.; Malmberg, K.; Pathak, P.; Gerstein, H.C. Stress hyperglycemia and prognosis of stroke in nondiabetic and diabetic patients: A systematic overview. *Stroke* **2001**, *32*, 2426–2432. [CrossRef]
16. Rom, S.; Zuluaga-Ramirez, V.; Gajghate, S.; Seliga, A.; Winfield, M.; Heldt, N.A.; Kolpakov, M.A.; Bashkirova, Y.V.; Sabri, A.K.; Persidsky, Y. Hyperglycemia-driven neuroinflammation compromises BBB leading to memory loss in both diabetes mellitus (DM) type 1 and type 2 mouse models. *Mol. Neurobiol.* **2019**, *56*, 1883–1896. [CrossRef]
17. Desilles, J.P.; Syvannarath, V.; Ollivier, V.; Journé, C.; Delbosc, S.; Ducroux, C.; Boisseau, W.; Louedec, L.; Di Meglio, L.; Loyau, S.; et al. Exacerbation of thromboinflammation by hyperglycemia precipitates cerebral infarct growth and hemorrhagic transformation. *Stroke* **2017**, *48*, 1932–1940. [CrossRef]
18. Robbins, N.M.; Swanson, R.A. Opposing effects of glucose on stroke and reperfusion injury: Acidosis, oxidative stress, and energy metabolism. *Stroke* **2014**, *45*, 1881–1886. [CrossRef]
19. Won, S.J.; Tang, X.N.; Suh, S.W.; Yenari, M.A.; Swanson, R.A. Hyperglycemia promotes tissue plasminogen activator-induced hemorrhage by Increasing superoxide production. *Ann. Neurol.* **2011**, *70*, 583–590. [CrossRef]
20. Poppe, A.Y.; Majumdar, S.R.; Jeerakathil, T.; Ghali, W.; Buchan, A.M.; Hill, M.D. Canadian Alteplase for Stroke Effectiveness Study Investigators. Admission hyperglycemia predicts a worse outcome in stroke patients treated with intravenous thrombolysis. *Diabetes Care* **2009**, *32*, 617–622. [CrossRef]
21. Kim, J.T.; Jahan, R.; Saver, J.L. SWIFT Investigators. Impact of glucose on outcomes in patients treated with mechanical thrombectomy: A post hoc analysis of the solitaire flow restoration with the intention for thrombectomy study. *Stroke* **2016**, *47*, 120–127. [CrossRef]
22. Goyal, N.; Tsivgoulis, G.; Pandhi, A.; Dillard, K.; Katsanos, A.H.; Magoufis, G.; Chang, J.J.; Zand, R.; Hoit, D.; Safouris, A.; et al. Admission hyperglycemia and outcomes in large vessel occlusion strokes treated with mechanical thrombectomy. *J. Neurointerv. Surg.* **2018**, *10*, 112–117. [CrossRef] [PubMed]
23. Osei, E.; den Hertog, H.M.; Berkhemer, O.A.; Fransen, P.S.S.; Roos, Y.B.W.E.M.; Beumer, D.; van Oostenbrugge, R.J.; Schonewille, W.J.; Boiten, J.; Zandbergen, A.A.M.; et al. MR CLEAN Investigators. Admission glucose and effect of intra-arterial treatment in patients with acute ischemic stroke. *Stroke* **2017**, *48*, 1299–1305. [CrossRef] [PubMed]
24. Chamorro, Á.; Brown, S.; Amaro, S.; Hill, M.D.; Muir, K.W.; Dippel, D.W.J.; van Zwam, W.; Butcher, K.; Ford, G.A.; den Hertog, H.M.; et al. HERMES Collaborators. Glucose modifies the effect of endovascular thrombectomy in patients with acute stroke. *Stroke* **2019**, *50*, 690–696. [CrossRef] [PubMed]
25. Marik, P.E.; Bellomo, R. Stress hyperglycemia: An essential survival response! *Crit. Care* **2013**, *17*, 305. [CrossRef] [PubMed]
26. Li, F.; Ren, Y.; Cui, X.; Liu, P.; Chen, F.; Zhao, H.; Han, Z.; Huang, Y.; Ma, Q.; Luo, Y. Postoperative hyperglycemia predicts symptomatic intracranial hemorrhage after endovascular treatment in patients with acute anterior circulation large artery occlusion. *J. Neurol. Sci.* **2020**, *409*, 116588. [CrossRef] [PubMed]
27. Yong, M.; Kaste, M. Dynamic of hyperglycemia as a predictor of stroke outcome in the ECASS-II trial. *Stroke* **2008**, *39*, 2749–2755. [CrossRef]
28. Putaala, J.; Sairanen, T.; Meretoja, A.; Lindsberg, P.J.; Tiainen, M.; Liebkind, R.; Strbian, D.; Atula, S.; Artto, V.; Rantanen, K.; et al. Post-thrombolytic hyperglycemia and 3-month outcome in acute ischemic stroke. *Cerebrovasc. Dis.* **2011**, *31*, 83–92. [CrossRef]
29. Yoo, D.S.; Chang, J.; Kim, J.T.; Choi, M.J.; Choi, J.; Choi, K.H.; Park, M.S.; Cho, K.H. Various blood glucose parameters that indicate hyperglycemia after intravenous thrombolysis in acute ischemic stroke could predict worse outcome. *PLoS ONE* **2014**, *9*, e94364. [CrossRef]
30. Merlino, G.; Sponza, M.; Gigli, G.L.; Lorenzut, S.; Vit, A.; Gavrilovic, V.; Pellegrin, A.; Cargnelutti, D.; Valente, M. Prior use of antiplatelet therapy and outcomes after endovascular therapy in acute ischemic stroke due to large vessel occlusion: A single-center experience. *J. Clin. Med.* **2018**, *7*, 518. [CrossRef]
31. Chen, X.; Liu, Z.; Miao, J.; Zheng, W.; Yang, Q.; Ye, X.; Zhuang, X.; Peng, F. High Stress hyperglycemia ratio predicts poor outcome after mechanical thrombectomy for ischemic stroke. *J. Stroke Cerebrovasc. Dis.* **2019**, *28*, 1668–1673. [CrossRef] [PubMed]

32. Zhu, B.; Pan, Y.; Jing, J.; Meng, X.; Zhao, X.; Liu, L.; Wang, Y.; Wang, Y.; Wang, Z. Stress hyperglycemia and outcome of non-diabetic patients after acute ischemic stroke. *Front. Neurol.* **2019**, *10*, 1003. [CrossRef]
33. Adams, H.P., Jr.; Bendixen, B.H.; Kappelle, L.J.; Biller, J.; Love, B.B.; Gordon, D.L.; Marsh, E.E., 3rd. Classification of subtype of acute ischemic stroke. Definitions for use in a multicenter clinical trial. TOAST. Trial of Org 10172 in Acute Stroke Treatment. *Stroke* **1993**, *24*, 35–41. [CrossRef] [PubMed]
34. Brott, T.; Adams, H.P., Jr.; Olinger, C.P.; Marler, J.R.; Barsan, W.G.; Biller, J.; Spilker, J.; Holleran, R.; Eberle, R.; Hertzberg, V.; et al. Measurements of acute cerebral infarction: A clinical examination scale. *Stroke* **1989**, *20*, 864–870. [CrossRef]
35. Brown, D.L.; Johnston, K.C.; Wagner, D.P.; Haley, E.C., Jr. Predicting major neurological improvement with intravenous recombinant tissue plasminogen activator treatment of stroke. *Stroke* **2004**, *35*, 147–150. [CrossRef] [PubMed]
36. Saposnik, G.; Di Legge, S.; Webster, F.; Hachinski, V. Predictors of major neurologic improvement after thrombolysis in acute stroke. *Neurology* **2005**, *65*, 1169–1774. [CrossRef]
37. Yaghi, S.; Hinduja, A.; Bianchi, N. Predictors of major improvement after intravenous thrombolysis in acute ischemic stroke. *Int. J. Neurosci.* **2016**, *126*, 67–69. [CrossRef] [PubMed]
38. van Swieten, J.C.; Koudstaal, P.J.; Visser, M.C.; Schouten, H.J.; van Gijn, J. Interobserver agreement for the assessment of handicap in stroke patients. *Stroke* **1988**, *19*, 604–607. [CrossRef]
39. Hacke, W.; Kaste, M.; Fieschi, C.; Toni, D.; Lesaffre, E.; von Kummer, R.; Boysen, G.; Bluhmki, E.; Höxter, G.; Mahagne, M.H.; et al. Intravenous thrombolysis with recombinant tissue plasminogen activator for acute hemispheric stroke. The European Cooperative Acute Stroke Study (ECASS). *JAMA* **1995**, *274*, 1017–1025. [CrossRef]
40. Hacke, W.; Kaste, M.; Bluhmki, E.; Brozman, M.; Dávalos, A.; Guidetti, D.; Larrue, V.; Lees, K.R.; Medeghri, Z.; Machnig, T.; et al. Thrombolysis with alteplase 3 to 4.5 hours after acute ischemic stroke. *N. Engl. J. Med.* **2008**, *359*, 1317–1329. [CrossRef]
41. Chen, R.; Ovbiagele, B.; Feng, W. Diabetes and Stroke: Epidemiology, Pathophysiology, Pharmaceuticals and Outcomes. *Am. J. Med. Sci.* **2016**, *351*, 380–386. [CrossRef] [PubMed]
42. Melamed, E. Reactive hyperglycaemia in patients with acute stroke. *J. Neurol. Sci.* **1976**, *29*, 267–275. [CrossRef]
43. Sewdarsen, M.; Jialal, I.; Vythilingum, S.; Govender, G.; Rajput, M.C. Stress hyperglycaemia is a predictor of abnormal glucose tolerance in Indian patients with acute myocardial infarction. *Diabetes Res.* **1987**, *6*, 47–49.
44. Capes, S.E.; Hunt, D.; Malmberg, K.; Gerstein, H.C. Stress hyperglycaemia and increased risk of death after myocardial infarction in patients with and without diabetes: A systematic overview. *Lancet* **2000**, *355*, 773–778. [CrossRef]
45. Christensen, H.; Boysen, G. Blood glucose increases early after stroke onset: A study on serial measurements of blood glucose in acute stroke. *Eur. J. Neurol.* **2002**, *9*, 297–301. [CrossRef] [PubMed]
46. Johnston, K.C.; Bruno, A.; Pauls, Q.; Hall, C.E.; Barrett, K.M.; Barsan, W.; Fansler, A.; Van de Bruinhorst, K.; Janis, S.; Durkalski-Mauldin, V.L.; et al. Intensive vs standard treatment of hyperglycemia and functional outcome in patients with acute ischemic stroke: The SHINE randomized clinical trial. *JAMA* **2019**, *322*, 326–335. [CrossRef]
47. Muller, C.; Cheung, N.W.; Dewey, H.; Churilov, L.; Middleton, S.; Thijs, V.; Ekinci, E.I.; Levi, C.; Lindley, R.; Donnan, G.; et al. Treatment with exenatide in acute ischemic stroke trial protocol: A prospective, randomized, open label, blinded end-point study of exenatide vs. standard care in post stroke hyperglycemia. *Int. J. Stroke* **2018**, *13*, 857–862. [CrossRef]

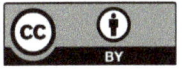

© 2020 by the authors. Licensee MDPI, Basel, Switzerland. This article is an open access article distributed under the terms and conditions of the Creative Commons Attribution (CC BY) license (http://creativecommons.org/licenses/by/4.0/).

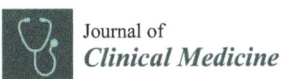

Article

Fasting Normoglycemia after Intravenous Thrombolysis Predicts Favorable Long-Term Outcome in Non-Diabetic Patients with Acute Ischemic Stroke

Marcin Wnuk [1,2,*], Justyna Derbisz [1,2], Leszek Drabik [3,4], Maciej Malecki [2,5] and Agnieszka Slowik [1,2]

1. Department of Neurology, Jagiellonian University Medical College, 30-688 Krakow, Poland; justyna.derbisz@gmail.com (J.D.); agnieszka.slowik@uj.edu.pl (A.S.)
2. The University Hospital in Krakow, 30-688 Krakow, Poland; maciej.malecki@uj.edu.pl
3. Department of Pharmacology, Jagiellonian University Medical College, 31-531 Krakow, Poland; leszek.drabik@uj.edu.pl
4. John Paul II Hospital, 31-202 Krakow, Poland
5. Department of Metabolic Diseases, Jagiellonian University Medical College, 30-688 Krakow, Poland
* Correspondence: marcin.wnuk@uj.edu.pl

Abstract: Background: Only a few studies evaluated the role of fasting glucose levels after intravenous thrombolysis (IVT) in patients with acute ischemic stroke (AIS). Importantly, formal analysis concerning the prognostic role of fasting glucose levels in these patients with and without diabetes mellitus (DM) was not performed. Therefore, we assessed whether fasting normoglycemia (FNG) next morning after AIS treated with IVT was associated with 90-day functional outcome in diabetic and non-diabetic patients. Methods: We retrospectively analyzed 362 AIS patients treated with IVT at The University Hospital in Krakow. FNG was defined as glucose below 5.5 mmol/L. A favorable outcome was defined as modified Rankin score (mRS) of 0–2 at day 90 after AIS onset. Results: At 3-month follow-up, FNG was associated with favorable outcome (87.5% vs. 60.8%, $p < 0.001$) and decreased risk of death (3.1% vs. 18.1%, $p = 0.002$). Independent predictors of a favorable outcome for the whole group were: younger age (HR 0.92, 95%CI 0.89–0.95), lower NIHSS score after IVT (HR 0.70, 95%CI 0.65–0.76), lower maximal systolic blood pressure within 24 h after IVT (HR 0.92, 95%CI 0.89–0.95) and FNG (HR 4.12, 95%CI 1.38–12.35). Association between FNG and mortality was found in univariable (HR 1.47, 95%CI 0.04–0.62) but not in multivariable analysis (HR 0.23, 95%CI 0.03–1.81). In subgroup analyses, FNG was an independent predictor of favorable outcome (HR 5.96, 95%CI 1.42–25.1) only in patients without DM. Conclusions: FNG next morning after IVT is an independent protective factor for a favorable long-term outcome in non-diabetic AIS patients.

Keywords: stroke; thrombolysis; fasting hyperglycemia; fasting normoglycemia; long-term outcome

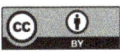

1. Introduction

The prognostic significance of admission glucose levels in patients with acute ischemic stroke (AIS) treated with intravenous thrombolysis (IVT) is well established [1]. Hyperglycemia on admission has been associated with worse functional outcomes and increased mortality within 3 months after IVT in patients with or without diabetes mellitus (DM) [2].

However, only a few studies so far have evaluated the role of fasting glucose levels after IVT in patients with AIS [3,4]. Fasting hyperglycemia the next day or 2–5 days after IVT was associated with worse 3-month functional outcomes and increased mortality [3,4]. Importantly, the association with outcome was stronger for fasting glucose levels than for admission ones [3]. Diabetes mellitus was not found to be correlated with a 90-day poor clinical outcome as assessed with modified Rankin scale (mRS); however, the formal analysis concerning the prognostic role of fasting glucose levels in AIS patients treated with IVT according to the presence of DM was not performed [3,4]. To the best of our knowledge, no studies so far evaluated the impact of fasting glucose next morning after IVT in diabetic and non-diabetic patients on a 90-day clinical outcome.

The recent Stroke Hyperglycemia Insulin Network Effort (SHINE) trial, performed in AIS patients with concomitant hyperglycemia, evaluated the impact of intensive versus standard insulin therapy during the first 72 h from symptom onset on a 90-day functional outcome [5]. Although the analysis, adjusted for IVT or mechanical thrombectomy (MT) use, did not show any significant difference in long-term prognosis, it occurred that DM was present in around 80% of patients in both treated subgroups, and, consequently, the results may not be generalizable for a whole stroke population, including patients without pre-existent DM [5].

Therefore, the aim of the present study was to search whether fasting normoglycemia (FNG) the next day after IVT was associated with long-term outcomes in a large cohort of AIS patients according to the presence of DM.

2. Materials and Methods

The data supporting the results of this study are available from the corresponding author upon reasonable request from any qualified investigator.

2.1. Patients

The study was designed as a retrospective analysis of the prospectively collected data of 1209 AIS patients from the Krakow Stroke Data Bank, the registry conducted in the single stroke center, The University Hospital in Krakow, from the year 2007. Finally, the study included 362 AIS patients (29.9%), all of Caucasian origin, treated with IVT between June 2014 and December 2018. We collected the data on demographics, the presence of vascular risk factors, etiology of AIS and National Institutes of Health Stroke Scale (NIHSS) on admission and after IVT. The diagnosis of DM was made as described previously [6]. In brief, patients were diagnosed with DM based on the previous medical history or the use of insulin or antidiabetic oral drugs before the onset of stroke [6].

The outcome was measured with mRS at day 90 from AIS onset, and a favorable outcome was defined as an mRS score of 0–2, similarly to the previous studies investigating the prognostic role of fasting hyperglycemia [3,4]. Additionally, an excellent outcome was defined as an mRS score of 0–1 at day 90 after AIS onset. We also evaluated 3-month mortality. Bleeding brain complications due to IVT were defined in accordance with the ECASS-1 classification [7]. As higher systolic blood pressure (SBP) was found to increase the risk of symptomatic intracranial hemorrhage in the previous stroke registries [8,9], we additionally noted the maximal SBP value within 24 h after IVT.

2.2. Glucose Measurements

We evaluated serum glucose levels in each patient the next morning after IVT and overnight fasting. Fasting normoglycemia and hyperglycemia were defined as the glucose levels below 5.5 mmol/L (100 mg%) and equal or above this value, respectively, in accordance with the American Diabetes Association's Standards of Care [10]. Patients with hyperglycemia greater than 10 mmol/L were treated with four subcutaneous insulin injections daily with doses adjusted to the current level of glucose [11].

The study was approved by the Jagiellonian University Ethical Committee (KBET 54/B/2007). All patients gave informed consent to participate in the study, which was either written or verbal in the presence of at least two physicians in case of inability to use the dominant hand because of AIS.

2.3. Statistics

The continuous variables were presented as mean and standard deviation (SD), and in the case of categorical data, counts and percentages were shown. Continuous variables were tested for normality with the use of the Shapiro–Wilk test and then compared, as appropriate, by a Student's t-test or by the Mann–Whitney U test. The multivariable logistic regression model comprised only those variables that showed a *p*-value of <0.1 in the univariable analysis. We considered a *p*-value of 0.05 (two-sided) as statistically significant and performed all statistical analyses with the use of STATISTICA version 13 (Statsoft Inc, Tulsa, OK, USA).

3. Results

3.1. Patient Characteristics

The characteristics of 362 AIS patients treated with IVT were summarized in Table 1. Among patients, 108 (29.8%) underwent additionally MT.

Patients with FNG were younger, had lower Body Mass Index (BMI), lower NIHSS score before and after treatment with IVT and lower maximal SBP within 24 h after IVT in comparison to those with fasting hyperglycemia (Table 1).

3.2. Association between FNG and Favorable Outcome

3.2.1. All Patients

A favorable outcome applied to 231 (63.8%) patients at 3-month follow-up. Patients with favorable outcome were younger (median, interquartile range IQR 70 (59–79) vs. 78 (69–83) years, $p < 0.001$), less often women (43.7% vs. 59.5%, $p = 0.005$), less often suffered from hypertension (77.5% vs. 95.0%, $p < 0.001$), had lower fasting glucose levels (median, IQR 6.4 (5.5–7.9) vs. 6.9 (6.1–8.6) mmol/L, $p = 0.004$), lower NIHSS score on admission (mean ± standard deviation (SD), 9.7 ± 6.0 vs. 16.3 ± 6.0, $p < 0.001$) and after IVT (mean ± SD, 4.5 ± 4.3 vs. 16.0 ± 7.6, $p < 0.001$), lower value of maximal SBP within 24 h after IVT (145 (126–160) vs. 146 (137–165) mmHg, $p = 0.048$) and less often experienced bleeding brain complications (10.0% vs. 41.3%, $p < 0.001$) compared with the remainder (Supplemental Table S1, for subgroup of patients treated only with IVT and without MT see also Supplemental Table S2).

Patients with FNG had a higher prevalence of a favorable 3-month outcome than those with fasting hyperglycemia (Table 1, Figure 1). The independent predictors of favorable long-term outcome for the whole group were: younger age, lower NIHSS score after IVT, lower maximal SBP and FNG (Table 2). In the subgroup of patients treated only with IVT (without MT), favorable long-term outcome was predicted by age and NIHSS score after IVT. The association between FNG and outcome for these patients was found in the univariable analysis (Supplemental Figure S1, Supplemental Table S3). The optimal cutoff value of glucose for predicting mRS 0–2 was 5.49 mmol/L. Sensitivity and specificity using this cutoff value were 86.7% and 59.2%, respectively.

Table 1. Baseline characteristics of patients according to glycemia < 5.5 mmol/L and diabetes mellitus (DM).

	Whole Group			With DM			Without DM		
	Glucose < 5.5 mmol/L n = 69	Glucose ≥ 5.5 mmol/L n = 293	p-Value	Glucose < 5.5 mmol/L n = 12	Glucose ≥ 5.5 mmol/L n = 93	p-Value	Glucose < 5.5 mmol/L n = 57	Glucose ≥ 5.5 mmol/L n = 200	p-Value
Age (years)	70 (54–78)	73 (64–82)	0.005	78 (71–80)	74 (65–82)	0.331	65 (53–75)	72 (64–82)	<0.001
Women, n (%)	30 (43.5)	147 (50.2)	0.317	4 (33.3)	47 (50.5)	0.360	26 (45.6)	100 (50.0)	0.559
BMI (kg/m^2)	25.8 (23.4–27.8)	27.1 (24.4–30.1)	0.013	24.9 (23.4–27.0)	29.1 (26.1–31.8)	0.001	25.9 (23.4–28.7)	25.9 (23.9–29.4)	0.578
Hypertension, n (%)	54 (78.3)	250 (85.3)	0.150	11 (91.7)	87 (93.5)	0.584	43 (75.4)	163 (81.5)	0.311
Ischemic heart disease, n (%)	14 (20.3)	70 (23.9)	0.523	3 (25.0)	30 (32.3)	0.749	11 (19.3)	40 (20.0)	0.907
Atrial fibrillation, n (%)	16 (23.2)	90 (30.7)	0.216	3 (25.0)	36 (38.7)	0.528	13 (22.8)	54 (27.0)	0.525
Hypercholesterolemia, n (%)	29 (42.0)	88 (30.0)	0.055	7 (58.3)	30 (32.3)	0.108	22 (38.6)	58 (29.0)	0.167
Smoking, n (%)	12 (17.7)	43 (15.2)	0.736	1 (8.3)	10 (10.8)	1.00	11 (19.3)	33 (17.2)	0.812
Previous stroke, n (%)	12 (17.4)	54 (18.40)	0.840	2 (16.7)	21 (22.6)	1.00	10 (17.5)	33 (16.5)	0.852
Stroke etiology, n (%)			0.172			0.534			0.077
- large-vessel disease	10 (14.5)	39 (13.3)		4 (33.3)	14 (15.0)		6 (10.5)	25 (12.5)	
- small-vessel disease	2 (2.9)	1 (0.3)		0 (0.0)	1 (1.1)		2 (3.5)	0 (0.0)	
- cardioembolic	19 (27.5)	100 (34.1)		3 (25.0)	38 (40.9)		16 (28.1)	62 (31.0)	
- other	5 (7.3)	12 (4.1)		0 (0.0)	2 (2.1)		5 (8.8)	10 (5.0)	
- undetermined	33 (47.8)	141 (48.1)		5 (41.7)	38 (40.9)		28 (49.1)	103 (51.5)	
Mechanical thrombectomy, n (%)	26 (37.7)	82 (28.0)	0.113	1 (8.3)	33 (35.5)	0.978	25 (43.9)	49 (24.5)	0.004
Time from stroke onset to thrombolysis (min)	138 (99–176)	135 (95–183)	0.655	115 (91–156)	135 (96–185)	0.243	140 (100–190)	135 (94–180)	0.998
NIHSS score on admission	10.3 ± 6.6	12.3 ± 6.8	0.026	8.7 ± 4.9	12.3 ± 6.4	0.060	10.7 ± 6.1	12.3 ± 7.0	0.122
NIHSS score after r-tPA	6.3 ± 6.6	9.0 ± 7.9	0.012	7.0 ± 5.1	8.4 ± 7.0	0.665	6.1 ± 6.9	9.3 ± 8.3	0.010
Post-MT hemorrhagic brain complications, n (%)			0.810			0.718			0.892
- no complication	58 (84.1)	229 (78.2)		11 (91.7)	73 (78.5)		47 (82.5)	156 (78.0)	
- HI type 1	4 (5.8)	21 (7.2)		1 (8.3)	6 (6.4)		3 (5.3)	15 (7.5)	
- HI type 2	4 (5.8)	20 (6.8)		0 (0.0)	7 (7.5)		4 (7.0)	13 (6.5)	
- PH type 1	2 (2.9)	12 (4.1)		0 (0.0)	4 (4.3)		2 (3.5)	8 (4.0)	
- PH type 2	1 (1.5)	11 (3.8)		0 (0.0)	3 (3.2)		1 (1.7)	8 (4.0)	

Table 1. Cont.

	Whole Group			With DM			Without DM		
	Glucose < 5.5 mmol/L $n = 69$	Glucose $\geq$ 5.5 mmol/L $n = 293$	p-Value	Glucose < 5.5 mmol/L $n = 12$	Glucose $\geq$ 5.5 mmol/L $n = 93$	p-Value	Glucose < 5.5 mmol/L $n = 57$	Glucose $\geq$ 5.5 mmol/L $n = 200$	p-Value
Maximal SBP within 24 h after r-tPA (mmHg)	140 (120–150)	147 (135–164)	0.002	140 (125–150)	148 (135–160)	0.285	140 (120–150)	146 (134–165)	0.005
Maximal DBP within 24 h after r-tPA (mmHg)	80 (71–83)	80 (70–90)	0.101	80 (70–80)	80 (70–90)	0.459	80 (72–85)	80 (71–90)	0.124
Fasting glucose (mmol/L)	5.0 (4.7–5.3)	6.9 (6.2–8.6)	<0.001	4.4 (3.6–4.7)	8.1 (6.5–11.5)	<0.001	5.2 (4.9–5.3)	6.7 (6.1–7.8)	<0.001
Creatinine (μmol/L)	78 (69–98)	82 (68–97)	0.572	103 (72–122)	83 (64–99)	0.177	74 (67–95)	82 (69–92)	0.202
mRS 0–1, 90 days, n (%)	53 (82.8)	153 (53.1)	<0.001	7 (63.6)	42 (45.6)	0.259	46 (86.8)	111 (56.6)	<0.001
mRS 0–2, 90 days, n (%)	56 (87.5)	175 (60.8)	<0.001	8 (72.7)	54 (58.7)	0.368	48 (90.6)	121 (61.7)	<0.001
Death (mRS = 6), 90 days, n (%)	2 (3.1)	52 (18.1)	0.002	1 (9.1)	15 (16.3)	1.000	1 (1.9)	37 (18.9)	0.001

Values are presented as n (%), mean ± standard deviation, or median and interquartile range. Abbreviations: BMI—body mass index, DBP—diastolic blood pressure, DM—diabetes mellitus, HI—hemorrhagic infarction, mRS—modified Rankin scale, MT—mechanical thrombectomy, NIHSS—National Institutes of Health Stroke Scale, PH—parenchymal hematoma, r-tPA—recombinant tissue plasminogen activator and SBP—systolic blood pressure.

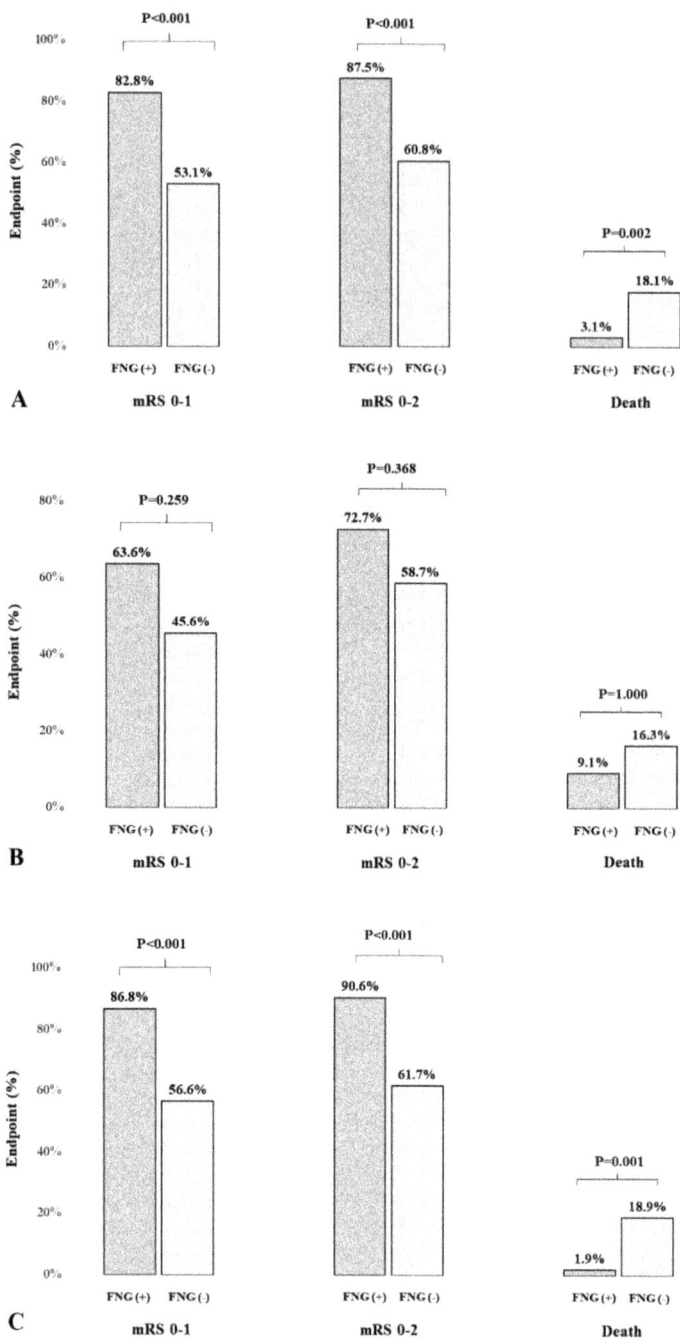

Figure 1. The proportion of patients with a favorable (mRS 0–2) or excellent (mRS 0–1) outcome and those who died (mRS = 6) according to the presence of fasting normoglycemia in the whole group (**A**) and patients with (**B**) and without diabetes mellitus (**C**).

Table 2. The multivariable logistic regression model for a favorable (mRS 0–2) and excellent (mRS 0–1) 3-month clinical outcome.

	Favorable Outcome (mRS 0–2)					
	Univariable			Multivariable		
90-day favorable clinical outcome, diabetic + non-diabetic patients	HR	95% CI	p-Value	HR	95% CI	p-Value
Age (per 1 year)	0.95	0.94–0.97	<0.001	0.92	0.89–0.95	<0.001
Sex (female)	0.53	0.34–0.83	0.005	-	-	-
BMI (per 1 unit)	0.96	0.92–1.02	0.163	-	-	-
Atrial fibrillation	0.57	0.35–0.91	0.019	-	-	-
NIHSS score after r-tPA (per 1 point)	0.73	0.69–0.78	<0.001	0.70	0.65–0.76	<0.001
Maximal SBP within 24 h after r-tPA (per 1 mmHg)	0.99	0.98–0.99	0.053	0.92	0.89–0.95	0.037
Mechanical thrombectomy	0.67	0.42–1.07	0.091	-	-	-
Hemorrhagic brain complications (ECASS 1–3)	0.16	0.09–0.28	<0.001	-	-	-
Fasting glucose < 5.5 mmol/L	4.52	2.08–9.83	<0.001	4.12	1.38–12.35	0.011
90-day favorable clinical outcome, diabetic patients						
Age (per 1 year)	0.96	0.92–0.99	0.352	0.87	0.80–0.95	0.002
Sex (female)	0.92	0.42–2.03	0.841	-	-	-
BMI (per 1 unit)	0.89	0.81–0.98	0.018	-	-	-
Atrial fibrillation	0.48	0.21–1.08	0.075	-	-	-
Previous stroke	0.41	0.16–1.06	0.067	-	-	-
NIHSS score after r-tPA (per 1 point)	0.77	0.70–0.85	<0.001	0.64	0.54–0.77	<0.001
Hemorrhagic brain complications (ECASS 1–3)	0.25	0.09–0.68	0.007	-	-	-
Creatinine (per 1 μmol/L)	0.98	0.97–0.99	0.019	0.97	0.94–0.99	0.018
Fasting glucose < 5.5 mmol/L	1.88	0.47–1.54	0.375	-	-	-
90-day favorable clinical outcome, non-diabetic patients						
Age (per 1 year)	0.95	0.93–0.98	<0.001	0.94	0.90–0.98	0.01
Sex (female)	0.40	0.23–0.69	0.011	-	-	-
BMI (per 1 unit)	1.02	0.95–1.09	0.585	-	-	-
Hypertension	0.18	0.07–0.47	<0.001	-	-	-
Maximal SBP within 24 h after r-tPA (per 1 mmHg)	0.99	0.98–0.99	0.012	1.03	1.01–1.05	0.007
NIHSS score after r-tPA (per 1 point)	0.71	0.66–0.77	<0.001	0.68	0.62–0.75	<0.001
Hemorrhagic brain complications (ECASS 1–3)	0.13	0.07–0.25	<0.001	-	-	-
Fasting glucose < 5.5 mmol/L	5.95	2.27–15.6	<0.001	5.96	1.42–25.1	0.015

Table 2. *Cont.*

90-day excellent clinical outcome, diabetic + non-diabetic patients	Excellent Outcome (mRS 0–1)					
	Univariable			Multivariable		
	HR	95% CI	*p*-Value	HR	95% CI	*p*-Value
Sex (female)	0.59	0.38–0.90	0.015	-	-	-
BMI (per 1 unit)	0.96	0.96–1.01	0.126	-	-	-
Atrial fibrillation	0.63	0.40–0.99	0.049	-	-	-
NIHSS score after r-tPA (per 1 point)	0.73	0.69–0.77	<0.001	0.71	0.66–0.76	<0.001
Maximal SBP within 24 h after r-tPA (per 1 mmHg)	0.99	0.98–0.99	0.014	-	-	-
Mechanical thrombectomy	0.53	0.33–0.84	0.007	-	-	-
Hemorrhagic brain complications (ECASS 1–3)	0.17	0.10–0.30	<0.001	-	-	-
Fasting glucose < 5.5 mmol/L	4.25	2.13–8.47	<0.001	3.47	1.32–9.14	0.012
90-day excellent clinical outcome, diabetic patients						
Age (per 1 year)	0.98	0.94–1.02	0.226	-	-	-
Sex (female)	1.52	0.70–3.32	0.289	-	-	-
BMI (per 1 unit)	0.89	0.81–0.98	0.019	-	-	-
NIHSS score after r-tPA (per 1 point)	0.70	0.62–0.80	<0.001	0.69	0.60–0.79	<0.001
Mechanical thrombectomy	0.42	0.18–1.00	0.050	-	-	-
Hemorrhagic brain complications (ECASS 1–3)	0.27	0.09–0.81	0.019	-	-	-
Creatinine (per 1 µmol/L)	0.99	0.97–0.99	0.040	0.98	0.96–0.99	0.021
Fasting glucose < 5.5 mmol/L	2.08	0.57–7.61	0.267	-	-	-
90-day excellent clinical outcome, non-diabetic patients						
Age (per 1 year)	0.95	0.93–0.97	<0.001	0.96	0.93–0.99	0.02
Sex (female)	0.37	0.22–0.63	<0.001	0.34	0.14–0.87	0.024
BMI (per 1 unit)	1.03	0.96–1.10	0.474	-	-	-
Hypertension	0.21	0.09–0.49	<0.001	-	-	-
Maximal SBP within 24 h after r-tPA (per 1 mmHg)	0.98	0.97–0.99	<0.001	-	-	-
NIHSS score after r-tPA (per 1 point)	0.72	0.67–0.78	<0.001	0.71	0.65–0.77	<0.001
Mechanical thrombectomy	0.59	0.34–1.03	0.065	-	-	-
Hemorrhagic brain complications (ECASS 1–3)	0.14	0.07–0.28	<0.001	-	-	-
Fasting glucose < 5.5 mmol/L	5.03	2.16–11.7	<0.001	3.47	1.10–12.2	0.035

Abbreviations, see Table 1; ECASS—The European Cooperative Acute Stroke Study.

3.2.2. Subgroup Analyses According to Diabetes

Patients without DM who presented with FNG in comparison to those with fasting hyperglycemia were younger, had lower NIHSS score after IVT, lower fasting glucose levels, lower maximal SBP and more often underwent additionally MT (Table 1). In non-diabetic patients, variables that predicted a favorable 3-month outcome were: younger age, lower NIHSS score after IVT, lower maximal SBP and FNG (Table 2). In the subgroup of non-diabetic patients treated only with IVT, a favorable 3-month outcome was predicted by age, NIHSS score after IVT, maximal SBP and FNG (Supplemental Table S3).

Patients with DM and FNG in comparison to those with fasting hyperglycemia had a lower BMI and lower fasting glucose levels (Table 1). The presence of FNG was not an independent predictor of favorable long-term outcome in diabetic patients in contrast to a younger age, lower NIHSS score after IVT and lower creatinine concentration (Table 2). In the subgroup of diabetic patients treated only with IVT, a favorable long-term outcome was predicted by age, BMI and NIHSS score after IVT (Supplemental Table S3).

3.3. Association between FNG and Excellent Outcome

3.3.1. All Patients

Patients with FNG had a higher prevalence of an excellent 3-month outcome than those with fasting hyperglycemia (Table 1, Figure 1).

An excellent outcome occurred in 206 (56.9%) patients. Patients with excellent outcome were younger (median, IQR, 69.5 (59–78) vs. 77 (68–83) years, $p < 0.001$), less often women (43.7% vs. 56.9%, $p = 0.015$), less often suffered from hypertension (76.2% vs. 93.8%, $p < 0.001$) and atrial fibrillation (25.2% vs. 34.9%, $p = 0.049$), less often underwent MT (24.3% vs. 37.7%, $p = 0.007$), had lower NIHSS score on admission (mean ± SD, 9.1 ± 5.7 vs. 16.0 ± 6.0, $p < 0.001$) and after IVT (mean ± SD, 3.9 ± 3.8 vs. 14.8 ± 7.6, $p < 0.001$), a lower maximal SBP within 24 h after IVT (median, IQR 145 (126–159) vs. 146.5 (136–166) mmHg, $p = 0.019$), lower fasting glucose levels (median, IQR 6.3 (5.5–7.7) vs. 7.0 (6.1–8.8) mmol/L, $p < 0.001$) and less often experienced bleeding brain complications (9.2% vs. 37.0%, $p < 0.001$) compared with the remainder (Supplemental Table S1). In the multivariable logistic regression model, the excellent outcome was predicted by lower NIHSS score after IVT and the presence of FNG (Table 2). In the subgroup of patients treated only with IVT and without MT, an excellent 3-month outcome was predicted by age, NIHSS score after IVT and FNG (Supplemental Table S3).

3.3.2. Subgroup Analyses According to Diabetes

For non-diabetic patients, independent predictors of excellent outcome were lower age, female sex, lower NIHSS score after IVT and FNG (Table 2). In the subgroup of non-diabetic patients treated only with IVT, an excellent 3-month outcome was predicted by age and NIHSS score after IVT (Supplemental Table S3).

An excellent outcome for diabetics was predicted by a lower NIHSS score after IVT and lower creatinine concentration but not by FNG (Table 2). In the subgroup of patients with diabetes treated with IVT and without MT, the independent predictors of excellent outcome were BMI, NIHSS score after IVT and creatinine concentration (Supplemental Table S3).

3.4. Association between FNG and Mortality

At a 3-month follow-up, 54 (14.9%) patients died. Patients with FNG had a lower risk of death than those with fasting hyperglycemia (Table 1, Figure 1). The association between FNG and mortality was found in the univariable model for the whole group and the subgroup of patients treated only with IVT (Table 3, Supplemental Table S4). The factors that independently predicted the risk of death were older age, higher NIHSS score after IVT and hemorrhagic brain complications for the whole group, and age and NIHSS score after IVT in the subgroup of patients treated only with IVT and without MT (Table 3, Supplemental Table S4).

Table 3. The multivariable logistic regression model for the risk of death.

90-Day Risk of Death, Diabetic + Non-Diabetic Patients	Univariable			Multivariable		
	HR	95% CI	*p*-Value	HR	95% CI	*p*-Value
Age (per 1 year)	1.05	1.02–1.08	<0.001	1.07	1.03–1.11	<0.001
Sex (female)	1.48	0.82–2.66	0.189	-	-	-
BMI (per 1 unit)	1.07	0.94–1.08	0.870	-	-	-
NIHSS score after r-tPA (per 1 point)	1.24	1.17–1.31	<0.001	1.22	1.15–1.29	<0.001
Hemorrhagic brain complications (ECASS 1–3)	6.70	3.59–12.5	<0.001	2.66	1.19–5.91	0.017
Maximal SBP within 24 h after r-tPA (per 1 mmHg)	1.01	1.01–1.03	0.014	-	-	-
Hypertension	3.85	1.16–12.78	0.028	-	-	-
Atrial fibrillation	2.02	1.11–3.67	0.021	-	-	-
Platelets (per 10⁵/μL)	0.65	0.40–1.04	0.071	-	-	-
Fasting glucose < 5.5 mmol/L	1.47	0.04–0.62	0.009	0.23	0.03–1.81	0.164
90-day risk of death, diabetic patients						
Age (per 1 year)	1.03	0.98–1.09	0.254	-	-	-
Sex (female)	1.12	0.39–3.26	0.832	-	-	-
BMI (per 1 unit)	1.11	1.00–1.25	0.057	-	-	-
NIHSS score after r-tPA (per 1 point)	1.24	1.12–1.38	<0.001	1.27	1.12–1.42	<0.001
Hemorrhagic brain complications (ECASS 1–3)	4.06	1.30–12.7	0.016	-	-	-
Atrial fibrillation	3.70	1.22–11.2	0.021	5.12	1.31–20.1	0.019
Platelets count (per 10⁵/μL)	0.37	0.12–1.11	0.075	-	-	-
Fasting glucose < 5.5 mmol/L	0.51	0.06–4.31	0.539	-	-	-
90-day risk of death, non-diabetic patients						
Age (per 1 year)	1.06	1.02–1.09	<0.001	1.07	1.02–1.11	0.005
Sex (female)	1.67	0.83–3.38	0.153	-	-	-
BMI (per 1 unit)	0.94	0.85–1.03	0.190	-	-	-
NIHSS score after r-tPA (per 1 point)	1.24	1.16–1.33	<0.001	1.20	1.12–1.29	<0.001
Hemorrhagic brain complications (ECASS 1–3)	8.29	3.92–17.6	<0.001	2.93	1.12–7.69	0.029
Maximal SBP within 24 h after r-tPA (per 1 mmHg)	1.02	1.01–1.04	0.001	-	-	-
Hypertension	5.44	1.27–23.4	0.023	-	-	-
Fasting glucose < 5.5 mmol/L	0.08	0.01–0.62	0.015	0.07	0.01–2.10	0.125

Abbreviations, see Tables 1 and 2.

4. Discussion

Our study is the first to show that the association between FNG and long-term functional outcome after AIS treated with IVT is limited to the patients without pre-existent DM. This association was present even when the group of AIS patients was restricted to those who were treated only with IVT and without MT. Although this observation might be biased by a small sample size of patients with DM, our results were similar to the conclusions coming from our previous study performed on AIS patients who underwent MT [6]. Similarly, in the recent study of more than one thousand Chinese AIS patients, it was found that admission glucose levels independently predicted worse clinical outcomes after IVT only in patients without DM [12]. Non-diabetic patients seemed to be less adjusted to increased glucose levels than diabetics. This observation also came from a large cohort of more than 20,000 patients in whom fasting or random hyperglycemia increased the risk of transfer to an intensive care unit or in-hospital mortality only in non-diabetics [13]. Moreover, the pathophysiological mechanisms underlying the response to hyperglycemia in patients with and without DM might be different as glucose levels affected enlargement of infarct size in non-diabetic patients in contrast to diabetics [14]. Interestingly, in non-diabetic patients, female sex decreased the chance of a long-term excellent outcome. This observation stayed in line with previous research showing that after adjustment for age, women suffered from more severe AIS on admission and had a worse 3-month functional outcome [15].

Our study revealed that FNG after IVT resulted in a 3 or 4-fold increase in the chance of an excellent or favorable long-term outcome, respectively, at 3-month follow-up in AIS patients. Our results stayed in accordance with previous studies performed on smaller patient populations, which showed that fasting hyperglycemia after IVT increased the risk of worse outcome 3 months after AIS onset [3,4]. However, in our study, the effect size of fasting glucose levels was higher than previously reported. Data coming from a greater study that used a more complex parameter termed the stress hyperglycemia ratio but based on fasting glucose and glycated hemoglobin levels also indirectly supported the role of fasting hyper- or normoglycemia as prognostic factors in AIS patients treated with IVT [16]. In our study, fasting glucose levels influenced long-term outcomes, as did other well-known risk factors such as age and NIHSS score [17], both on admission and after IVT [17,18]. Interestingly, the lower maximal SBP within 24 h after IVT also independently affected the 3-month favorable outcome after AIS. Similarly, the Chinese study of 433 patients treated with IVT supported the prognostic role of lower SBP and revealed that maintaining its levels below 159.5 mmHg increased the probability of a favorable 3-month outcome [19].

We found that FNG decreased the chance of death within 3 months after AIS in patients treated with IVT in univariable analysis. In the previous studies, there was either no analysis concerning the association with mortality performed [4] or, similar to our findings, fasting glucose levels did not independently predict the risk of death in the multivariable analysis [3]. One of the possible explanations of the lack of association between FNG and mortality may be a small number of patients who died at the 3-month follow-up. Other factors might also exhibit a more important risk for long-term mortality after IVT, such as age or bleeding brain complications rate, as was shown in the Pomeranian Stroke Register in Poland during the 3-year post-AIS observation period [20].

Patients with normoglycemia were younger, had lower BMI and less often suffered from DM, suggesting that insulin resistance might play a key role in mediating the risk of a long-term unfavorable outcome [21]. On the other hand, in the Japanese trial of 4655 AIS patients, it was found that the association of insulin resistance with outcome was also maintained in non-diabetic and non-obese patients [22]. Finally, neither BMI nor the presence of DM predicted outcome in the multivariable logistic regression model in our study for the whole group of AIS patients treated with IVT.

Our study has important limitations. First, the character of the study was retrospective. Moreover, we did not monitor for a change in glucose levels in the forthcoming days after IVT. We also did not gather the information on whether patients developed DM after hospitalization. Second, the subgroup analyses, especially according to the DM, may be biased by the small sample size. Third, the confounders, such as age, NIHSS score and SBP value, had a significant influence on the outcome of this study. Fourth, the study included only patients of Caucasian origin; therefore, its results may not be generalized to the patients of other ethnicities. Fifth, the results reported here may not reflect a cause-effect relationship.

5. Conclusions

In conclusion, although FNG is an infrequent finding in patients with AIS treated with IVT, it increases the chance of a favorable and even an excellent 3-month outcome in non-diabetics. It seems reasonable to undertake future studies to develop the prognostic scales in AIS patients treated with IVT with FNG as one of the important factors.

Supplementary Materials: The following are available online at https://www.mdpi.com/article/10.3390/jcm10143005/s1, Supplemental Table S1. Baseline characteristics of patients according to modified Rankin scale (mRS). Supplemental Table S2. Baseline characteristics of patients treated only with intravenous thrombolysis (without mechanical thrombectomy) according to modified Rankin scale (mRS). Supplemental Table S3. Multivariable logistic regression model for favorable (mRS 0–2) and excellent (mRS 0–1) 3-month clinical outcome in patients treated only with intravenous thrombolysis (without mechanical thrombectomy). Supplemental Table S4. Multivariable logistic regression model for the risk of death in patients treated only with intravenous thrombolysis (without mechanical thrombectomy). Supplemental Figure S1. Patients treated only with intravenous thrombolysis (without mechanical thrombectomy) with favorable (mRS 0–2) or excellent (mRS 0–1) outcome and those who died according to the presence of fasting normoglycemia in the whole group (A), in the subgroup with (B), and without diabetes mellitus (C).

Author Contributions: M.W. (conceptualization, draft writing and editing), J.D. (data curation), L.D. (formal analysis, methodology and draft editing), M.M. (supervision and draft review), A.S. (supervision and draft review). All authors have read and agreed to the published version of the manuscript.

Funding: This research received no external funding.

Institutional Review Board Statement: The study was approved by the Jagiellonian University Ethical Committee (KBET 54/B/2007) and conducted according to the guidelines of the Declaration of Helsinki.

Informed Consent Statement: All patients gave informed consent to participate in the study, which was either written or verbal in the presence of at least two physicians in case of inability to use the dominant hand because of acute ischemic stroke.

Data Availability Statement: The data supporting the results of this study are available from the corresponding author upon reasonable request from any qualified investigator.

Conflicts of Interest: The authors declare no conflict of interest.

References

1. Poppe, A.; Majumdar, S.; Jeerakathil, T.; Ghali, W.; Buchan, A.; Hill, M. Admission Hyperglycemia Predicts a Worse Outcome in Stroke Patients Treated with Intravenous Thromobolysis. *Diabetes Care* **2009**, *32*, 3–8. [CrossRef] [PubMed]
2. Tsivgoulis, G.; Katsanos, A.H.; Mavridis, D.; Lambadiari, V.; Roffe, C.; MacLeod, M.J.; Sevcik, P.; Cappellari, M.; Nevšímalová, M.; Toni, D.; et al. Association of baseline hyperglycemia with outcomes of patients with and without diabetes with acute ischemic stroke treated with intravenous thrombolysis: A propensity score-matched analysis from the SITS-ISTR registry. *Diabetes* **2019**, *68*, 1861–1869. [CrossRef] [PubMed]
3. Osei, E.; Fonville, S.; Zandbergen, A.A.M.; Koudstaal, P.J.; Dippel, D.W.J.; den Hertog, H.M. Impaired fasting glucose is associated with unfavorable outcome in ischemic stroke patients treated with intravenous alteplase. *J. Neurol.* **2018**, *265*, 1426–1431. [CrossRef]
4. Cao, W.; Ling, Y.; Wu, F.; Yang, L.; Cheng, X.; Dong, Q. Higher fasting glucose next day after intravenous thrombolysis is independently associated with poor outcome in acute ischemic stroke. *J. Stroke Cerebrovasc. Dis.* **2015**, *24*, 100–103. [CrossRef] [PubMed]
5. Johnston, K.C.; Bruno, A.; Pauls, Q.; Hall, C.E.; Barrett, K.M.; Barsan, W.; Fansler, A.; Van De Bruinhorst, K.; Janis, S.; Durkalski-Mauldin, V.L. Intensive vs Standard Treatment of Hyperglycemia and Functional Outcome in Patients with Acute Ischemic Stroke: The SHINE Randomized Clinical Trial. *JAMA J. Am. Med. Assoc.* **2019**, *322*, 326–335. [CrossRef]

6. Wnuk, M.; Popiela, T.; Drabik, L.; Brzegowy, P.; Lasocha, B.; Wloch-Kopec, D.; Pulyk, R.; Jagiella, J.; Wiacek, M.; Kaczorowski, R.; et al. Fasting Hyperglycemia and Long-term Outcome in Patients with Acute Ischemic Stroke Treated with Mechanical Thrombectomy. *J. Stroke Cerebrovasc. Dis.* **2020**, *29*, 104774. [CrossRef] [PubMed]
7. Trouillas, P.; Von Kummer, R. Classification and pathogenesis of cerebral hemorrhages after thrombolysis in ischemic stroke. *Stroke* **2006**, *37*, 556–561. [CrossRef]
8. Wahlgren, N.; Ahmed, N.; Eriksson, N.; Aichner, F.; Bluhmki, E.; Dávalos, A.; Erilä, T.; Ford, G.A.; Grond, M.; Hacke, W.; et al. Multivariable Analysis of Outcome Predictors and Adjustment of Main Outcome Results to Baseline Data Profile in Randomized Controlled Trials. *Stroke* **2008**, *39*, 3316–3322. [CrossRef]
9. Ahmed, N.; Wahlgren, N.; Brainin, M.; Castillo, J.; Ford, G.A.; Kaste, M.; Lees, K.R.; Toni, D. Relationship of Blood Pressure, Antihypertensive Therapy, and Outcome in Ischemic Stroke Treated With Intravenous Thrombolysis. *Stroke* **2009**, *40*, 2442–2449. [CrossRef]
10. American Diabetes Association. Standards of medical care in diabetes 2014. *Diabetes Care* **2014**, *37*, S81–S90.
11. Powers, W.J.; Rabinstein, A.A.; Ackerson, T.; Adeoye, O.M.; Bambakidis, N.C.; Becker, K.; Biller, J.; Brown, M.; Demaerschalk, B.M.; Hoh, B.; et al. 2018 Guidelines for the Early Management of Patients With Acute Ischemic Stroke: A Guideline for Healthcare Professionals From the American Heart Association/American Stroke Association. *Stroke* **2018**, *49*, e46–e110. [CrossRef]
12. Fang, H.; Pan, Y.; Wang, Y.; Wang, C.; Wang, Y.; Zhong, L. Prognostic value of admission hyperglycemia on outcomes of thrombolysis in ischemic stroke patients with or without diabetes. *Chin. Med. J.* **2020**, *133*, 2244–2246. [CrossRef]
13. Tayek, C.J. Diabetes patients and non-diabetic patients intensive care unit and hospital mortality risks associated with sepsis. *World J. Diabetes* **2012**, *3*, 29. [CrossRef] [PubMed]
14. Shimoyama, T.; Kimura, K.; Uemura, J.; Saji, N.; Shibazaki, K. Elevated glucose level adversely affects infarct volume growth and neurological deterioration in non-diabetic stroke patients, but not diabetic stroke patients. *Eur. J. Neurol.* **2014**, *21*, 402–410. [CrossRef] [PubMed]
15. Fraticelli, L.; Freyssenge, J.; Claustre, C.; Buisson, M.; Bischoff, M.; Nighoghossian, N.; Derex, L.; El Khoury, C. Sex-Related Differences in Management and Outcome of Acute Ischemic Stroke in Eligible Patients to Thrombolysis. *Cerebrovasc. Dis.* **2019**, *47*, 196–204. [CrossRef]
16. Ngiam, J.N.; Cheong, C.W.S.; Leow, A.S.T.; Wei, Y.-T.; Thet, J.K.X.; Lee, I.Y.S.; Sia, C.-H.; Tan, B.Y.Q.; Khoo, C.-M.; Sharma, V.K.; et al. Stress Hyperglycaemia is Associated with Poor Functional Outcomes in Patients with Acute Ischaemic Stroke after Intravenous Thrombolysis. *QJM Int. J. Med.* **2020**, 1–5. [CrossRef] [PubMed]
17. Bandettini di Poggio, M.; Finocchi, C.; Brizzo, F.; Altomonte, F.; Bovis, F.; Mavilio, N.; Serrati, C.; Malfatto, L.; Mancardi, G.L.; Balestrino, M. Management of acute ischemic stroke, thrombolysis rate, and predictors of clinical outcome. *Neurol. Sci.* **2019**, *40*, 319–326. [CrossRef]
18. Wu, Z.; Zeng, M.; Li, C.; Qiu, H.; Feng, H.; Xu, X.; Zhang, H.; Wu, J. Time-dependence of NIHSS in predicting functional outcome of patients with acute ischemic stroke treated with intravenous thrombolysis. *Postgrad. Med. J.* **2019**, *95*, 181–186. [CrossRef] [PubMed]
19. Wu, L.; Huang, X.; Wu, D.; Zhao, W.; Wu, C.; Che, R.; Zhang, Z.; Jiang, F.; Bian, T.; Yang, T.; et al. Relationship between Post-Thrombolysis Blood Pressure and Outcome in Acute Ischemic Stroke Patients Undergoing Thrombolysis Therapy. *J. Stroke Cerebrovasc. Dis.* **2017**, *26*, 2279–2286. [CrossRef]
20. Chwojnicki, K.; Kozera, G.; Sobolewski, P.; Fryze, W.; Nyka, W.M. Intravenous thrombolysis and three-year ischemic stroke mortality. *Acta Neurol. Scand.* **2017**, *135*, 540–545. [CrossRef] [PubMed]
21. Perova, N.V.; Ozerova, I.N.; Aleksandrovich, O.V.; Metel'skaia, V.A.; Shal'nova, S.A. Clinical value of insulin resistance in fasting normoglycemia. *Kardiologiia* **2011**, *51*, 49–54. [PubMed]
22. Ago, T.; Matsuo, R.; Hata, J.; Wakisaka, Y.; Kuroda, J.; Kitazono, T.; Kamouchi, M. Insulin resistance and clinical outcomes after acute ischemic stroke. *Neurology* **2018**, *90*, E1470–E1477. [CrossRef] [PubMed]

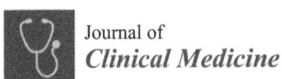

Article

RP11-362K2.2:RP11-767I20.1 Genetic Variation Is Associated with Post-Reperfusion Therapy Parenchymal Hematoma. A GWAS Meta-Analysis

Elena Muiño [1,†], Jara Cárcel-Márquez [1,†], Caty Carrera [2], Laia Llucià-Carol [1], Cristina Gallego-Fabrega [1,3], Natalia Cullell [1,4], Miquel Lledós [1], José Castillo [5], Tomás Sobrino [5], Francisco Campos [5], Emilio Rodríguez-Castro [6], Mònica Millán [7], Lucía Muñoz-Narbona [7], Alejandro Bustamante [7], Elena López-Cancio [8], Marc Ribó [9], José Álvarez-Sabín [10], Jordi Jiménez-Conde [11], Jaume Roquer [11], Eva Giralt-Steinhauer [11], Carolina Soriano-Tárraga [11], Cristófol Vives-Bauza [12], Rosa Díaz Navarro [13], Silvia Tur [13], Victor Obach [14], Juan F. Arenillas [15], Tomás Segura [16], Gemma Serrano-Heras [17], Joan Martí-Fàbregas [3], Raquel Delgado-Mederos [3], Pol Camps-Renom [3], Luis Prats-Sánchez [3], Daniel Guisado [3], Marina Guasch [3], Rebeca Marin [3], Alejandro Martínez-Domeño [3], Maria del Mar Freijo-Guerrero [18], Francisco Moniche [19], Juan Antonio Cabezas [19], Mar Castellanos [20], Jerzy Krupinsky [21,22], Daniel Strbian [23], Turgut Tatlisumak [24,25], Vincent Thijs [26,27], Robin Lemmens [28], Agnieszka Slowik [29], Joanna Pera [29], Laura Heitsch [30,31], Laura Ibañez [32], Carlos Cruchaga [32], Rajat Dhar [31], Jin-Moo Lee [31], Joan Montaner [19], Israel Fernández-Cadenas [1,*], on behalf of International Stroke Genetic Consortium and the Spanish Stroke Genetic Consortium

Citation: Muiño, E.; Cárcel-Márquez, J.; Carrera, C.; Llucià-Carol, L.; Gallego-Fabrega, C.; Cullell, N.; Lledós, M.; Castillo, J.; Sobrino, T.; Campos, F.; et al. *RP11-362K2.2:RP11-767I20.1* Genetic Variation Is Associated with Post-Reperfusion Therapy Parenchymal Hematoma. A GWAS Meta-Analysis. *J. Clin. Med.* **2021**, *10*, 3137. https://doi.org/10.3390/jcm10143137

Academic Editor: Hyo Suk Nam

Received: 7 June 2021
Accepted: 14 July 2021
Published: 16 July 2021

Publisher's Note: MDPI stays neutral with regard to jurisdictional claims in published maps and institutional affiliations.

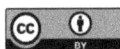

Copyright: © 2021 by the authors. Licensee MDPI, Basel, Switzerland. This article is an open access article distributed under the terms and conditions of the Creative Commons Attribution (CC BY) license (https://creativecommons.org/licenses/by/4.0/).

1. Stroke Pharmacogenomics and Genetics Group, Institut de Recerca de l'Hospital de la Santa Creu i Sant Pau, 08041 Barcelona, Spain; elena.muinho@gmail.com (E.M.); jara.carcel@gmail.com (J.C.-M.); laialluciacarol@gmail.com (L.L.-C.); cristina.gallego.fabrega@gmail.com (C.G.-F.); natalia.cullell@gmail.com (N.C.); miquel.lledos@gmail.com (M.L.)
2. Neurovascular Research Laboratory, Vall d'Hebron Institut de Recerca, Universitat Autònoma de Barcelona, 08025 Barcelona, Spain; catycarrerav@gmail.com
3. Department of Neurology, Hospital de la Santa Creu i Sant Pau, IIB-Sant Pau, 08025 Barcelona, Spain; jmarti@santpau.cat (J.M.-F.); rdelgado@santpau.cat (R.D.-M.); pcamps@santpau.cat (P.C.-R.); LPratsS@santpau.cat (L.P.-S.); DGuisado@santpau.cat (D.G.); MGuasch@santpau.cat (M.G.); rmarin@santpau.cat (R.M.); amartinezd@santpau.cat (A.M.-D.)
4. Stroke Pharmacogenomics and Genetics, Fundació MútuaTerrassa per la Docència i la Recerca, 08221 Terrassa, Spain
5. Clinical Neurosciences Research Laboratories, Health Research Institute of Santiago de Compostela (IDIS), 15706 Santiago de Compostela, Spain; jose.castillo.sanchez@sergas.es (J.C.); Tomas.Sobrino.Moreiras@sergas.es (T.S.); francisco.campos.perez@sergas.es (F.C.)
6. Department of Neurology, Hospital Clínico Universitario de Santiago, 15706 Santiago de Compostela, Spain; emiliorcastro@gmail.com
7. Department of Neuroscience, Hospital Germans Trias i Pujol, 08025 Badalona, Spain; mmillan.germanstrias@gencat.cat (M.M.); luciamunozn@gmail.com (L.M.-N.); alebustamanterangel@gmail.com (A.B.)
8. Stroke Unit, Hospital Universitario Central de Asturias, 33011 Oviedo, Spain; elenacancio@gmail.com
9. Stroke Unit, Hospital Universitario Valle de Hebrón, 08025 Barcelona, Spain; marcriboj@hotmail.com
10. Department of Neurology, Hospital Universitario Valle de Hebrón, Universidad Autónoma de Barcelona, 08025 Barcelona, Spain; josalvar@vhebron.net
11. Department of Neurology, Neurovascular Research Group, Instituto de Investigaciones Médicas Hospital del Mar-Hospital del Mar, 08025 Barcelona, Spain; jjimenez@imim.es (J.J.-C.); jroquer@hospitaldelmar.cat (J.R.); egiralt@imim.es (E.G.-S.); csoriano@imim.es (C.S.-T.)
12. Neurobiology Laboratory, Instituto de Investigación Sanitaria de Palma, 07120 Mallorca, Spain; cristofol.vives@ssib.es
13. Department of Neurology, Hospital Universitari Son Espases, 07120 Mallorca, Spain; rosam.diaz@ssib.es (R.D.N.); silvia.tur@ssib.es (S.T.)
14. Department of Neurology, Hospital Clínic i Provincial de Barcelona, 08025 Barcelona, Spain; VOBACH@clinic.cat
15. Department of Neurology, Hospital Clínico Universitario, University of Valladolid, 47003 Valladolid, Spain; juanfarenillas@gmail.com
16. Department of Neurology, Complejo Hospitalario Universitario de Albacete, 02006 Albacete, Spain; tseguram@gmail.com

17 Experimental Research Unit, Complejo Hospitalario Universitario de Albacete, 02006 Albacete, Spain; gemmas@sescam.jccm.es
18 Neurovascular Unit, Biocruces Bizkaia Health Research Institute, 48903 Bilbao, Spain; marimar.freijoguerrero@osakidetza.eus
19 Department of Neurology, Virgen del Rocío, Instituto de Biomedicina de Sevilla, 41013 Seville, Spain; pmoniche@gmail.com (F.M.); juancaro.jacr@gmail.com (J.A.C.); joan.montaner@vhir.org (J.M.)
20 Department of Neurology, Complejo Hospitalario Universitario A Coruña, 15006 A Coruña, Spain; Maria.del.Mar.Castellanos.Rodrigo@sergas.es
21 School of Healthcare Science, Manchester Metropolitan University, Manchester M15 6BH, UK; jkrupinski@mutuaterrassa.es
22 Neurology Unit, Hospital Universitari Mútua Terrassa, 08221 Terrassa, Spain
23 Department of Neurology, Helsinki University Hospital, FI-00029 Helsinki, Finland; daniel.strbian@hus.fi
24 Department of Clinical Neuroscience, Institute of Neurosciences and Physiology, Sahlgrenska Academy at University of Gothenburg, 41345 Gothenburg, Sweden; turgut.tatlisumak@neuro.gu.se
25 Department of Neurology, Sahlgrenska University Hospital, 41345 Gothenburg, Sweden
26 Stroke Division, Florey Institute of Neuroscience and Mental Health, University of Melbourne, Heidelberg VIC 3072, Australia; vincent.thijs@austin.org.au
27 Department of Neurology, Austin Health, Heidelberg VIC 3072, Australia
28 Department of Neurology, University Hospitals Leuven, Campus Gasthuisberg, 3000 Leuven, Belgium; robin.lemmens@uzleuven.be
29 Department of Neurology, Jagiellonian University Medical College, 31-007 Kraków, Poland; slowik@neuro.cm-uj.krakow.pl (A.S.); pera@su.krakow.pl (J.P.)
30 Division of Emergency Medicine, Washington University School of Medicine, St. Louis, MO 63110-1010, USA; lheitsch@wustl.edu
31 Department of Neurology, Washington University School of Medicine, St. Louis, MO 63110-1010, USA; dharr@wustl.edu (R.D.); leejm@wustl.edu (J.-M.L.)
32 Department of Psychiatry, Washington University School of Medicine, St. Louis, MO 63110-1010, USA; ibanezl@wustl.edu (L.I.); cruchagac@wustl.edu (C.C.)
* Correspondence: israelcadenas@yahoo.es
† E.M. and J.C.-M. contributed equally to this work.

Abstract: Stroke is one of the most common causes of death and disability. Reperfusion therapies are the only treatment available during the acute phase of stroke. Due to recent clinical trials, these therapies may increase their frequency of use by extending the time-window administration, which may lead to an increase in complications such as hemorrhagic transformation, with parenchymal hematoma (PH) being the more severe subtype, associated with higher mortality and disability rates. Our aim was to find genetic risk factors associated with PH, as that could provide molecular targets/pathways for their prevention/treatment and study its genetic correlations to find traits sharing genetic background. We performed a GWAS and meta-analysis, following standard quality controls and association analysis (fastGWAS), adjusting age, NIHSS, and principal components. FUMA was used to annotate, prioritize, visualize, and interpret the meta-analysis results. The total number of patients in the meta-analysis was 2034 (216 cases and 1818 controls). We found rs79770152 having a genome-wide significant association (beta 0.09, p-value 3.90×10^{-8}) located in the *RP11-362K2.2:RP11-767I20.1* gene and a suggestive variant (rs13297983: beta 0.07, p-value 6.10×10^{-8}) located in *PCSK5* associated with PH occurrence. The genetic correlation showed a shared genetic background of PH with Alzheimer's disease and white matter hyperintensities. In addition, genes containing the ten most significant associations have been related to aggregated amyloid-β, tau protein, white matter microstructure, inflammation, and matrix metalloproteinases.

Keywords: hemorrhagic transformation; parenchymal hematoma; GWAS; single nucleotide variants

1. Introduction

Stroke is the second most common cause of death worldwide, and the third most common cause of disability [1]. For ischemic strokes, the only treatments available during the acute phase are the reperfusion therapies such as thrombolysis and mechanical thrombectomy.

Ischemic strokes may present hemorrhagic transformation (HT). This may be early, associated with reperfusion of the occluded vessel; or late, which is thought to be related to increased permeability and blood flow [2].

HT is a well-recognized complication following reperfusion therapies. HT could be classified, according to the European Cooperative Acute Stroke Study (ECASS) criteria, into petechial infarction without space-occupying effect (HI) and hematoma/coagulum with mass effect (PH) [2].

HT may result in neurological deterioration [3], and the presence of a PH independently predicts early and late mortality, with a hazard ratio of late mortality of 7.9, with a 95% confidence interval (CI) of 2.9–21.4 [4]. Nevertheless, petechial changes may indicate that reperfusion occurred when the ischemic tissue was still at least partially viable.

Patients exhibiting an early HI did not have a higher risk of neurological deterioration compared with patients without hemorrhagic transformation. Among patients treated with rtPA, HI was even loosely associated with early improvement. Overall, three-month mortality and disability were also not influenced by HI [2].

The percentage of HT in studies of stroke patients varies from 6.4% to 43% [3], and the use of reperfusion therapies has favored the increase in this incidence. Moreover, clinical trials such as WAKE-UP [5], DAWN [6], or DEFUSE 3 [7] will allow a major use of these therapies, extending the time-window administration, which may lead to an increase in HT. It is therefore of utmost importance to identify those patients at higher risk of suffering a PH, as this is the subtype of HT that causes the highest morbidity and mortality [2,4].

There is a genetic predisposition for HTs following intravenous thrombolysis (IVT). This genetic contribution has been explored through candidate genes [8,9] or more recently through a Genome Wide Association Study (GWAS), carried out by our own group [10]. In this last study, we found that single nucleotide variants (SNVs) in the ZBTB46 gene were associated with PH in patients who underwent IVT [10]. For this purpose, we studied the extreme phenotype, patients with PH vs. patients without HT, excluding patients with petechial infarction (HI) subtype.

We decided to carry out a new analysis by including in the control group those patients who had a HI, to ensure that the findings achieved are exclusively attributed to the PH subtype due to reperfusion therapies, including patients that underwent mechanical thrombectomy or intra-arterial fibrinolysis, increasing our sample size, and with it, our statistical power.

Currently, articles using GWAS to understand different diseases are complemented by the study of genetic correlations with other traits to find common genetic architecture [11]. Knowing which traits share a genetic correlation allows a better understanding of diseases and the realization of further studies to find variants associated with them by increasing its statistical power, such as multitrait analysis of GWAS (MTAG). As example, the article performing a MTAG of small vessel occlusion strokes and intracerebral hemorrhage, due to these traits sharing a genetic background, allows us to find new loci associated with these diseases [12].

In the article we mentioned above, published by our group, we found that PH shared a genetic background with deep intracerebral hemorrhage (ICH), lobar ICH, and white matter hyperintensities (WMH) [10]. After Bonferroni correction, only lobar ICH remained significantly correlated.

Therefore, the aim of our study was to find genetic risk factors associated exclusively with PH, including patients with different reperfusion treatments. PH occurrence is still an important problem in the reperfusion strategy for stroke patients. Hence the importance of finding molecules that could be used as biomarkers to guide the therapeutic decision or potential therapeutic targets to prevent the appearance of this life-threatening complication. We also wanted to assess whether the same genetic correlations found in our previous paper were still found and whether we could find any new ones.

In this work we found a genome-wide significant locus associated with PH, regardless of the reperfusion treatment performed. Moreover, we found that there is a genetic correlation of PH with Alzheimer's disease and white matter hyperintensities (WMH). In fact, the study of nominally significant genomic loci in the meta-analysis has shown that pathways related to aggregated amyloid-β, tau protein, and inflammatory pathways could be related to PH occurrence.

2. Materials and Methods

This is an observational case-control study, conducted in a discovery and replication cohort, with subsequent meta-analysis of both results, in order to find SNVs associated with PH.

2.1. Subjects

2.1.1. Discovery Cohort

The participants included in the discovery cohort were part of the Genetic Study in Ischemic Stroke Patients treated with recombinant tissue plasminogen activator (r-tPA) (GenoTPA) [9], Genetic contribution to Functional Outcome and Disability after Stroke (GODS) [13], the Genotyping Recurrence Risk of Stroke (GRECOS) [14], and Genetics of Early Neurological Instability After Ischemic Stroke (GENISIS) [15] studies. These studies have, in common, the recruitment of patients with ischemic stroke between 2002 and 2020.

From these four studies, (n = 4667), 161 cases (patients with PH after reperfusion therapy) and 1236 controls (patients without PH after reperfusion therapy) fulfilled the inclusion and exclusion criteria, incorporated in a total of 8 batches (Table 1). All of the subjects of the discovery cohort had a Spanish origin.

Table 1. Discovery cohort.

Study	Total	Cases	Controls	Arrays	Batches	Country
GenoTPA [9]	240	34	180	HumanOmni1-Quad BeadChip (Illumina)	1	Spain
GODS [13]	993	28	342	HumanCoreExome (Illumina)	1	Spain
GRECOS [14]	214	3	0	HumanCoreExome (Illumina)	1	Spain
GENISIS [15]	3220	96	714	HumanCoreExome (Illumina)	5	Spain
Total	4667	161	1236		8	Spain

GenoTPA: Genetic Study in Ischemic Stroke Patients treated with recombinant tissue plasminogen activator (r-tPA); GODS: Genetic contribution to Functional Outcome and Disability after Stroke; GRECOS: Genotyping Recurrence Risk of Stroke study; GENISIS: Genetics of Early Neurological Instability After Ischemic Stroke.

2.1.2. Replication Cohort

The participants included in the replication cohort were part of the Genetic Study in Ischemic Stroke Patients treated with tPA (GenoTPA) [9], BAse de Datos de ICtus del hospital del MAR (BASICMAR) (Stroke database of the Hospital del Mar) [16], Leuven Stroke Genetics Study (LSGS) [17], Helsinki 2000 Ischemic Stroke Genetics Study, and Genetics of Early Neurological Instability After Ischemic Stroke (GENISIS) [15] studies.

From these five studies, the imputed genotype was available from a total of 1064 patients, 112 cases and 913 controls, incorporated in a total of 7 batches (Table 2).

For a detailed description of the different studies included in the discovery and replication cohorts see Supplemental Methods.

2.1.3. Variables

Detailed clinical-epidemiological data was collected from each patient, including age, sex, vascular risk factors such as hypertension, diabetes mellitus (DM), dyslipidemia (DLP), smoking habits, history of atrial fibrillation (AF), physical examination including stroke severity assessed with the National Institutes of Health Stroke Scale (NIHSS) at initial evaluation and the modified Rankin Score (mRS) prior to stroke, systolic (SBP) and diastolic blood pressure (DBP), initial glycaemia, TOAST classification, or treatment decisions. In Supplemental Methods, there is detailed information about variable definition.

CT scans were obtained prior to reperfusion procedure (baseline), and 24 h after, or whenever a neurological deterioration detected by the clinician was observed, to assess the presence of HT and its degree. All brain images were reviewed by a radiologist or neuro-radiologist.

Table 2. Replication cohort.

Study	Total	Cases	Controls	Arrays	Batches	Country
GenoTPA [9]	157	36	121	HumanOmni1-Quad BeadChip (Illumina)	1	Spain
BASICMAR	91	8	83	Human Omni Quad 5M (Illumina)	1	Spain
LSGS	45	8	37	Human Omni Quad 5M (Illumina)	1	Belgium
HELSINKI2000	164	12	152	HumanCoreExome (Illumina)	1	Finland
	70	2	68	HumanCoreExome (Illumina)	1	Finland
GENISIS [15]	53	4	49	HumanCoreExome (Illumina)	1	Poland
	484	42	403	HumanCoreExome (Illumina)	1	Spain
Total	1064	112	913		7	Spain

GenoTPA: Genetic Study in Ischemic Stroke Patients treated with recombinant tissue plasminogen activator (r-tPA); BASICMAR: BAse de Datos de ICtus del hospital del MAR; LSGS: Leuven Stroke Genetics Study; HELSINKI2000: Helsinki 2000 Ischemic Stroke Genetics Study; and Genetics of Early Neurological Instability After Ischemic Stroke studies.

HT was classified, according to the ECASS criteria, into petechial infarction without space-occupying effect (HI) with two subtypes, HI1 (small petechiae) and HI2 (more confluent petechiae); and hematoma/coagulum with mass effect (PH) divided into PH1 when affecting ≤30% of the infarct bed with mild mass effect and PH2, when affecting >30% of the infarct bed with significant mass effect or remote hemorrhage [2].

As the aim of our study was to find SNV associated with the risk of PH (PH1 and PH2) after reperfusion treatment, patients without HT or with HI (HI1 and HI2) were chosen as controls, and patients with PH were chosen as cases. Remote hemorrhages were excluded from the study, as their etiology has not yet been clarified and the biological mechanisms underlying remote hemorrhages are probably different compared to the other HTs [18].

2.1.4. Eligibility Criteria

For the association study, patients >18 years of age with an ischemic stroke that underwent reperfusion therapy (ITV, including mechanical thrombectomy or intra-arterial fibrinolysis as second intention), who presented with PH, were considered as cases. Controls were selected as patients >18 years with ischemic stroke that underwent reperfusion therapy, who did not present HT or who presented with HI.

Exclusion criteria: patients not receiving reperfusion therapy, who suffered a remote PH or unknown HT phenotype.

2.1.5. Standard Protocol Approvals and Patient Consent

This study was approved by the local ethics committee of each participant and an informed consent document was signed by every patient or their relatives.

2.2. Genotyping

DNA samples were genotyped on commercial arrays from Illumina (San Diego, CA, USA) (Tables 1 and 2).

2.2.1. Quality Control

For detailed quality controls performed see Supplemental Methods.

Briefly, SNV missing in a large proportion of the subjects, non-biallelic SNV, ambiguous, monomorphic or duplicated SNV, or SNV that violates the Hardy–Weinberg (dis)equilibrium (HWE) law were deleted.

Individuals with high rates of genotype missingness, sex discrepancy or unknown sex, family members or duplicated samples, non-European individuals, and patients with outlier heterozygosity rates ($n = 814$) were removed.

After all these QCs, the total number of patients was 141 cases and 1003 controls in the discovery cohort. To ensure that there were no duplicate samples between the discovery and replication cohorts, patients with a pihat > 0.8 were removed from replication cohort. The number of patients with information for the covariates introduced in the analysis were 1139, 140 cases and 999 controls.

Finally, 895 patients (76 cases and 819 controls) passed the QC and had information for the covariates in the analysis, constituting the replication cohort.

Studies genotyped on the same platforms were combined in the discovery cohort. For the replication cohorts data were already imputed [10].

2.2.2. Genome Build

All genomic coordinates are given in NCBI Build 37/UCSC hg19.

2.3. Imputation

Imputation was performed with the Michigan Imputation Server Pipeline using Minimac4, following their instructions (https://imputationserver.readthedocs.io/en/latest (accessed on 1 May 2021)). HRC r1.1 2016 (GRCh37/hg19) was the reference panel used, with European population and, for phasing, Eagle v2.4 was used.

After imputation, QC were performed. We removed SNV with $r^2 < 0.6$ and MAF < 0.1%. After merging all cohorts, SNVs that were not present in at least 90% of the individuals were removed.

2.4. Genome-Wide Association Analysis and Meta-Analysis

We performed a linear regression-based association analysis using fastGWAS [19]. Those SNV with minor allele count (MAC) < 6 were subsequently removed. For the discovery cohort, we adjusted for the first two principal components (PC) (Figure 1), age and the variables remaining significant in the multivariable logistic regression (p-value < 0.05) and that we had information on the replication cohort: NIHSS. For the replication cohort, the analysis was adjusted for the three first PC (Figure 1), and the same clinical variables as in the discovery analysis: age and NIHSS.

Due to the small sample size of the discovery cohort, in order to increase statistical power, we carried out a meta-analysis of the results of the discovery and replication cohort with the metal software (http://csg.sph.umich.edu/abecasis/metal (accessed on 5 May 2021)), weighted by the number of individuals contributing to each result [20]. Genomic control correction was applied to both input files and then to the meta-analysis results.

A p-value $< 5 \times 10^{-8}$ was considered genome-wide significant and a p-value $< 1 \times 10^{-5}$ a nominal genome-wide association.

2.5. Functional Annotation of Associated Variants

FUMA (Functional Mapping and Annotation of Genome-Wide Association Studies) was used to annotate, prioritize, visualize, and interpret the meta-analysis results (https://fuma.ctglab.nl (accessed on 6 May 2021)) [21]. This platform also permits the realization of an ANNOVAR enrichment test; MAGMA gene analysis, gene-set analysis and gene-property analysis; identification of expression quantitative trait loci (eQTL), chromatin interaction data, and mapping. It also provides information about the RegulomeBD score. This score, that provides information on the probability of affect binding and expression of target gene, goes from 1 (most likely) to 7 (least likely). As a reference panel, we used UKB release2b 10k European population.

To search for traits to which the genes closest to the most significant SNVs have been related, we used the GWAS Catalog (https://www.ebi.ac.uk/gwas (accessed on 6 May 2021)).

For finding gene ontology (GO) terms of the genes of interest, we performed a search in Ensembl (https://www.ensembl.org/index.html (accessed on 6 May 2021)).

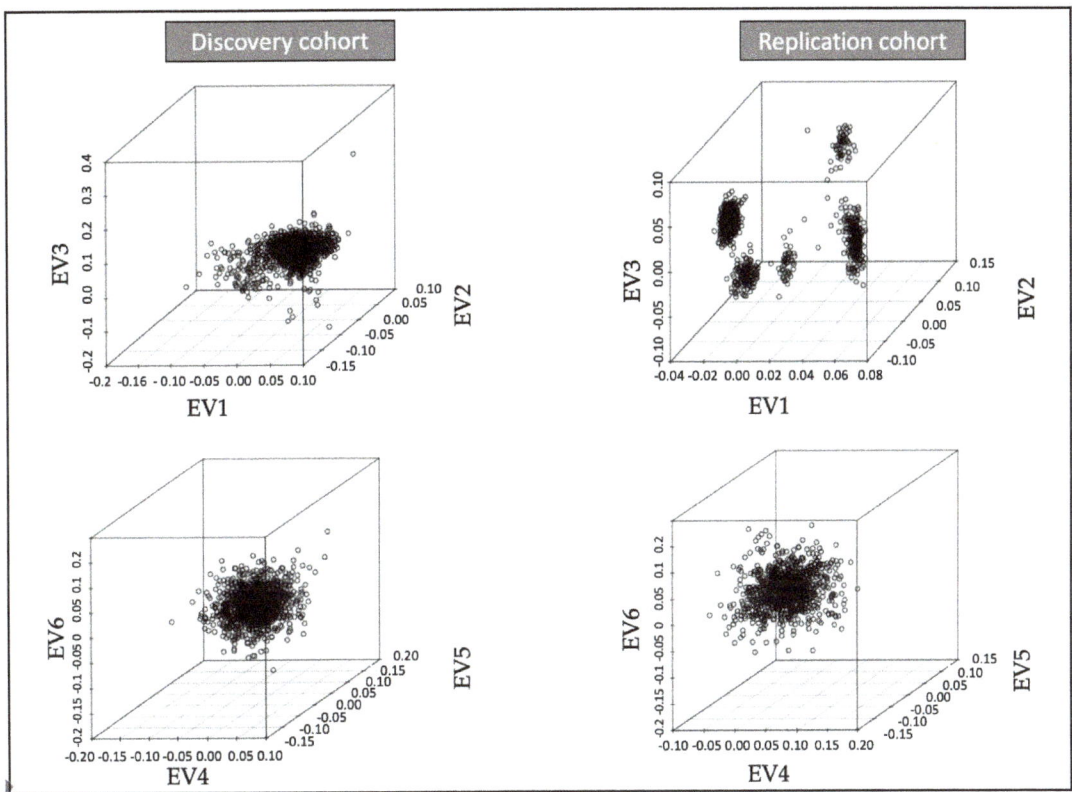

Figure 1. Principal component analysis (PCA) representation for discovery and replication cohorts. EV: eigenvector.

2.6. Estimation of Genetic Correlations

We used GNOVA (GeNetic cOVariance Analyzer) to estimate genetic covariance and correlation between traits. For this estimation, GNOVA only requires the genetic information available in the summary statistics of the traits of interest.

We tested genetic correlation for traits that have been related with HT: any ischemic strokes (AIS, n = 440,328), large artery atherosclerosis strokes (LAS, n = 301,663), cardioembolic strokes (CES, n = 362,661), and small vessel occlusion strokes (SVO, n = 348,946) using MEGASTROKE European data [22], deep intracerebral hemorrhage (n = 2075) [23], lobar intracerebral hemorrhage (n = 1148) [23], white matter hyperintensities (WMH, n = 11,226) [24], Alzheimer's disease (AD, n = 63,926) [11], total cholesterol (n = 94,595) [25], LDL (n = 94,595) [25], HDL (n = 94,595) [25], triglycerides (n = 94,595) [25], sistolic blood pressure (SBP, n = 757,601) [26], diastolic blood pressure (DBP, n = 757,601) [26], and diabetes mellitus 2 (DM2) (n = 69,033) [27].

2.7. Statistical Analyses

R version 3.6.3 and Bioconductor packages were used to perform the statistical analysis. To study whether there were significant differences (p-value < 0.05) between cases and controls in the discovery and replication cohorts, for quantitative variables with a normal distribution, we used t-test and a Mann–Whitney U for non-normal quantitative or ordinal variables. The Chi-square test was used for categorical variables.

Multivariable logistic regression was conducted following a forward stepwise approach to select clinical variables as covariates for the association study. First, univariable logistic regression was performed to study the association between the available variables and the occurrence of PH. Then, they were added to the multivariable logistic regression model according to their *p*-value, from the most significant to the least.

Variables with more than 10% missing values (less than 1030 observations) were not taken into account for the multivariate model (DLP, smoking habits, mRS, SBP, DBP, intra-arterial fibrinolysis, and mechanical thrombectomy), as the results of subsequent statistical analyses might be biased [28] and the analysis underpowered.

2.8. Data Availability

The data that supports the findings of this study is available from the corresponding author upon reasonable request.

3. Results

3.1. Descriptive Analysis of the Cohorts

3.1.1. Discovery

A total of 1144 patients with an ischemic stroke, and who were treated with reperfusion treatment, met the inclusion criteria and passed the QC; a total of 1139, with 140 cases and 999 controls, had information for the covariates of the analysis. A total of 10,058,599 SNP passed QC and were evaluated.

There was a total of 141 cases with PH (12%) and 1003 controls (88%). Of these controls, 840 had no hemorrhagic transformation (84%) and 163 had HI (16%). Cases were 77 ± 12 years old (median ± interquartile range -IQR-), 52% were males, 13% (11/88) received intra-arterial fibrinolysis, and none received mechanical thrombectomy. Controls were 75 ± 16 years old (median ± IQR), 55% were males, 5% (28/620) received intra-arterial fibrinolysis, and 6% (17/286) mechanical thrombectomy. In the univariable analysis, the variables significantly associated with PH were a higher NIHSS, higher mean mRS (0.83 vs. 0.46 in controls), higher percentage of intra-arterial fibrinolysis, and lower percentage of strokes of atherothrombotic etiology. The detailed descriptive analysis can be found in Table 3.

The final sample for the analysis with information for all the covariates included in the association test was 1139 patients, with 140 cases and 999 controls.

In the multivariate analysis with age and the first two PCs, only NIHSS remains significant (p-value 5.36×10^{-3}). Variables with a miss rate >10% or those that were not collected in the replication cohort were excluded from this analysis.

3.1.2. Replication

A total of 895 patients with an ischemic stroke undergoing reperfusion treatment, met the inclusion criteria and passed the QC. A total of 7,224,265 SNP after QCs were evaluated.

There was a total of 76 cases with PH (8%) and 819 controls (92%). Cases were 76 ± 11 years old (median ± IQR) and 53% were males. Controls were 72 ± 17 years old (median ± IQR) and 52% were males. In the univariable analysis, the variables significantly associated with PH were a higher age, a higher proportion of AF and CES, and a higher NIHSS. The detailed descriptive analysis can be found in Table 4.

The final sample for the analysis with covariates was 895 patients, 76 cases and 819 controls.

3.2. GWAS

We did not observe any SNV that reached the GWAS significance threshold (p-value $< 5 \times 10^{-8}$) in the discovery analysis.

The Manhattan and quantile-quantile (QQ) plots, obtained from the discovery and replication cohorts association study, can be visualized in the supplementary Figures S1 and S2, respectively. We did not observe an overall inflation of *p*-values; genomic inflation factor λ was 1.007 in the discovery cohort and 0.999 in the replication.

Table 3. Descriptive analysis of discovery cohort.

Variables (Number of Observations)	Controls (n = 1003)	Cases (n = 141)	p-Value	OR (95% IC)
Age (n= 1142)	75 ± 16	77 ± 12	6.70×10^{-2}	
Sex (n = 1144), male	55% (548/1003)	52% (73/141)	5.29×10^{-1}	0.89 (0.62–1.29)
HTN (n = 1138)	64% (634/998)	65% (91/140)	7.79×10^{-1}	1.07 (0.73–1.58)
DM (n = 1143)	22% (225/1002)	30% (42/141)	5.64×10^{-2}	1.46 (0.97–2.19)
DLP (n = 821)	38% (279/728)	37% (34/93)	8.21×10^{-1}	0.93 (0.57–1.48)
AF (n = 1140)	37% (299/999)	38% (53/141)	7.93×10^{-2}	1.41 (0.96–2.07)
SH (n = 788)	21% (148/698)	18% (16/90)	3.93×10^{-1}	0.8 (0.42–1.44)
NIHSS (n = 1141)	**14 ± 11**	**17 ± 9**	$\mathbf{4.11 \times 10^{-4}}$	
mRS (n = 587)	**0 ± 1**	**0 ± 1**	$\mathbf{1.84 \times 10^{-2}}$	
Gly (n = 1104)	119 ± 44	127 ± 49	1.02×10^{-1}	
SBP (n = 705)	153 ± 35	158 ± 37	2.50×10^{-1}	
DBP (n = 731)	80 ± 20	80 ± 20	4.47×10^{-1}	
IA (n = 708)	**5% (28/620)**	**13% (11/88)**	$\mathbf{5.12 \times 10^{-3}}$	**3.01 (1.30–6.55)**
TM (n = 336)	6% (17/286)	0% (0/50)	8.72×10^{-2}	0 (0–1.36)
CES (n = 1115)	46% (451/977)	55% (76/138)	5.57×10^{-2}	1.43 (0.98–2.08)
LAS (n = 1115)	**20% (193/977)**	**9% (11/138)**	$\mathbf{3.91 \times 10^{-4}}$	**0.35 (0.17–0.67)**
SVO (n = 1115)	1% (12/977)	1% (2/138)	6.88×10^{-1}	1.18 (0.13–5.40)

OR (95% IC): odds ratio (95% confidence interval -CI-). HTN: hypertension, DLP: dyslipidemia, AF: atrial fibrillation, SH: smoking habits, NIHSS: National Institutes of Health Stroke Scale, mRS: modified Rankin Score, Gly: initial glycaemia, SBP: systolic blood pressure, DBP: diastolic blood pressure; IA: intra-arterial fibrinolysis, TM: mechanical thrombectomy, CES: cardioembolic stroke, LAS: large artery atherosclerosis stroke, SVO: small vessel occlusion stroke. For quantitative variables, information is expressed as median ± interquartile range. For categorical variables in frequency (%). Variables significantly associated with PH (p-value < 0.05) are highlighted in bold.

Table 4. Descriptive analysis of the replication cohort.

Variables (Number of Observations)	Controls (n = 819)	Cases (n = 76)	p-Value	OR (95% IC)
Age (n = 895)	72 ± 17	76 ± 11	9.82×10^{-3}	
Sex (n = 895), male	52% (425/819)	53% (40/76)	1	1.03 (0.63–1.7)
DM (n = 643)	18% (103/586)	16% (9/57)	8.56×10^{-1}	0.88 (0.37–1.89)
AF (n = 770)	32% (223/700)	49% (34/70)	7.40×10^{-3}	2.02 (1.19–3.42)
NIHSS (n = 895)	11 ± 11	16 ± 8	6.33×10^{-6}	
Gly (n = 464)	120 ± 42	135 ± 52	1.35×10^{-1}	
CES (n = 670)	60% (365/604)	77% (51/66)	7.36×10^{-3}	2.22 (1.20–4.36)

OR (95% IC): odds ratio (95% confidence interval). AF: atrial fibrillation, NIHSS: National Institutes of Health Stroke Scale, Gly: initial glycaemia, CES: cardioembolic stroke. For quantitative variables, information is expressed as median ± interquartile range. For categorical variables, in frequency (%).

3.3. Meta-Analysis

With the meta-analysis, we found a genomic locus with a significant genome-wide association (p-value $<5 \times 10^{-8}$). This genomic locus is constituted by 57 SNV in our meta-analysis (Supplementary Table S1). Its leading SNV is 12:59127963:A:G (rs79770152) and it is an intronic variant located in the RP11-362K2.2:RP11-767I20.1 gene, with a p-value of 3.90×10^{-8} (MAF: 0.09; Beta coefficient: 0.09, standard error (SE): 0.015).

In addition, a total of 28 genomic loci with nominal SNV were found (p-value $< 1.00 \times 10^{-5}$) (Supplementary Table S2). One of these loci contains a leading SNV that almost reaches statistical significance at genome-wide level, 9:78563802:G:T (rs13297983). It is an intronic variant located in the gene PCSK5 with a p-value of 6.10×10^{-8} (MAF: 0.07; Beta coefficient: 0.097, SE: 0.017).

None of these two SNVs are eQTL or present chormatin interactions regarding the databases available in FUMA. Table 5 shows the description of the top ten genomic loci with the most significant SNV and Figure 2 the Manhattan plot.

One of the SNV belonging to one of this top ten genomic loci (17:72393744:A:G, rs4348170, p-value 1.60×10^{-6}) has been associated in another GWAS with interleukin levels [28]. If we perform a GWAS Catalog search for the genes closest to the leading SNVs of these genomic loci, we find that variants of PCSK5 have been associated with diffuse plaques of aggregated amyloid-β peptide in the brain, measurement of tau protein in the form of paired helical filaments, apolipoproteina B, or LDL levels regarding the consumption of alcohol. KLF5 with neutrophil and monocyte count or lymphocyte percentage of leukocytes. TGFBR3 with multiple sclerosis and pulse pressure measurement. C15orf48 with urinary albumin to creatinine ratio, glomerular filtration rate, and albuminuria. RNA5SP448 with LDL and interleukin 12 measurement. SEMA3A with white matter microstructure measurement, cortical thickness, major depression, and alcohol dependence or DNA methylation. EIF3H with neurofibrillary tangles.

Gene-based analysis performed with FUMA took into account a total of 18317 protein coding genes. Therefore, the significant p-value corrected for multiple comparisons was 2.73×10^{-6}. None of the genes reached statistical significance. The most significant associations were SLC30A4 (p-value 1.82×10^{-5}) and C15orf48 (p-value 4.58×10^{-5}), both in chromosome 15 (Figure 3).

3.4. MAGMA Analysis and GO Terms

FUMA platform performs MAGMA gene-set analysis for curated gene sets and gene ontology (GO) terms obtained from MsigDB. The only significant association after adjusting for the Bonferroni method was the GO term (molecular function) myosin V binding (adjusted p-value 2.04×10^{-3}), which definition is the interaction selectively and non-covalently with a class V myosin. Supplementary Table S3 shows the top ten of the most significant curated gene sets and GO terms.

The most relevant GO terms could be visualized on Table 5.

3.5. Genetic Correlations

Genetic correlation analysis detected a shared genetic background among PH presence and Alzheimer' Disease and white matter hyperintensities (WMH) with a raw p-value < 0.05 (Table 6). None of the traits reached a significant p-value adjusted for multiple comparisons (p-value adjusted with Bonferroni method: 4.16×10^{-3}).

Table 5. The ten genomic loci with its leading SNV.

ID	Rs	p-Value	Beta (SE)	MAF	Nearest Gene	Func	RDB	eQTL	GO Terms
12:59127963:A:G	rs79770152	Metal: 3.90×10^{-8} DC: 2.18×10^{-5} RC: 3.79×10^{-5}	0.0895 (0.0152) (++)	9%	RP11-362K2.2;RP11-767I20.1	ncRNA (intronic)	7		
9:78563802:G:T	rs13297983	Metal: 6.10×10^{-8} DC: 7.80×10^{-7} RC: 1.00×10^{-3}	0.0968 (0.0166) (++)	7%	PCSK5	Intronic	7		Renin secretion into blood stream, proteolysis, heart development
13:73655521:G:T	rs1537385	Metal: 1.69×10^{-7} DC: 1.11×10^{-4} RC: 4.09×10^{-5}	−0.1096 (0.0195) (−−)	4%	KLF5	Intergenic	3a		Angiogenesis
10:10130938:A:G	rs35246078	Metal: 1.87×10^{-7} DC: 1.50×10^{-4} RC: 3.57×10^{-5}	0.1091 (0.0195) (++)	7%	RP5-933E2.1	Intergenic	6		
4:148508838:G:T	rs61170156	Metal: 1.28×10^{-6} DC: 2.20×10^{-5} RC: 1.45×10^{-3}	0.0670 (0.0129) (++)	17%	RP11-752L20.5	ncRNA (intronic)	5	TMEM184C (thyroid), GPRC5C, CD300C, BTBD17, KIF19, FDXR, MRP57	
1:92310874:A:G	rs6686126	Metal: 1.37×10^{-6} DC: 9.87×10^{-3} RC: 3.13×10^{-6}	0.0868 (0.0167) (++)	7%	TGFBR3	Intronic	2b		Blood vessel development, heart morphogenesis, organ regeneration
15:45737253:A:C	rs72711259	Metal: 1.58×10^{-6} DC: 2.12×10^{-2} RC: 6.62×10^{-7}	0.0731 (0.0142) (++)	12%	C15orf48	Intronic	7	SLC28A2 (rectum, colon, esofagus and gastroesophagus junction, tibial nerve, testis, thyroid, cervical spinal cord), SQRDL (thyroid), SLC30A4, SHF (cervical spinal cord), DUOX1 (cerebellum), SORD, SPATA5L1 (adipose tissue, whole blood, artery tibial, esofagus and gastroesophagus junction, skeletal muscle, thyroid), SLC28A2, SPATA5L1, RP11-96O20.4, GATM (artery tibial, skeletal muscle), TRIM69 (thyroid)	Nucleus, mitochondrion
17:72393744:A:G	rs4348170	Metal: 1.60×10^{-6} DC: - RC: 2.55×10^{-7}	0.1077 (0.0209) (?+)	10%	RNA5SP448	Intergenic	NA	BTBD17, FDXR (brain cortex), CD300C, FDXR, GPRC5C (adrenal gland), KIF19, MRP57 (liver)	

Table 5. Cont.

ID	Rs	p-Value	Beta (SE)	MAF	Nearest Gene	Func	RDB	eQTL	GO Terms
7:83857204:C:T	rs7802925	Metal: 2.09×10^{-6} DC: 4.73×10^{-6} RC: 6.89×10^{-3}	−0.0907 (0.0178) (−−)	6%	SEMA3A	Intronic	5		Apoptotic process, neuron migration, nerve development
8:117535199:C:T	rs16888486	Metal: 2.19×10^{-6} DC: 2.71×10^{-3} RC: 3.10×10^{-5}	−0.1023 (0.0201) (++)	6%	EIF3H	Intergenic	7	UTP23 (whole blood)	Gene expression, extracellular vesicular exosome

ID: SNV identifier; rs: RefSNP; Beta (SE): β coefficient and standard error, between brackets the direction of the SNV in the discovery and replication cohort; MAF: minor allele frequency; Func: functional consequence of the SNV on the gene obtained from ANNOVAR; RDB: RegulomeDB score which is the categorical score (from 1a to 7), 1a is the highest score that the SNV has the most biological evidence to be regulatory element; eQTL: expression quantitative trait loci, here appears the gene which expression the SNV modifies; GO terms: the most relevant gene ontology terms. +: positive effect of the β coefficient; −: negative effect of the β coefficient; ?: the SNV was not evaluated; the first symbol corresponds to discovery and the second to replication cohorts.

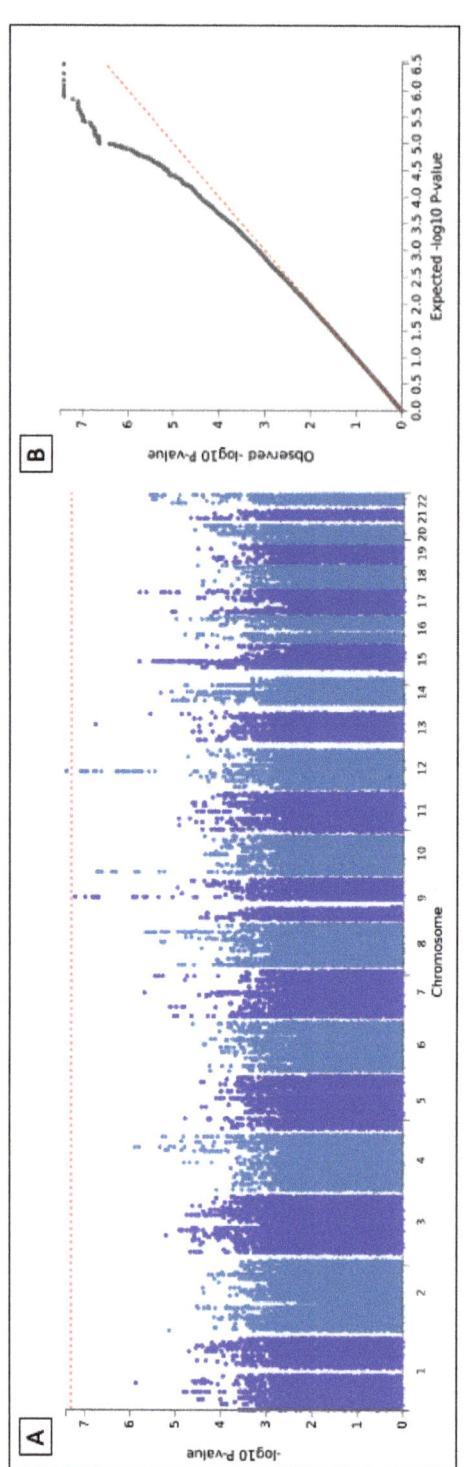

Figure 2. Manhattan and QQ plot of the meta-analysis. (**A**) Manhattan plot. SNVs were represented by dots and plotted based on their genome-wide association study *p*-values. Red line shows genome-wide significance (*p*-value $< 5 \times 10^{-8}$). (**B**) QQ plot of the *p*-values obtained after the association testing. The x-axis represents the expected $-\log_{10}$ *p*-value under the null hypothesis and lambda is the median of the resulting chi-squared test statistics divided by the expected median of the chi-squared distribution under the null hypothesis.

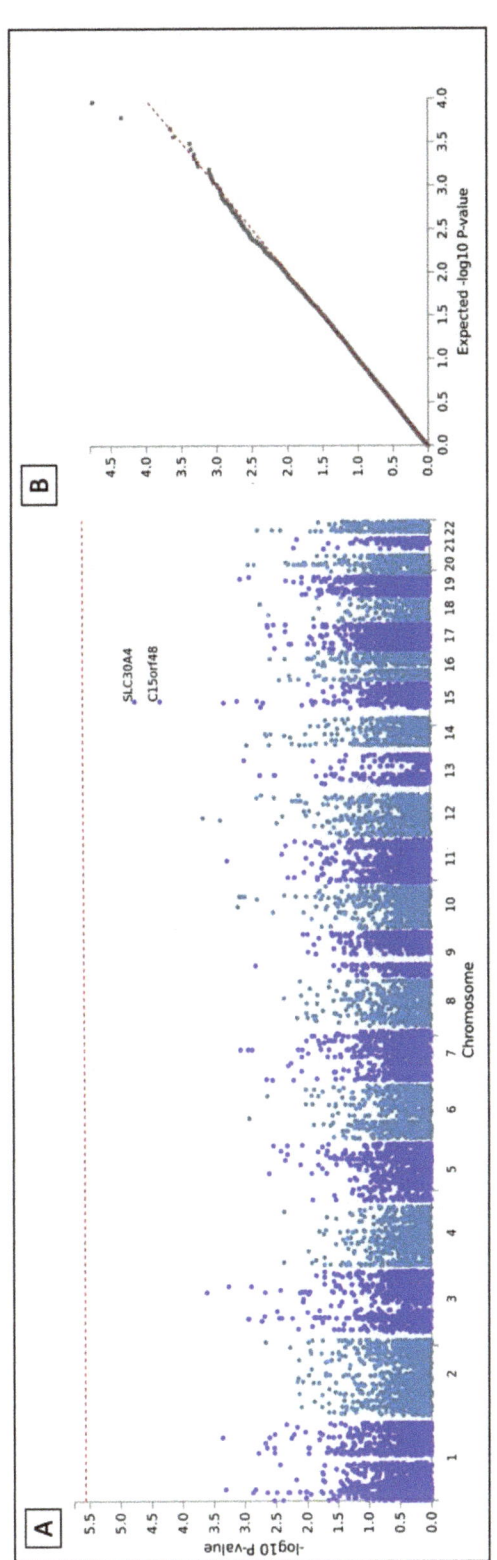

Figure 3. Manhattan and QQ plot of the gene-based meta-analysis. (**A**) Manhattan plot. Genes were represented by dots and plotted based on their *p*-values. Red line shows the considered significant *p*-value ($p < 5 \times 10^{-8}$). (**B**) QQ plot of the *p*-values obtained after the association testing. The x-axis represents the expected $-\log_{10}$–*p*-value under the null hypothesis and lambda is the median of the resulting chi-squared test statistics divided by the expected median of the chi-squared distribution under the null hypothesis.

Table 6. Results of the genetic correlation (GNOVA).

Trait	Rho	Rho SE	Corr	p-Value
Alzheimer's Disease	0.049	0.021	0.200	2.15×10^{-2}
White Matter Hyperintensities	−0.100	0.047	−2.257	3.46×10^{-2}
Deep ICH	0.089	0.80	0.141	2.66×10^{-1}
ICH	0.070	0.082	0.199	3.03×10^{-1}
SVO	−0.006	0.008	−0.067	4.90×10^{-1}
SBP	−0.007	0.013	−0.021	6.06×10^{-1}
Lobar ICH	0.031	0.080	0.189	6.96×10^{-1}
CES	−0.002	0.008	−0.021	7.96×10^{-1}
AIS	−0.002	0.008	−0.017	8.32×10^{-1}
DBP	−0.003	0.013	−0.009	8.41×10^{-1}
LAS	−0.001	0.009	−0.006	9.46×10^{-1}
AS	−0.0005	0.008	−0.005	2.66×10^{-1}

Rho: the genetic covariance estimate; rho SE: standard error of the estimate of rho; Corr: the genetic correlation estimate. ICH: intracerebral hemorrhage; SVO: small vessel occlusion stroke; SBP: systolic blood pressure; CES: cardioembolic stroke; AIS: any ischemic stroke; DBP: diastolic blood pressure; LAS: large artery atherosclerosis stroke; AS: all strokes. Traits with p-values < 0.05 are highlighted in bold.

4. Discussion

This is an observational case-control study in order to find genetic risk factors and biological mechanisms associated with brain parenchymal hemorrhagic transformation after reperfusion treatment in ischemic stroke.

In a previous work by our group, we explored which SNVs were associated with hemorrhagic transformation through a GWAS, analyzing extreme phenotypes: PH vs. non hemorrhagic transformation in patients undergoing only IVT [10]. This led to the finding that rs7648433, located in *ZBTB46* gene, was associated with this phenotype and it has been implicated in mechanisms such as shear stress and atherosclerosis in other studies.

In the current study, we analyzed patients undergoing IVT and including, additionally, patients with intra-arterial fibrinolysis or mechanical thrombectomy. We wanted to obtain more generalized results, as these therapies are widely used and their window time administration has recently been increased [5–7]. This longer time-window administration may lead to an increase of hemorrhagic complications, one of the major problems of these treperfusion therapies. Understanding why a patient may develop PH including patients underwent any type of reperfusion treatment may be of great interest, as this subtype is the one with the highest rates of morbi-mortality [2,4].

In addition, we have added other HT subtypes different from PH to the group of controls (HI). This strategy is interesting to find genetic risk factors associated exclusively to PH in contrast to our previous work [10], as we are avoiding any possible genetic risk factor that could be associated to both, HI and PH.

Including HI patients and all reperfusion therapies, we could increase the number of cases respect to previous studies, increasing our statistical power and analyzing the major genetic study performed in this field. In our previous work, we analyzed 1904 patients and in our present study, we were able to analyze 2034 patients.

The differences in these sample sizes are due to the slight increase in the number of cohorts introduced, the generalization of the study to patients who had undergone intra-arterial fibrinolysis or mechanical thrombectomy as a second intention, and the different QC carried out.

Although we did not find statistically significant SNVs after adjusting for multiple comparisons in our discovery cohort, the meta-analysis did allow us to detect rs79770152 with a *p*-value 3.90×10^{-8}, an intronic variant located in the *RP11-362K2.2:RP11-767I20.1* genes, which are uncharacterized genes. We found that the lncRNAs are supposed to likely exert their functions in other genomic locations (trans-regulation) [29].

Another SNV very close to be genome-wide significant was rs13297983 with a *p*-value 6.10×10^{-8}, an intronic variant located in the gene *PCSK5*.

From these leading SNVs of the first ten loci, we can point out that there is one with the most biological evidence to be a regulatory element: rs6686126, an intronic variant located in TGFBR3. In addition, some of these SNVs are eQTL which regulate the expression of different genes in tissues such as the brain, arteries, and peripheral nerves. None of these two SNVs most significant are eQTL or present chromatin interactions regarding the databases available in FUMA.

All the leading SNVs that constituted the top ten most significant variants, followed the same direction of effect in the discovery and replication cohorts. Except rs4348170, which was not present in the discovery cohort. Furthermore, some of the GO terms were related with angiogenesis or neuronal development. This is noteworthy, since the blood vessel is of relevance in the PH and neuronal apoptosis in the prognosis.

Interestingly, several of the genes from the genes included in these loci have been associated in other GWAS studies to aggregated amyloid-β peptide and tau protein such as *PCSK5* or *EIF3H* [30]. *SEMA3A* has been associated with cortical thickness and white matter microstructure measurement [31], parameters related to cognitive impairment. *SEMA3A* gene was also found in the GWAS performed previously by our group (*p*-value: 7.85×10^{-8}) [10].

We have also found that Alzheimer's disease, the leading cause of dementia characterized by amyloid-β and tau aggregates, shares a genetic background with a predisposition to PH in patients undergoing reperfusion treatment (raw *p*-value < 0.05). Moreover, we found that WMH also share a genetic background with PH. In previous results from our group, we also observed this genetic correlation with WMH and also with ICH that has not been observed in the current work [10]. We could hypothesize that the lack of this association could be due to the fact that it shares genetic background with HT but not so much with PH, or simply due to a lack of statistical power.

The effect of IVT on overall HT in patients with dementia is controversial in the literature [32]. Some authors conclude that ITV did not increase the risk of HT in the patients with dementia compared to the controls without dementia, that underwent IVT [32].

Our results suggest that dementia might play a role in the development of PH due to Alzheimer's disease and WMH share a genetic background with PH, although these associations did not remain significant after adjusting for multiple comparisons. Besides, we found SNVs (from the genes *PCSK5*, *EIF3H*, and *SEMA3A*) related to amyloid-β, tau protein, cortical thickness, or WMH. Moreover, the occurrence and localization of cerebral microbleeds (CMBs) associated with IVT-related hemorrhagic complications could indicate an underlying cerebral amyloid angiopathy [33]. This pathology is characterized by the presence of amyloid-β aggregated in the vascular walls of the brain, leading to dementia and a predisposition to ICH. That could indicate that patients who may develop amyloid angiopathy in the future may have an increased risk of HT. However, we did not find a genetic correlation between ICH or ICH subtypes with PH occurrence in our study.

PCSK5 [34] and *RNA5SP448* [35] has been found to be associated with LDL levels, a molecule that has been shown to promote inflammation [36]. Actually, it has been found that lower LDL cholesterol levels had been associated with HT [3]. *KLF5* has been associated with neutrophil and monocyte count or lymphocyte percentage of leukocytes [37], and *RNA5SP448* with interleukin 12 [38]. Both interleukins and the neutrophil-to-lymphocyte ratio (NLR) have been shown to be a marker associated with inflammation; a high NLR can predict HT [39]. This suggests that inflammation may play an important role in the development of PH. Actually, it has been observed that r-tPA mobilizes immune cells that exacerbate hemorrhagic transformation in stroke [40].

TGFBR3 has been associated with pulse pressure measurement. Besides, the SNV found with nominal significance: 1:92310874:A:G, an intronic variant located in TGFBR3, has a RegulomeBD score of 2b. In addition, blood pressure variability was found to be correlated with HT [41]. Nevertheless, we failed to find a genetic correlation between SBP and DBP with PH.

It is also worth noting that myosin V binding was the GO term significantly associated with PH. Myosin V is primarily found in the central nervous system serving as neuronal marker [42] and has been linked to recycling endosomes and exocytosis of secretory MMP2 and MMP9 which have been widely associated with TH [43–45].

Regarding limitations, one of the most important is the small sample size of both the discovery and replication cohorts, even though it is one of the largest made in this topic. This is probably the root cause of not finding significant SNVs in the discovery cohort. For this reason, to increase our statistical power, we performed the meta-analysis that showed a genome-wide significant SNV and another that was almost significant. Another limitation is the lack of replication in an independent cohort. However, the same direction of effect observed for the most significant SNVs in the discovery and replication cohorts indicates that the results are consistent.

Another limitation is the Spanish origin of all the patients from the discovery cohort, this might make it difficult to generalize the results to other populations. To overcome this limitation, the replication cohort included patients from Poland and Finland. Likewise, the lack of values for the variable of the time elapsed between the onset of symptoms and the administration of treatment may limit our results. Furthermore, the fact that we did not have any patient with mechanical thrombectomy who presented PH limits the generalization of our results to this subgroup of patients. Therefore, studies with a larger sample size, incorporating more variables, and more patients subjected to mechanical thrombectomy will be necessary to establish more robust conclusions.

5. Conclusions

With this meta-analysis, we have found a new locus significantly associated with the risk of PH in patients treated with the different types of reperfusion therapies used in the clinical practice. Correlation analysis has shown us shared background genetics between PH and Alzheimer's disease and WMH. Moreover, the analysis of the most significant genomic loci supports this relationship, as the nearest genes associated with the leading SNVs have been related to aggregated amyloid-β, tau protein, or white matter microstructure. However, also of great interest is that other traits related to these SNVs pointed to the importance that inflammation may play in the risk of developing PH. Further studies are needed to test these hypotheses.

Supplementary Materials: The following are available online at https://www.mdpi.com/article/10.3390/jcm10143137/s1, Figure S1: Manhattan and QQ plot of the discovery cohort; Figure S2: Manhattan and QQ plot of the discovery cohort; Table S1: SNVs belonging to the genomic locus with the leading SNP being significant at GWAS level; Table S2: Description of the GWAS significant locus and the 28 nominal significant loci; and Table S3: Top ten of the most significant curated gene sets and gene ontology terms obtained from MsigDB.

Author Contributions: Conception and design of the work and writing—original draft preparation: E.M., J.C.-M. and I.F.-C.; Writing—review and editing: All authors. All authors have read and agreed to the published version of the manuscript.

Funding: This work was supported by grants from the Instituto de Salud Carlos III (PI 11/0176), Generación Project, Maestro Project (PI18/01338), INVICTUS+ network, Epigenesis Project (Marató de TV3), FEDER funds. E. Muiño is supported by a Río Hortega Contract (CM18/00198) from the Instituto de Salud Carlos III. J. Cárcel-Márquez is supported by an AGAUR Contract (agència de gestió d'ajuts universitaris i de recerca; FI_DGR 2020, grant number 2020FI_B1 00157) co-financed with Fons Social Europeu (FSE). C. Gallego-Fabrega is supported by a Sara Borrell Contract (CD20/00043) from Instituto de Salud Carlos III and Fondo Europeo de Desarrollo Regional (ISCIII-FEDER). M. Lledós is supported by a PFIS Contract (Contratos Predoctorales de Formación en Investigación en Salud) from the Instituto de Salud Carlos III. I (FI19/00309). Fernández-Cadenas (CP12/03298), Tomás Sobrino (CPII17/00027), and Francisco Campos (CPII19/00020) are supported by a research contract from Miguel Servet Program from the Instituto de Salud Carlos III.

Institutional Review Board Statement: The study was conducted according to the guidelines of the Declaration of Helsinki, and approved by the local Ethics Committee of every hospital participant.

Informed Consent Statement: Informed consent was obtained from all subjects involved in the study.

Data Availability Statement: The data presented in this study are available on request from the corresponding author.

Acknowledgments: We are grateful to Lucía Muñoz (Hospital Germans Trias i Pujol), Anna Penalba (Vall d'Hebron Research Institute), Uxue Lascano (IMIM-Hospital del Mar), Carmen Jimenez (Hospital Universitari Son Espases), Elisa Cortijo (Hospital Clínico Universitario), Esther Sarasola Diez (Hospital de Basurto), Carmen Gubern (Josep Trueta University Hospital), Aki Havulinna (Institute for Molecular Medicine Finland), Veikko Salomaa (Institute for Molecular Medicine Finland), and Antoni Ferens (Jagiellonian University) for their contribution to patient recruitment; and to Agustin Ruiz and Oscar Sotolongo (Fundació ACE) for their technical support.

Conflicts of Interest: The authors declare no conflict of interest.

References

1. Feigin, V.L.; Norrving, B.; Mensah, G.A. Global Burden of Stroke. *Circ. Res.* **2017**, *120*, 439–448. [CrossRef]
2. Fiorelli, M.; Bastianello, S.; von Kummer, R.; del Zoppo, G.J.; Larrue, V.; Lesaffre, E.; Ringleb, A.P.; Lorenzano, S.; Manelfe, C.; Bozzao, L. Hemorrhagic Transformation within 36 Hours of a Cerebral Infarct. *Stroke* **1999**, *30*, 2280–2284. [CrossRef]
3. Pande, S.D.; Win, M.M.; Khine, A.A.; Zaw, E.M.; Manoharraj, N.; Lolong, L.; Tin, A.S. Haemorrhagic Transformation Following Ischaemic Stroke: A Retrospective Study. *Sci. Rep.* **2020**, *10*, 5319. [CrossRef] [PubMed]
4. D'Amelio, M.; Terruso, V.; Famoso, G.; Di Benedetto, N.; Realmuto, S.; Valentino, F.; Ragonese, P.; Savettieri, G.; Aridon, P. Early and Late Mortality of Spontaneous Hemorrhagic Transformation of Ischemic Stroke. *J. Stroke Cerebrovasc. Dis.* **2014**, *23*, 649–654. [CrossRef]
5. Thomalla, G.; Simonsen, C.Z.; Boutitie, F.; Andersen, G.; Berthezene, Y.; Cheng, B.; Cheripelli, B.; Cho, T.-H.; Fazekas, F.; Fiehler, J.; et al. MRI-Guided Thrombolysis for Stroke with Unknown Time of Onset. *N. Engl. J. Med.* **2018**, *379*, 611–622. [CrossRef] [PubMed]
6. Nogueira, R.G.; Jadhav, A.P.; Haussen, D.C.; Bonafe, A.; Budzik, R.F.; Bhuva, P.; Yavagal, D.R.; Ribo, M.; Cognard, C.; Hanel, R.A.; et al. Thrombectomy 6 to 24 h after Stroke with a Mismatch between Deficit and Infarct. *N. Engl. J. Med.* **2018**, *378*, 11–21. [CrossRef]
7. Albers, G.W.; Marks, M.P.; Kemp, S.; Christensen, S.; Tsai, J.P.; Ortega-Gutierrez, S.; McTaggart, R.A.; Torbey, M.T.; Kim-Tenser, M.; Leslie-Mazwi, T.; et al. Thrombectomy for Stroke at 6 to 16 h with Selection by Perfusion Imaging. *N. Engl. J. Med.* **2018**, *378*, 708–718. [CrossRef] [PubMed]
8. del Río-Espínola, A.; Fernández-Cadenas, I.; Giralt, D.; Quiroga, A.; Gutiérrez-Agulló, M.; Quintana, M.; Fernández-Álvarez, P.; Domingues-Montanari, S.; Mendióroz, M.; Delgado, P.; et al. A Predictive Clinical-Genetic Model of Tissue Plasminogen Activator Response in Acute Ischemic Stroke. *Ann. Neurol.* **2012**, *72*, 716–729. [CrossRef]
9. Carrera, C.; Cullell, N.; Torres-Águila, N.; Muiño, E.; Bustamante, A.; Dávalos, A.; López-Cancio, E.; Ribó, M.; Molina, C.A.; Giralt-Steinhauer, E.; et al. Validation of a Clinical-Genetics Score to Predict Hemorrhagic Transformations after RtPA. *Neurology* **2019**, *93*, e851–e863. [CrossRef]
10. Carrera, C.; Cárcel-Márquez, J.; Cullell, N.; Torres-Águila, N.; Muiño, E.; Castillo, J.; Sobrino, T.; Campos, F.; Rodríguez-Castro, E.; Llucia-Carol, L.; et al. Single Nucleotide Variations in ZBTB46 Are Associated with Post-Thrombolytic Parenchymal Haematoma. *Brain* **2021**. [CrossRef]
11. Kunkle, B.W.; Grenier-Boley, B.; Sims, R.; Bis, J.C.; Damotte, V.; Naj, A.C.; Boland, A.; Vronskaya, M.; van der Lee, S.J.; Amlie-Wolf, A.; et al. Genetic Meta-Analysis of Diagnosed Alzheimer's Disease Identifies New Risk Loci and Implicates Aβ, Tau, Immunity and Lipid Processing. *Nat. Genet.* **2019**, *51*, 414–430. [CrossRef]

12. Chung, J.; Marini, S.; Pera, J.; Norrving, B.; Jimenez-Conde, J.; Roquer, J.; Fernandez-Cadenas, I.; Tirschwell, D.L.; Selim, M.; Brown, D.L.; et al. Genome-Wide Association Study of Cerebral Small Vessel Disease Reveals Established and Novel Loci. *Brain* **2019**, *142*, 3176–3189. [CrossRef] [PubMed]
13. Mola-Caminal, M.; Carrera, C.; Soriano-Tárraga, C.; Giralt-Steinhauer, E.; Díaz-Navarro, R.M.; Tur, S.; Jiménez, C.; Medina-Dols, A.; Cullell, N.; Torres-Aguila, N.P.; et al. PATJ Low Frequency Variants Are Associated with Worse Ischemic Stroke Functional Outcome: A Genome-Wide Meta-Analysis. *Circ. Res.* **2019**, *124*, 114–120. [CrossRef]
14. Fernández-Cadenas, I.; Mendióroz, M.; Giralt, D.; Nafria, C.; Garcia, E.; Carrera, C.; Gallego-Fabrega, C.; Domingues-Montanari, S.; Delgado, P.; Ribó, M.; et al. GRECOS Project (Genotyping Recurrence Risk of Stroke). *Stroke* **2017**, *48*, 1147–1153. [CrossRef]
15. Heitsch, L.; Ibanez, L.; Carrera, C.; Pera, J.; Jimenez-Conde, J.; Slowik, A.; Strbian, D.; Fernandez-Cadenas, I.; Montaner, J.; Lee, J.-M. Meta-Analysis of Transethnic Association (MANTRA) Reveals Loci Associated with Neurological Instability after Acute Ischemic Stroke. In Proceedings of the International Stroke Conference, Houston, TX, USA, 21–24 February 2017.
16. Roquer, J.; Rodríguez-Campello, A.; Gomis, M.; Jiménez-conde, J.; Cuadrado-godia, E.; Vivanco, R.; Giralt, E.; Sepúlveda, M.; Pont-Sunyer, C.; Cucurella, G.; et al. Acute Stroke Unit Care and Early Neurological Deterioration in Ischemic Stroke. *J. Neurol.* **2008**, *255*, 1012–1017. [CrossRef] [PubMed]
17. Robberecht, W.; Vanhees, L.; Lemmens, R.; Pandolfo, M.; Thijs, V.; Goris, A. Variant on 9p21 Strongly Associates with Coronary Heart Disease, but Lacks Association with Common Stroke. *Eur. J. Hum. Genet.* **2009**, *4*, 1287–1293. [CrossRef]
18. Charidimou, A.; Pasi, M. Microbleeds Evolution and Remote Hemorrhage Post-TPA: Red Meets White Revisited. *Neurology* **2019**, *92*, 307–308. [CrossRef] [PubMed]
19. Jiang, L.; Zheng, Z.; Qi, T.; Kemper, K.E.; Wray, N.R.; Visscher, P.M.; Yang, J. A Resource-Efficient Tool for Mixed Model Association Analysis of Large-Scale Data. *Nat. Genet.* **2019**, *51*, 1749–1755. [CrossRef]
20. Willer, C.J.; Li, Y.; Abecasis, G.R. METAL: Fast and Efficient Meta-Analysis of Genomewide Association Scans. *Bioinformatics* **2010**, *26*, 2190–2191. [CrossRef] [PubMed]
21. Watanabe, K.; Taskesen, E.; Van Bochoven, A.; Posthuma, D. Functional Mapping and Annotation of Genetic Associations with FUMA. *Nat. Commun.* **2017**, *8*, 1826. [CrossRef]
22. Malik, R.; Chauhan, G.; Traylor, M.; Sargurupremraj, M.; Okada, Y.; Mishra, A.; Rutten-Jacobs, L.; Giese, A.K.A.-K.; van der Laan, S.W.S.W.; Gretarsdottir, S.; et al. Multiancestry Genome-Wide Association Study of 520,000 Subjects Identifies 32 Loci Associated with Stroke and Stroke Subtypes. *Nat. Genet.* **2018**, *50*, 524–537. [CrossRef]
23. Woo, D.; Falcone, G.J.; Devan, W.J.; Brown, W.M.; Biffi, A.; Howard, T.D.; Anderson, C.D.; Brouwers, H.B.; Valant, V.; Battey, T.W.K.; et al. Meta-Analysis of Genome-Wide Association Studies Identifies 1q22 as a Susceptibility Locus for Intracerebral Hemorrhage. *Am. J. Hum. Genet.* **2014**, *94*, 511–521. [CrossRef]
24. Traylor, M.; Tozer, D.J.; Croall, I.D.; Lisiecka Ford, D.M.; Olorunda, A.O.; Boncoraglio, G.; Dichgans, M.; Lemmens, R.; Rosand, J.; Rost, N.S.; et al. Genetic Variation in PLEKHG1 Is Associated with White Matter Hyperintensities (n = 11,226). *Neurology* **2019**, *92*, E749–E757. [CrossRef]
25. Willer, C.J.; Schmidt, E.M.; Sengupta, S.; Peloso, G.M.; Gustafsson, S.; Kanoni, S.; Ganna, A.; Chen, J.; Buchkovich, M.L.; Mora, S.; et al. Discovery and Refinement of Loci Associated with Lipid Levels. *Nat. Genet.* **2018**, *176*, 139–148. [CrossRef]
26. Evangelou, E.; Warren, H.R.; Mosen-Ansorena, D.; Mifsud, B.; Pazoki, R.; Gao, H.; Ntritsos, G.; Dimou, N.; Cabrera, C.P.; Karaman, I.; et al. Genetic Analysis of over One Million People Identifies 535 New Loci Associated with Blood Pressure Traits. *Nat. Genet.* **2018**, *50*, 1412–1425. [CrossRef]
27. Morris, A.P.; Voight, B.F.; Teslovich, T.M.; Ferreira, T.; Segre, A.V.; Steinthorsdottir, V.; Strawbridge, R.J.; Khan, H.; Grallert, H.; Mahajan, A.; et al. Large-Scale Association Analysis Provides Insights into the Genetic Architecture and Pathophysiology of Type 2 Diabetes. *Nat. Genet.* **2012**, *44*, 981–990. [CrossRef] [PubMed]
28. Bennett, D.A. How Can I Deal with Missing Data in My Study? *Aust. N. Z. J. Public Health* **2001**, *25*, 464–469. [CrossRef]
29. Müller, R.; Weirick, T.; John, D.; Militello, G.; Chen, W.; Dimmeler, S.; Uchida, S. ANGIOGENES: Knowledge Database for Protein-Coding and Noncoding RNA Genes in Endothelial Cells. *Sci. Rep.* **2016**, *6*, 1–8. [CrossRef] [PubMed]
30. Wang, H.; Yang, J.; Schneider, J.A.; De Jager, P.L.; Bennett, D.A.; Zhang, H.Y. Genome-Wide Interaction Analysis of Pathological Hallmarks in Alzheimer's Disease. *Neurobiol. Aging* **2020**, *93*, 61–68. [CrossRef] [PubMed]
31. van der Meer, D.; Frei, O.; Kaufmann, T.; Shadrin, A.A.; Devor, A.; Smeland, O.B.; Thompson, W.K.; Fan, C.C.; Holland, D.; Westlye, L.T.; et al. Understanding the Genetic Determinants of the Brain with MOSTest. *Nat. Commun.* **2020**, *11*, 1–9. [CrossRef] [PubMed]
32. Alshekhlee, A.; Li, C.C.; Chuang, S.Y.; Vora, N.; Edgell, R.C.; Kitchener, J.M.; Kale, S.P.; Feen, E.; Piriyawat, P.; Callison, R.C.; et al. Does Dementia Increase Risk of Thrombolysis?: A Case-Control Study. *Neurology* **2011**, *76*, 1575–1580. [CrossRef] [PubMed]
33. Braemswig, T.B.; Villringer, K.; Turc, G.; Erdur, H.; Fiebach, J.B.; Audebert, H.J.; Endres, M.; Nolte, C.H.; Scheitz, J.F. Predictors of New Remote Cerebral Microbleeds after IV Thrombolysis for Ischemic Stroke. *Neurology* **2019**, *92*, E630–E638. [CrossRef] [PubMed]
34. De Vries, P.S.; Brown, M.R.; Bentley, A.R.; Sung, Y.J.; Winkler, T.W.; Ntalla, I.; Schwander, K.; Kraja, A.T.; Guo, X.; Franceschini, N.; et al. Multiancestry Genome-Wide Association Study of Lipid Levels Incorporating Gene-Alcohol Interactions. *Am. J. Epidemiol.* **2019**, *188*, 1033–1054. [CrossRef]

35. Noordam, R.; Bos, M.M.; Wang, H.; Winkler, T.W.; Bentley, A.R.; Kilpeläinen, T.O.; de Vries, P.S.; Sung, Y.J.; Schwander, K.; Cade, B.E.; et al. Multi-Ancestry Sleep-by-SNP Interaction Analysis in 126,926 Individuals Reveals Lipid Loci Stratified by Sleep Duration. *Nat. Commun.* **2019**, *10*, 5121. [CrossRef]
36. Puig, N.; Montolio, L.; Camps-Renom, P.; Navarra, L.; Jiménez-Altayó, F.; Jiménez-Xarrié, E.; Sánchez-Quesada, J.L.; Benitez, S. Electronegative LDL Promotes Inflammation and Triglyceride Accumulation in Macrophages. *Cells* **2020**, *9*, 583. [CrossRef]
37. Chen, M.H.; Raffield, L.M.; Mousas, A.; Sakaue, S.; Huffman, J.E.; Moscati, A.; Trivedi, B.; Jiang, T.; Akbari, P.; Vuckovic, D.; et al. Trans-Ethnic and Ancestry-Specific Blood-Cell Genetics in 746,667 Individuals from 5 Global Populations. *Cell* **2020**, *182*, 1198–1213. [CrossRef]
38. Ahola-Olli, A.V.; Würtz, P.; Havulinna, A.S.; Aalto, K.; Pitkänen, N.; Lehtimäki, T.; Kähönen, M.; Lyytikäinen, L.P.; Raitoharju, E.; Seppälä, I.; et al. Genome-Wide Association Study Identifies 27 Loci Influencing Concentrations of Circulating Cytokines and Growth Factors. *Am. J. Hum. Genet.* **2017**, *100*, 40–50. [CrossRef]
39. Zhang, R.; Wu, X.; Hu, W.; Zhao, L.; Zhao, S.; Zhang, J.; Chu, Z.; Xu, Y. Neutrophil-to-Lymphocyte Ratio Predicts Hemorrhagic Transformation in Ischemic Stroke: A Meta-Analysis. *Brain Behav.* **2019**, *9*, 1–9. [CrossRef]
40. Shi, K.; Zou, M.; Jia, D.M.; Shi, S.; Yang, X.; Liu, Q.; Dong, J.F.; Sheth, K.N.; Wang, X.; Shi, F.D. TPA Mobilizes Immune Cells That Exacerbate Hemorrhagic Transformation in Stroke. *Circ. Res.* **2021**, *128*, 62–75. [CrossRef]
41. Kim, T.J.; Park, H.K.; Kim, J.M.; Lee, J.S.; Park, S.H.; Jeong, H.B.; Park, K.Y.; Rha, J.H.; Yoon, B.W.; Ko, S.B. Blood Pressure Variability and Hemorrhagic Transformation in Patients with Successful Recanalization after Endovascular Recanalization Therapy: A Retrospective Observational Study. *Ann. Neurol.* **2019**, *85*, 574–581. [CrossRef] [PubMed]
42. Langford, G.M.; Molyneaux, B.J. Myosin V in the Brain: Mutations Lead to Neurological Defects. *Brain Res. Rev.* **1998**, *28*, 1–8. [CrossRef]
43. Montaner, J.; Molina, C.A.; Monasterio, J.; Abilleira, S.; Arenillas, J.F.; Ribó, M.; Quintana, M.; Alvarez-Sabín, J. Matrix Metalloproteinase-9 Pretreatment Level Predicts Intracranial Hemorrhagic Complications after Thrombolysis in Human Stroke. *Circulation* **2003**, *107*, 598–603. [CrossRef] [PubMed]
44. Cuadrado, E.; Ortega, L.; Hernández-Guillamon, M.; Penalba, A.; Fernández-Cadenas, I.; Rosell, A.; Montaner, J. Tissue Plasminogen Activator (t-PA) Promotes Neutrophil Degranulation and MMP-9 Release. *J. Leukoc. Biol.* **2008**, *84*, 207–214. [CrossRef]
45. Zheng, L.; Xiong, Y.; Liu, J.; Yang, X.; Wang, L.; Zhang, S.; Liu, M.; Wang, D. MMP-9-Related MicroRNAs as Prognostic Markers for Hemorrhagic Transformation in Cardioembolic Stroke Stroke Patients. *Front. Neurol.* **2019**, *10*, 1–7. [CrossRef] [PubMed]

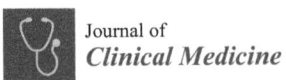

Article

Reperfusion Therapies for Acute Ischemic Stroke in COVID-19 Patients: A Nationwide Multi-Center Study

Justina Jurkevičienė [1,*], Mantas Vaišvilas [1], Rytis Masiliūnas [2], Vaidas Matijošaitis [3], Antanas Vaitkus [3], Dovilė Geštautaitė [3], Saulius Taroza [4], Paulius Puzinas [5], Erika Galvanauskaitė [6], Dalius Jatužis [2] and Aleksandras Vilionskis [7]

1. Stroke Centre, Republican Vilnius University Hospital, 04130 Vilnius, Lithuania; mantas.vaisvilas@rvul.lt
2. Center of Neurology, Vilnius University, 08661 Vilnius, Lithuania; rytis.masiliunas@santa.lt (R.M.); dalius.jatuzis@santa.lt (D.J.)
3. Department of Neurology, Lithuanian University of Health Sciences, 50009 Kaunas, Lithuania; vaidas.matijosaitis@kaunoklinikos.lt (V.M.); antanas.vaitkus@kaunoklinikos.lt (A.V.); dovile.gestautaite@kaunoklinikos.lt (D.G.)
4. Laboratory of Behavioral Medicine (Palanga), Neuroscience Institute, Lithuanian University of Health Sciences, 00135 Palanga, Lithuania; saulius.taroza@lsmuni.lt
5. Department of Neurology, Republican Panevėžys Hospital, 35144 Panevėžys, Lithuania; pauliuspuzinas@gmail.com
6. Department of Neurology, Republican Šiauliai Hospital, 76231 Šiauliai, Lithuania; erika.galvanauskaite@siauliuligonine.lt
7. Clinic of Neurology and Neurosurgery, Vilnius University, 03101 Vilnius, Lithuania; aleksandras.vilionskis@rvul.lt
* Correspondence: justina.jurkeviciene@rvul.lt

Abstract: (1) Background: Acute ischemic stroke (AIS) is a possible complication of the coronavirus disease 2019 (COVID-19). Safety and efficacy data on reperfusion therapies (RT)—intravenous thrombolysis and endovascular treatment (EVT)—in stroke patients with COVID-19 is lacking. (2) Methods: We performed a retrospective nationwide multi-center pair-matched analysis of COVID-19 patients with AIS who underwent RT. We included adult COVID-19 patients with AIS who were treated with RT between 16 March 2020 and 30 June 2021. All subjects were paired with non-infected controls, matched for age, sex, stroke arterial vascular territory, and RT modality. The primary outcome measure was a favorable functional outcome defined by the modified Rankin scale (mRS 0–2). (3) Results: Thirty-one subjects and thirty-one matched controls were included. The median baseline National Institutes of Health Stroke Scale (NIHSS) score was higher in the COVID-19 group (16 vs. 12, $p = 0.028$). Rates of ischemic changes and symptomatic intracerebral hemorrhages did not differ significantly between the two groups at 24 h after RT. The median NIHSS 24 h after reperfusion remained significantly higher in the COVID-19 group (16 vs. 5, $p = 0.003$). MRS 0–2 at discharge was significantly less common in COVID-19 patients (22.6% vs. 51.8%, $p = 0.018$). Three-month mortality was 54.8% in the COVID-19 group versus 12.9% in controls ($p = 0.001$). (4) Conclusion: Reperfusion therapies on AIS in COVID-19 patients appear to be safe; however, functional outcomes are significantly worse, and 3-month mortality is higher.

Keywords: COVID-19; ischemic stroke; thrombolysis; thrombectomy; Lithuania; reperfusion therapies; outcomes; safety

1. Introduction

In December 2019, a cluster of patients with pneumonia caused by a novel severe acute respiratory coronavirus 2 (SARS-CoV-2) was first described in Wuhan, China [1]. Due to the vast spread of the virus across the globe, a pandemic was declared in March 2020. Ever since, a growing number of publications regarding extrapulmonary manifestations of coronavirus disease (COVID-19) arose. Neurologic manifestations of both the central and the peripheral nervous system described included COVID-19 encephalitis, acute disseminated encephalomyelitis, epileptic seizures, neuromuscular symptoms, acute demyelinating polyneuropathies, and their variants, as well as acute cerebrovascular syndromes [2–8]. It has been postulated that COVID-19 patients are at an increased risk for stroke, although the true causality is yet uncertain [9].

The first COVID-19 case in Lithuania was confirmed in late February 2020, followed shortly by the introduction of a strict nationwide lockdown. Despite thousands of daily new confirmed cases and the need for allocation of specific healthcare resources, emergency stroke services were operating in all major stroke centers across the country throughout the pandemic at full capacity [10,11]. Both intravenous thrombolysis (IVT) and endovascular treatment (EVT) were used continuously for acute ischemic stroke (AIS) in COVID-19 patients. However, data on the safety of reperfusion therapies (RT) in the COVID-19 population is scarce, and potential adverse effects of RTs could be life-threatening. Therefore, we sought to evaluate the safety and outcomes of reperfusion therapies in COVID-19 patients with AIS in a nationwide pair-matched retrospective study.

2. Materials and Methods

We conducted a multi-center retrospective pair-matched analysis of reperfusion therapy in COVID-19 patients with AIS across all six comprehensive stroke centers (CSCs) in Lithuania [12].

Data collection. The data were extracted retrospectively from electronic health records. We collected demographic data (age, gender), cardiovascular risk factors (hypertension, dyslipidemia, smoking, diabetes, atrial fibrillation, presence of symptomatic internal carotid artery (ICA) >70% or intracranial artery stenosis > 70% on computed tomography angiography), clinical (hypoxemia, body temperature, blood pressure on admission) and laboratory test data (white blood cell (WBC) and lymphocyte count, C reactive protein (CRP) and D-dimer levels on admission), head computed tomography (CT) findings (Alberta Stroke Programme Early CT Score (ASPECTS) on admission, ischemic changes on CT scan 24 h after RT), median timeliness metrics (onset-to-door (OTD), door-to-needle (DTN) and door-to-puncture (DTP) times), National Institute of Health Stroke Scale (NIHSS) on admission, at 24 h after reperfusion therapy, and on day 7 after stroke or at discharge (whichever occurred first) and reperfusion therapy data (treatment modality, Thrombolysis in Cerebral Infarction (TICI) score). Neurologic (symptomatic intracerebral hemorrhage (sICH), cerebral edema), COVID-19-related, and other complications (urinary tract infection, pulmonary embolism, myocardial infarction, acute heart failure, pulmonary edema, other organ dysfunction, or major bleeding) were collected. Patient functional outcomes corresponding to modified Rankin Scale (mRS) score at discharge, as well as in-hospital and 3-month mortality rates, were retrieved.

Patient selection. We included adult (18 years old or older) AIS patients with diagnosed acute COVID-19 infection prior to or on admission to a CSC, treated with reperfusion therapy (IVT, EVT, or both) between 16 March 2020 and 30 June 2021. Our patients had not received full vaccination doses. COVID-19 status was confirmed by a nasopharyngeal swab SARS-CoV-2 real-time polymerase chain reaction (RT-PCR). Patients who recovered from COVID-19 according to the epidemiological criteria at the time of index AIS were excluded from the analysis despite having a positive SARS-CoV2 RT-PCR test result.

Control group. Each patient from the subject group was weighted against a control. All control patients were treated in one of the 6 Lithuanian CSCs during the study period and were not concomitant with a COVID-19 infection. In addition, control subjects were matched for age (±5 years), gender, stroke arterial vascular territory, and type of reperfusion therapy (IVT, EVT, or both). To avoid selection bias, cases for this group were collected by independent stroke physicians, who were not part of this study, and were only informed about matching criteria.

Outcomes. The primary outcome measure was a favorable functional outcome, defined as the mRS score of 0–2 on the day of discharge.

Secondary outcome measures included: early neurological improvement, defined as reduction of NIHSS score by 4 points or more or score 0–1 at 24 h after reperfusion therapy; change in NIHSS score 24 h after reperfusion therapy; change in NIHSS score 7 days after stroke onset or on discharge (whichever occurred first); neurological complications of reperfusion therapy: sICH was classified using the Safe Implementation of Thrombolysis in Stroke-Monitoring Study (SITS-MOST) classification (parenchymal hemorrhage type 2, 22–36 h after treatment leading to neurologic deterioration 4 points or more on NIHSS from baseline or lowest NIHSS or leading to death as previously reported) [13], and cerebral edema; in-hospital mortality rate; mortality rate 3 months after stroke.

To investigate the effects of clinical and laboratory factors (evaluated on admission) on the likelihood of favorable functional outcome (mRS 0–2) on the day of discharge and of 3-month mortality after stroke and reperfusion therapies, multivariate logistic regression models were built.

Statistical analysis. Statistical analysis was performed using the IBM SPSS Statistics for Windows, Version 26 (IBM SPSS Statistics for Windows, IBM Corporation, Armonk, NY, USA). The Kolmogorov–Smirnov test was used to verify the normality of the distribution of continuous variables. The qualitative variables were expressed as absolute frequencies and percentages. For continuous data, the mean and standard deviation (SD) or median and interquartile range (IQR) were reported, as appropriate. The Student's t test (for normally distributed data) or the Mann–Whitney U test (for not normally distributed data) was used for the continuous variables and the Chi-square test for the categorical variables. $p < 0.05$ was considered to be statistically significant. The significant predictors (using a significance level of <0.1) in the univariate analysis were included in the multivariate analysis, and the entered method was applied for the logistic regression model to determine the predictors for a favorable functional outcome (mRS 0–2) on discharge and 3-month mortality after stroke. The odds ratio (OR) and 95% confidence interval (95% CI) were calculated.

3. Results

3.1. Demographic, Clinical, and Stroke-Related Data

Thirty-one pairs of subjects and matched controls were included in the study. The mean age was 74.0 years in COVID-19-positive AIS patients and 73.7 years in controls. Forty females (64.5%) comprised the entire cohort. Prevalence of stroke risk factors did not differ statistically significantly between the two groups. Fourteen (22.5%) patients underwent IVT, thirty (48.4%) patients were treated with EVT, and eighteen (29.1%) patients received bridging therapy. Fifty-six (90.3%) patients in the entire cohort were diagnosed with anterior circulation stroke. The detailed demographic data and stroke risk factors are displayed in Table 1.

The median NIHSS score on admission was significantly higher in the COVID-19 patient group compared to controls (16 [10–19] vs. 12.5 (5–15), $p = 0.028$). The timeliness metrics (OTD, DTN, and DTP times) did not differ significantly between the two groups. Albeit not significant, the OTD time was longer for COVID-19 patients as compared to controls (126 (83–218) vs. 95 (66–205) minutes, respectively). The ASPECTS score on admission also did not differ significantly.

As expected, the baseline body temperature was statistically significantly higher in COVID-19 patients compared to controls ($p = 0.025$), while the rate of hypoxemia and arterial blood pressure on admission did not differ significantly (Table 2). A significantly lower lymphocyte count ($p = 0.013$) and higher CRP values ($p < 0.001$) were observed in the COVID-19 group compared to controls, while total WBC count and D-dimer concentration on admission did not differ.

Table 1. Patient demographic data and stroke characteristics.

	Stroke Patients with COVID-19 (n = 31)	Control Group without COVID-19 (n = 31)	p Value
Female, n (%)	20 (64.5)	20 (64.5)	1.000
Mean Age, Years (SD)	74.0 (12.9)	73.7 (12.3)	0.912
Cardiovascular Risk Factors, n (%)			
Hypertension	29 (93.5)	26 (83.9)	0.425
Dyslipidemia	15 (48.4)	23 (74.2)	0.067
Smoking	5 (16.1)	2 (6.5)	0.229
Diabetes	6 (19.4)	2 (6.5)	0.255
Atrial Fibrillation	12 (38.7)	19 (61.3)	0.075
Symptomatic ICA Stenosis	6 (19.4)	2 (6.5)	0.255
Intracranial Artery Stenosis	3 (9.7)	5 (16.1)	0.707
Circulation of Stroke, n (%)			
Anterior Circulation	28 (90.3)	28 (90.3)	1.000
Posterior Circulation	3 (9.7)	3 (9.7)	1.000
Reperfusion Treatment, n (%)			
IVT	7 (22.5)	7 (22.5)	1.000
EVT	15 (48.4)	15 (48.4)	1.000
Bridging Therapy	9 (29.1)	9 (29.1)	1.000
Median Timeliness Metrics, min (IQR)			
Onset-To-Door Time	126 (83–218)	95 (66–205)	0.294
IVT	94 (81–137)	80 (55–105)	
EVT	245 (121–720)	154.5 (67.75–198.75)	
Bridging Therapy	101 (65–130.5)	84 (67.75–220)	
Door-To-Needle Time	40.5 (26–72.5)	36 (27–46)	0.626
Door-To-Puncture Time	101 (80.75–162.5)	116.5 (75.5–138.75)	1
Baseline NIHSS, Median (IQR)	16 (10–19)	12.5 (5–15)	**0.028**
ASPECTS, Median (IQR) [§]	9 (7.75–10)	10 (8–10)	0.229

SD—standard deviation, ICA—internal carotid artery, IV—Intravenous thrombolysis, EVT—endovascular treatment, mRS—modified Rankin Scale, IQR—interquartile range, NIHSS—National Institutes of Health Stroke Scale, ASPECTS—Alberta Stroke Programme Early CT Score. [§] Sample size differs for both subjects (n = 30), and control group (n = 27) due to missing data. Bold values denote statistical significance at the $p < 0.05$ level.

Table 2. Baseline clinical and laboratory data.

	Stroke Patients with COVID-19 (n = 31)	Control Group without COVID-19 (n = 31)	p Value
Clinical Data			
Hypoxemia, n (%) [†]	5 (16.1)	3 (9.7)	0.712
Median Body Temperature, °C (IQR)	36.6 (36.4–36.8)	36.5 (36.1–36.6)	**0.025**
Mean Systolic Blood Pressure, mmHg (SD)	159 (28.6)	168 (28.6)	0.214
Mean Diastolic Blood Pressure, mmHg (SD)	86 (21.8)	90 (14.9)	0.350
Laboratory Data			
Mean Total WBC Count, $\times 10^9$/L (SD)	8.8 (5.4)	8.7 (2.6)	0.473
Mean Lymphocyte Count, $\times 10^9$/L (SD)	1.5 (0.7)	2.1 (1.4)	**0.013**
Mean CRP, mg/L (SD)	44.3 (63.8)	5.3 (6.4)	**<0.001**
CRP > 5 mg/L, n (%)	23 (74.2)	8 (25.8)	**<0.001**
Median D-Dimer, μg/L (IQR)	675 (78–4898)	1048 (479–2065)	0.979

IQR—interquartile range, SD—standard deviation, WBC—white blood cells, CRP—C-reactive protein. [†] Defined as SpO2 < 93%. Bold values denote statistical significance at the $p < 0.05$ level.

3.2. Primary and Secondary Outcomes

Only 22.6% of COVID-19 patients with AIS in the subject cohort achieved favorable functional outcomes (mRS 0–2) on discharge as compared to 51.6% in the control group ($p = 0.018$) (Table 3).

Table 3. Patient treatment outcomes and complications.

	Stroke Patients with COVID-19 (n = 31)	Control Group without COVID-19 (n = 31)	p Value
TICI Score, n (%) [†]			0.190
2b/3	19 (79.2)	21 (95.5)	
0/1/2a	5 (20.8)	1 (4.5)	
Ischemic Changes on CT Scan 24 h After RT, n (%)	24 (77.4)	21 (67.7)	0.393
Stroke Severity, NIHSS, Median (IQR)			
24 h After Reperfusion Therapy	16 (5–24)	5 (2–13)	**0.003**
24 h Change From Baseline	0 (−3–3)	−2 (−7.25–0)	**0.029**
Day 7 or Discharge [‡]	15 (5–21)	4 (1–10)	**<0.001**
Overall Change From Baseline	−1 (−6–2)	−4 (−9–1)	**0.022**
Early Neurological Improvement, n (%) [§]	6 (19.4)	12 (38.7)	0.077
Functional Outcome at Discharge [‖]			
Median mRS (IQR)	4 (3–6)	2 (1–4)	**0.004**
mRS ≤ 2, n (%)	7 (22.6)	16 (51.6)	**0.018**
Complications, n (%)			
Symptomatic ICH	0 (0)	0 (0)	1.000
Cerebral Edema	7 (22.6)	6 (19.4)	0.755
Pneumonia [¥]	21 (67.7)	2 (8.0)	**<0.001**
Respiratory Failure [¥¥]	20 (64.5)	4 (22.2)	**0.007**
Other [¶]	8 (25.8)	9 (29.0)	0.776
Prolonged Stay in ICU (>1 day), n (%)	12 (38.7)	6 (19.4)	0.093
Mortality, n (%)			
In-Hospital	9 (29.0)	2 (6.5)	**0.043**
Day 90	17 (54.8)	4 (12.9)	**0.001**

TICI—thrombolysis in cerebral infarction, NIHSS—National Institutes of Health Stroke Scale, IQR—interquartile range, mRS—modified Rankin Scale, ICH—intracerebral hemorrhage, ICU—intensive care unit. [†] Only patients who had undergone mechanical thrombectomy (n = 46, data of 2 patients was missing). [‡] Whichever occurred first. [§] Defined as reduction of NIHSS score by 4 points or more or score 0–1 at 24 h after reperfusion therapy. [‖] Sample size differs for both subjects (n = 26) and control group (n = 29) due to missing data. [¥] Sample size differs for both subjects (n = 31) and control group (n = 25) due to missing data. [¥¥] Sample size differs for both subjects (n = 31) and control group (n = 18) due to missing data. [¶] Including urinary tract infection, pulmonary embolism, myocardial infarction, acute heart failure, pulmonary oedema, other organ dysfunction, major bleeding (excluding pneumonia and respiratory failure). Bold values denote statistical significance at the $p < 0.05$ level.

Significantly higher NIHSS scores 24 h after reperfusion therapy (16 (5–24) vs. 5 (2–13), $p = 0.003$) and on day 7 or discharge (15 (5–21) vs. 4 (1–10), $p < 0.001$) were evident in the COVID-19 group as compared to matched controls. The detail outcome data are shown in Table 3. Rate of cerebral edema after the reperfusion treatment did not differ between the two groups, and no sICHs were observed. Both in-hospital and 3 month mortality rates were significantly higher in the COVID-19 group compared to controls (29% and 54.8% vs. 6.5% and 12.9%, $p = 0.043$ and $p = 0.001$, respectively).

The analysis of in-hospital mortality patients in both groups showed severe stroke from onset (baseline NIHSS > 15). COVID-19-positive stroke patients who died in hospital: 5/9 (55.6%) underwent MTE and 4/9 (44.4%) underwent bridging therapy, 2/9 (22.2%) had unsuccessful MTE (TICI 1 and 2a), 7/9 (77.8%) had acute ischemic changes on CT scan 24 h after RT, 2/9 (22.2%) experienced reperfusion complications (small scattered petechiae and subarachnoid hemorrhage, confluent petechiae), 5/9 (55.6%) had various degree cerebral edema, 8/9 (88.9%) had pneumonia and respiratory failure, 2/9 (22.2%) had other somatic complications (sepsis, acute kidney failure and urinary tract infection), 2/2 (100%) control group stroke patients who died in hospital underwent MTE, and reperfusion therapy was successful (TICI 3) in both cases, Both patients had acute ischemic changes on CT scan 24 h after RT, both experienced reperfusion complications (hematoma within infarcted tissue, occupying <30%, intraventricular hemorrhage), both had cerebral edema, and both had pneumonia and respiratory failure and no other somatic complications.

3.3. COVID-19 Associated Complications

Severe respiratory failure was observed in 64.5% of COVID-19 patients during any time point of inpatient treatment, and it was significantly more common compared to controls, where only 22% of patients were in respiratory compromise ($p = 0.007$). Importantly, on admission, rates of respiratory failure did not differ between the two groups (hypoxemia rate 5 (16.1%) in COVID-19 group vs. 3 (9.7%) in controls, $p = 0.712$). Pneumonia complicated the disease course of 67.7% of COVID-19 patients as compared to 8% of controls ($p < 0.001$). Prolonged stay in ICU was observed in 38.7% of COVID-19 patients compared to 19.4% in control group ($p = 0.093$).

3.4. Multivariate Analysis

The accuracy of a favorable functional outcome prediction was 83.6%. The significant variables in the univariate analysis included age ($p = 0.028$), baseline NIHSS ($p < 0.001$), and COVID-19 infection ($p = 0.011$). In the multivariable model, only baseline NIHSS retained significance (OR 0.790; 95% CI 0.691–0.902) (Table 4).

Table 4. Logistic regression model on the likelihood of favorable functional outcome (mRS 0–2) on discharge ($n = 61$).

Covariates	Univariate Analysis	Multivariate Analysis	
	p Value	OR (95% CI)	p Value
Age	0.028	0.959 (0.899–1.022)	0.199
Baseline NIHSS	<0.001	0.790 (0.691–0.902)	**0.000**
COVID-19 Infection	0.011	0.312 (0.077–1.260)	0.102

OR—odds ratio, CI—confidence interval, NIHSS—National Institutes of Health Stroke Scale. Bold values denote statistical significance at the $p < 0.05$ level in multivariate analysis.

The accuracy of 3-month mortality after stroke and reperfusion therapy was 78.8%. The significant variables included age ($p = 0.022$), hypoxemia ($p = 0.079$), baseline NIHSS ($p = 0.001$), COVID-19 infection ($p = 0.001$), total WBC count ($p = 0.079$), and CRP concentration ($p = 0.093$). Increasing age and higher baseline NIHSS on admission were associated with a higher likelihood of 3-month mortality after stroke and reperfusion therapy. COVID-19 infection increased the likelihood of death 3 months after stroke and reperfusion therapy seven times (OR 6.696; 95% CI 1.029–43.584), while hypoxemia, total WBC count, and CRP concentration were not significant predictors (Table 5).

Table 5. Logistic regression model on the likelihood of 3-month mortality after stroke and reperfusion therapy ($n = 52$).

Covariates	Univariate Analysis	Multivariate Analysis	
	p Value	OR (95% CI)	p Value
Age	0.022	1.086 (1.002–1.178)	**0.045**
Hypoxemia (SpO2 < 93%)	0.079	1.861 (0.225–15.406)	0.565
Baseline NIHSS	0.001	1.184 (1.013–1.383)	**0.034**
COVID-19 infection	0.001	6.696 (1.029–43.584)	**0.047**
Total WBC count	0.079	1.126 (0.829–1.530)	0.447
CRP concentration	0.093	1.004 (0.990–1.018)	0.586

OR—odds ratio, CI—confidence interval, NIHSS—National Institutes of Health Stroke Scale, WBC—white blood cells, CRP—C-reactive protein. Bold values denote statistical significance at the $p < 0.05$ level in multivariate analysis.

4. Discussion

This is the first Lithuanian nationwide pair-matched multicenter study evaluating outcomes of COVID-19-positive AIS patients treated with reperfusion therapies. We demonstrated that COVID-19 stroke patients present with a significantly higher neurologic burden than non-infected controls. We also found that reperfusion therapies appear safe for COVID-19 stroke patients in relation to reperfusion-associated complications (symptomatic ICH and cerebral edema). Despite successful reperfusion, the COVID-19 stroke patients had significantly worse outcomes and a high 3-month mortality rate as compared to control patients. We additionally report 3-month mortality of COVID-19-positive patients with AIS representing distant sequalae of AIS. Hypoxia had a major role in our COVID-19 cohort and may have contributed to the high in-hospital and 3-month mortality rate.

Outcomes of COVID-19 patients with AIS seem to be universally unfavorable despite successful reperfusion. Although COVID-19 patients with mild stroke presentations seemed to have more favorable outcomes, in general, COVID-19 patients with AIS were more severely disabled, with a median NIHSS of 15 at discharge as compared to controls. This is in line with other studies reporting in-hospital mortality rates ranging from 31% to 60% [14–16]. The European multicenter EVT study provided data on 30-day mortality of 27% [17]. In contrast, we report insights on 3-month mortality even higher than previously reported [18].

In our study, the absolute majority of COVID-19 stroke patients had a more severe stroke despite no differences in ASPECTS scores between study groups on admission. These results are comparable to previous reports [18]. However, the true size of ischemic territory in COVID-19 patients may be larger than initially anticipated. Significantly lower ASPECTS scores and higher infarct volumes were observed for COVID-19 patients with AIS on MRI despite early imaging in a previous study [19]. In contrast, we used CT as our main screening modality. Although discordances between MRI and CT median ASPECTS scores in non-COVID-19 AIS have been documented, no impact to overall outcomes was observed [20]. Therefore, COVID-19-specific endothelial dysfunction may have a role in infarct core size expansion and contribute to poor outcomes.

Moreover, in our study, we demonstrated that COVID-19 stroke patients eligible for reperfusion therapies had prolonged onset-to-door times. Prolonged ODT in COVID-19 patients might be explained by human factors: first, the lack of available paramedical teams on-call could have delayed arrival to the hospital. Second, both stroke admission rates and prolonged ODT were previously reported owing to the reluctance of stroke patients to seek medical care, especially during the start of the pandemic when vaccination was not yet available [21]. However, the impact of prolonged ODT on stroke severity is debatable. Prolonged ODT might also be explained in part by the expanded intervention window for EVT according to the DAWN trial, demonstrating the undeniable benefits of EVT beyond 6 h for rigorously selected patients [22]. However, this approach was not validated for COVID-19 patients, but despite the lack of evidence, the DAWN criteria were applied according to best clinical practice and consensus statements valid at the time of therapy [23,24]. Second, data regarding the efficacy of EVT beyond 6 h in COVID-19 stroke patients are conflicting, since there are no studies specifically addressing this issue in the COVID-19 population. Studies specifically addressing reperfusion beyond 6 h are required to assess their safety and efficacy profile and more importantly, assess the impact of COVID-19 in these patients, especially in cases with respiratory compromise.

In our study, DTN and DTP times did not differ significantly between patients infected with COVID-19 and controls. Every stroke center was pre-notified about COVID-19 positivity in cases when information was available to the paramedical team and when stroke teams made safety preparations in advance. However, in most cases, COVID-19 status was unknown. Treatment of stroke and reperfusion therapy was considered a priority and did not cause delays in logistics in the emergency departments in either of the stroke centers.

Another aspect to consider is early neurological improvement after reperfusion therapy. In our cohort, successful reperfusion (TICI 2b or TICI 3) was observed in 79.2% of COVID-19 patients with AIS who underwent EVT, and in all but one patient (95.5%) in the control group. In addition, the rate of ischemic changes on CT scan 24 h after RT did not differ between COVID-19 and control groups. Despite successful and timely reperfusion, COVID-19 stroke patients did not improve neurologically 24 h after reperfusion. We acknowledge the possibility that some patients may have exhibited a higher neurological burden due to their severe general state and the need for intensive care due to COVID-19.

We did not calculate the ICU severity scores to represent the general state of these patients. However, NIHSS scores were evaluated either at 7 days or on discharge for every patient. At these time points, the absolute majority of patients were discharged from the ICU. Therefore, we believe that evaluation of NIHSS later in the disease course more accurately reflects the true neurologic burden. Moreover, a lack of early neurological improvement was observed in other studies owing to several factors. Early consecutive ischemic strokes or re-occlusions of the same vessel after successful or complete recanalization were observed at a higher than expected rate of 8% in a systematic study [25]. In our cohort, we have no data regarding early re-occlusions in COVID-19 stroke patients, since this was a retrospective study and we do not routinely perform CTA after successful reperfusion according to national guidelines, unless there is a high clinical suspicion of re-occlusion.

Another proposed explanation for no neurological improvement is the difference in clot composition in COVID-19 and non-COVID-19 patients. Wang et al. described several patients with excessive clot fragmentation and distal migration during thrombectomy. Moreover, once evaluated with thromboelastography, the thrombi showed features of high clot consolidation and reduced time of clot formation consistent with a severe procoagulant state [26]. Several other studies reported a hypercoagulable state in COVID-19 patients as compared to controls, which may attribute to both the devastating multivessel occlusions, clot fragmentation, consecutive ischemic strokes, or early re-occlusions of blood vessels that might contribute to poor outcomes [27]. Although we cannot confirm the different clot features for COVID-19 stroke patients in our study, other aspects of these patients are worth considering.

Hypoxia is a major contributing factor to poor outcomes in AIS patients. In our cohort, 64.5% of COVID-19 stroke patients suffered from respiratory failure. Almost one-third of COVID-19 patients with AIS required prolonged intubation due to severe respiratory system compromise. In a subgroup analysis of the former group (unpublished data), patients in whom the respiratory function was severely affected were those who showed no neurologic improvement 24 h after reperfusion. Most of these patients presented with LVOs and required EVT for reperfusion. Due to a relatively small sample size in our cohort, we could not perform a subgroup analysis with optimal statistical power, but a tendency toward more severe strokes in patients with severe respiratory compromise was observed. This is in line with previous reports. Two meta-analyses showed that severe COVID-19 disease is more often complicated by severe ischemic strokes [16,28]. It is proposed that patients with severe respiratory compromise can be deemed as high risk for poor outcomes and in-hospital mortality [15]. A stroke center in New York reported good early neurological improvement in COVID-19 stroke patients who underwent endovascular treatment. None of the COVID-19 stroke patients who dramatically improved showed signs of respiratory distress [29]. Respiratory function, although analyzed in AIS with COVID-19 cohorts, has not been widely addressed in the subpopulation of patients undergoing reperfusion therapies for AIS. In our study, we emphasize the importance of respiratory complications for AIS patients undergoing specialized treatment. Respiratory failure could be an important factor for early neurological deterioration or lack of improvement despite successful reperfusion. Novel strategies involving optimal management of respiratory compromise should be exploited to improve the outcomes for stroke patients undergoing reperfusion therapy.

Although available safety evidence is scarce, reperfusion in cases of AIS was recommended by an international panel of experts [23,24]. For IVT, various studies report sICH rates from 2.8% to 10% in COVID-19 stroke patients [30–33]. As for EVT, a European multicenter retrospective study of 93 COVID-19 stroke patients reported a rate of sICH of 5.4% [17]. In contrast, results from the largest to date EVT trial MR CLEAN reports sICH rates of 7.7%, although differences between the two studies' sample sizes have to be taken into account [34]. Results from our study are comparable to the aforementioned studies and provide additional insights into the safety of reperfusion therapies for COVID-19 stroke patients. All ICHs were asymptomatic in the COVID-19 group and did not differ statistically from controls. As given the information provided, reperfusion therapies appear to be safe and beneficial for some patients, but large prospective trials evaluating both the safety and efficacy of these treatments are warranted.

Risk factors associated with high dependency and mortality in COVID-19 AIS patients include older age, COVID-19 infection, and stroke severity on admission. The logistic regression model in our study showed only higher baseline NIHSS to be associated with worse functional outcomes. As for 3-month mortality, age, higher baseline NIHSS and COVID-19 infection were significant predictors in the logistic regression model. COVID-19 infection increased the likelihood of death 3 months after stroke and reperfusion therapy seven times. We acknowledge that the regression analysis model in our study may not reflect the true predictors of poor outcomes in COVID-19 AIS patients undergoing RT due to the retrospective nature of the study, data shortages, and a small sample size. Furthermore, we included to our univariate and multivariate logistic regression only patient history data and clinical and laboratory data evaluated on admission. Earlier, we argued that hypoxia is an important factor for the expansion of infarcted brain tissue and may be associated with poor outcomes given the high rates of severe respiratory failure in our study. This might explain the higher rates of in-hospital mortality. However, for the survivors, the causes of 3-month mortality rates remain to be validated.

Strengths. The strength of our study lies within a couple of points. First, the study was conducted across all Lithuanian stroke centers. Second, we added valuable insights to the available safety data of reperfusion therapies in AIS with COVID-19 demonstrating relative safety of all treatment modalities. We have performed one of the few studies reporting COVID-19 patients with AIS mortality at 3 months. As a result, it was possible to compare COVID-19 patients with AIS with controls demonstrating clear differences in mortality and functional outcomes, raising COVID-19 as a potential risk factor predicting poor outcomes in AIS patients.

Limitations. The major weaknesses of our study are the retrospective nature and a relatively small sample size, restricting subgroup analysis of reperfusion modalities and evaluation of outcomes within. Another weakness is the chosen pair-matched analysis method, which might not accurately represent the true demographic and stroke-specific data of the control patients. We could not perform a subgroup analysis of different treatment modalities that would have added additional safety and outcome data. The regression analysis model, albeit significant for some factors, we believe, does not reflect all predictors of poor outcomes in COVID-19 patients. Heterogeneity between different centers concerning treatment management of patients with AIS should be considered. Although we reported 3-month mortality rates, we could not compare functional outcomes of surviving COVID-19 stroke patients to the control group, which would provide additional information on distant effects of COVID-19 on AIS survivors.

5. Conclusions

In conclusion, reperfusion therapies on AIS in COVID-19 patients appear to be safe and should be used. COVID-19-positive AIS patients seem to have more debilitating strokes from onset. Despite successful and timely reperfusion, they tend to have poor functional outcomes with high in-hospital and 3-month mortality rates. For the surviving patients, studies to compare functional outcomes in the post-acute COVID phase between COVID-19 patients with AIS and non-infected stroke survivors are needed.

Author Contributions: Conceptualization, A.V. (Aleksandras Vilionskis), M.V. and J.J.; methodology, A.V. (Aleksandras Vilionskis), M.V., J.J., S.T. and V.M.; software, J.J.; validation, A.V. (Antanas Vaitkus), R.M. and D.J.; formal analysis, J.J.; investigation, J.J., M.V., A.V. (Aleksandras Vilionskis), S.T., V.M., E.G., P.P. and D.G.; data curation: J.J., M.V., A.V. (Aleksandras Vilionskis), D.G., V.M., S.T., E.G. and P.P.; writing—original draft preparation, J.J. and M.V.; writing—review and editing, A.V. (Aleksandras Vilionskis), R.M., D.J., S.T. and V.M.; supervision, D.J. and A.V. (Antanas Vaitkus). All authors have read and agreed to the published version of the manuscript.

Funding: This research received no external funding.

Institutional Review Board Statement: The study was conducted according to the guidelines of the Declaration of Helsinki and was approved by the Ethics Committee of the LITHUANIAN BIOETHICS COMMITTEE (protocol code Nr. L-21-06, 15 September 2021).

Informed Consent Statement: Patient consent was waived due to the retrospective nature of the study and the impossibility to obtain written consent from patients, who were discharged before the study had been started.

Data Availability Statement: Not applicable.

Acknowledgments: This publication is based upon work from IRENE COST Action—Implementation Research Network in Stroke Care Quality (CA18118), supported by COST (European Cooperation in Science and Technology; www.cost.eu, accessed on 22 April 2022).

Conflicts of Interest: The authors declare no conflict of interest.

References

1. Zhu, N.; Zhang, D.; Wang, W.; Li, X.; Yang, B.; Song, J.; Zhao, X.; Huang, B.; Shi, W.; Lu, R.; et al. A Novel Coronavirus from Patients with Pneumonia in China, 2019. *N. Engl. J. Med.* **2020**, *382*, 727–733. [CrossRef]
2. Mao, L.; Jin, H.; Wang, M. Neurologic Manifestations of Hospitalized Patients With Coronavirus Disease 2019 in Wuhan, China. *JAMA Neurol.* **2020**, *77*, 683–690. [CrossRef] [PubMed]
3. Sohal, S.; Mossammat, M. COVID-19 Presenting with Seizures. *IDCases* **2020**, *20*, 00782. [CrossRef] [PubMed]
4. Moriguchi, T.; Harii, N.; Goto, J.; Harada, D.; Sugawara, H.; Takamino, J.; Ueno, M.; Sakata, H.; Kondo, K.; Myose, N.; et al. A first case of meningitis/encephalitis associated with SARS-Coronavirus-2. *Int. J. Infect. Dis.* **2020**, *94*, 55–58. [CrossRef] [PubMed]
5. Vollono, C.; Rollo, E.; Romozzi, M.; Frisullo, G.; Servidei, S.; Borghetti, A.; Calabresi, P. Focal status epilepticus as unique clinical feature of COVID-19: A case report. *Seizure* **2020**, *78*, 109–112. [CrossRef] [PubMed]
6. Zanin, L.; Saraceno, G.; Panciani, P.P.; Renisi, G.; Signorini, L.; Migliorati, K.; Fontanella, M.M. SARS-CoV-2 can induce brain and spine demyelinating lesions. *Acta Neurochir.* **2020**, *162*, 1491–1494. [CrossRef]
7. Alberti, P.; Beretta, S.; Piatti, M.; Karantzoulis, A.; Piatti, M.L.; Santoro, P.; Viganò, M.; Giovannelli, G.; Pirro, F.; Montisano, D.A.; et al. Guillain-Barre syndrome related to COVID-19 infection. *Neurol.-Neuroimmunol. Neuroinflamm.* **2020**, *7*, e741. [CrossRef]
8. Gutierrez-Ortiz, C.; Mendez-Guerrero, A.; Rodrigo-Rey, S.; Pedro-Murillo, E.S.; Bermejo-Guerrero, L.; Gordo-Mañas, R.; de Aragón-Gómez, F.; Benito-León, J. Miller Fisher syndrome and polyneuritis cranialis in COVID-19. *Neurology* **2020**, *95*, 601–605. [CrossRef]
9. Merkler, A.E.; Parikh, N.S.; Mir, S. Risk of Ischemic Stroke in Patients With Coronavirus Disease 2019 (COVID-19) vs. Patients With Influenza. *JAMA Neurol.* **2020**, *77*, 1366–1372. [CrossRef]
10. Sveikata, L.; Melaika, K.; Wiśniewski, A.; Vilionskis, A.; Petrikonis, K.; Stankevičius, E.; Jurjans, K.; Ekkert, A.; Jatužis, D.; Masiliūnas, R. Interactive Training of the Emergency Medical Services Improved Prehospital Stroke Recognition and Transport Time. *Front. Neurol.* **2022**, *13*, 765165. [CrossRef]
11. Melaika, K.; Sveikata, L.; Wiśniewski, A.; Jaxybayeva, A.; Ekkert, A.; Jatužis, D.; Masiliūnas, R. Changes in Prehospital Stroke Care and Stroke Mimic Patterns during the COVID-19 Lockdown. *Int. J. Environ. Res. Public Health* **2021**, *18*, 2150. [CrossRef] [PubMed]
12. Masiliunas, R.; Vilionskis, A.; Bornstein, N.A.; Rastenyte, D.; Jatuzis, D. The impact of a comprehensive national policy on improving acute stroke patient care in Lithuania. *Eur. Stroke J.* **2022**, *1*, 239698732210891. [CrossRef]
13. Mazya, M.; Egido, J.A.; Ford, G.A.; Lees, K.R.; Mikulik, R.; Toni, D.; Wahlgren, N.; Ahmed, N. Predicting the risk of symptomatic intracerebral hemorrhage in ischemic stroke treated with intravenous alteplase: Safe Implementation of Treatments in Stroke (SITS) symptomatic intracerebral hemorrhage risk score. *Stroke* **2012**, *43*, 1524–1531. [CrossRef] [PubMed]
14. Escalard, S.; Maier, B.; Redjem, H.; Delvoye, F.; Hébert, S.; Smajda, S.; Ciccio, G.; Desilles, J.-P.; Mazighi, M.; Blanc, R.; et al. Treatment of Acute Ischemic Stroke due to Large Vessel Occlusion With COVID-19: Experience From Paris. *Stroke* **2020**, *51*, 2540–2543. [CrossRef]
15. Fridman, S.; Bres Bullrich, M.; Jimenez-Ruiz, A.; Costantini, P.; Shah, P.; Just, C.; Vela-Duarte, D.; Linfante, I.; Sharifi-Razavi, A.; Karimi, N.; et al. Stroke risk, phenotypes, and death in COVID-19: Systematic review and newly reported cases. *Neurology* **2020**, *95*, 3373–3385. [CrossRef] [PubMed]

16. Nannoni, S.; de Groot, R.; Bell, S.; Markus, H.S. Stroke in COVID-19: A systematic review and meta-analysis. *Int. J. Stroke* **2021**, *16*, 137–149. [CrossRef] [PubMed]
17. Cagnazzo, F.; Piotin, M.; Escalard, S.; Maier, B.; Ribo, M.; Requena, M.; Pop, R.; Hasiu, A.; Gasparotti, R.; Mardighian, D.; et al. European Multicenter Study of ET-COVID-19. *Stroke* **2021**, *52*, 31–39. [CrossRef]
18. Marti-Fabregas, J.; Guisado-Alonso, D.; Delgado-Mederos, R.; Martínez-Domeño, A.; Prats-Sánchez, L.; Guasch-Jiménez, M.; Cardona, P.; Núñez-Guillén, A.; Requena, M.; Rubiera, M.; et al. Impact of COVID-19 Infection on the Outcome of Patients With Ischemic Stroke. *Stroke* **2021**, *52*, 3908–3917. [CrossRef]
19. Escalard, S.; Chalumeau, V.; Escalard, C.; Redjem, H.; Delvoye, F.; Hébert, S.; Smajda, S.; Ciccio, G.; Desilles, J.-P.; Mazighi, M.; et al. Early Brain Imaging Shows Increased Severity of Acute Ischemic Strokes With Large Vessel Occlusion in COVID-19 Patients. *Stroke* **2020**, *51*, 3366–3370. [CrossRef]
20. Kim, J.T.; Cho, B.H.; Choi, K.-H.; Park, M.-S.; Kim, B.J.; Park, J.-M.; Kang, K.; Lee, S.J.; Kim, J.G.; Cha, J.K.; et al. Magnetic Resonance Imaging Versus Computed Tomography Angiography Based Selection for Endovascular Therapy in Patients With Acute Ischemic Stroke. *Stroke* **2019**, *50*, 365–372. [CrossRef]
21. Teo, K.C.; Leung, W.C.Y.; Wong, Y.-K.; Liu, R.K.C.; Chan, A.H.Y.; Choi, O.M.Y.; Kwok, W.-M.; Leung, K.-K.; Tse, M.-Y.; Cheung, R.T.F.; et al. Delays in Stroke Onset to Hospital Arrival Time During COVID-19. *Stroke* **2020**, *51*, 2228–2231. [CrossRef] [PubMed]
22. Nogueira, R.G.; Jadhav, A.P.; Haussen, D.C.; Bonafe, A.; Budzik, R.F.; Bhuva, P.; Yavagal, D.R.; Ribo, M.; Cognard, C.; Hanel, R.A.; et al. Thrombectomy 6 to 24 Hours after Stroke with a Mismatch between Deficit and Infarct. *N. Engl. J. Med.* **2018**, *378*, 11–21. [CrossRef] [PubMed]
23. Qureshi, A.I.; Abd-Allah, F.; Al-Senani, F.; Aytac, E.; Borhani-Haghighi, A.; Ciccone, A.; Wang, Y. Management of acute ischemic stroke in patients with COVID-19 infection: Report of an international panel. *Int. J. Stroke* **2020**, *15*, 540–554. [CrossRef] [PubMed]
24. Venketasubramanian, N.; Anderson, C.; Ay, H.; Aybek, S.; Brinjikji, W.; de Freitas, G.R.; Del Brutto, O.H.; Fassbender, K.; Fujimura, M.; Goldstein, L.B.; et al. Stroke Care during the COVID-19 Pandemic: International Expert Panel Review. *Cerebrovasc. Dis.* **2021**, *50*, 245–261. [CrossRef]
25. Al-Smadi, A.S.; Mach, J.C.; Abrol, S.; Luqman, A.; Chamiraju, P.; Abujudeh, H. Endovascular Thrombectomy of COVID-19-Related Large Vessel Occlusion: A Systematic Review and Summary of the Literature. *Curr. Radiol. Rep.* **2021**, *9*, 1–8. [CrossRef]
26. Wang, A.; Mandigo, G.K.; Yim, P.D.; Meyers, P.M.; Lavine, S.D. Stroke and mechanical thrombectomy in patients with COVID-19: Technical observations and patient characteristics. *J. Neurointerv. Surg.* **2020**, *12*, 648–653. [CrossRef]
27. Janardhan, V.; Janardhan, V.; Kalousek, V. COVID-19 as a Blood Clotting Disorder Masquerading as a Respiratory Illness: A Cerebrovascular Perspective and Therapeutic Implications for Stroke Thrombectomy. *J. Neuroimaging* **2020**, *30*, 555–561. [CrossRef]
28. Siow, I.; Lee, K.S.; Zhang, J.J.Y.; Saffari, S.E.; Ng, A.; Young, B. Stroke as a Neurological Complication of COVID-19: A Systematic Review and Meta-Analysis of Incidence, Outcomes and Predictors. *J. Stroke Cerebrovasc. Dis.* **2021**, *30*, 105549. [CrossRef]
29. Yaeger, K.A.; Fifi, J.T.; Lara-Reyna, J.; Rossitto, C.; Ladner, T.; Yim, B.; Hardigan, T.; Maragkos, G.A.; Shigematsu, T.; Majidi, S.; et al. Initial Stroke Thrombectomy Experience in New York City during the COVID-19 Pandemic. *AJNR Am. J. Neuroradiol.* **2020**, *41*, 1357–1360. [CrossRef]
30. Zhou, Y.; Hong, C.; Chang, J.; Xia, Y.; Jin, H.; Li, Y.; Mao, L.; Wang, Y.; Zhang, L.; Pan, C.; et al. Intravenous thrombolysis for acute ischaemic stroke during COVID-19 pandemic in Wuhan, China: A multicentre, retrospective cohort study. *J. Neurol. Neurosurg. Psychiatry* **2021**, *92*, 226–228. [CrossRef]
31. Sangalli, D.; Polonia, V.; Colombo, D.; Mantero, V.; Filizzolo, M.; Scaccabarozzi, C.; Salmaggi, A. A single-centre experience of intravenous thrombolysis for stroke in COVID-19 patients. *Neurol. Sci.* **2020**, *41*, 2325–2329. [CrossRef] [PubMed]
32. Sobolewski, P.; Antecki, J.; Brola, W.; Fudala, M.; Bieniaszewski, L.; Kozera, G. Systemic thrombolysis in ischaemic stroke patients with COVID-19. *Acta Neurol. Scand.* **2021**, *145*, 47–52. [CrossRef] [PubMed]
33. Cappellari, M.; Zini, A.; Sangalli, D.; Cavallini, A.; Reggiani, M.; Sepe, F.N.; Rifino, N.; Giussani, G.; Guidetti, D.; Zedde, M.; et al. Thrombolysis and bridging therapy in patients with acute ischaemic stroke and COVID-19. *Eur. J. Neurol.* **2020**, *27*, 2641–2645. [CrossRef] [PubMed]
34. Diener, H.C.; Nitschmann, S. Endovascular treatment for acute ischemic stroke: Multicenter Randomized Clinical Trial of Endovascular Treatment for Acute Ischemic Stroke in the Netherlands (MR CLEAN). *Internist* **2015**, *56*, 847–850. [CrossRef] [PubMed]

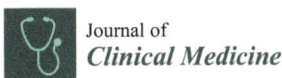

Article

Analysis of Frailty in Geriatric Patients as a Prognostic Factor in Endovascular Treated Patients with Large Vessel Occlusion Strokes

Marlena Schnieder [1,*], Mathias Bähr [1], Mareike Kirsch [2], Ilko Maier [1], Daniel Behme [3], Christian Heiner Riedel [4], Marios-Nikos Psychogios [5], Alex Brehm [5], Jan Liman [1,†] and Christine A. F. von Arnim [2,†]

1. Department of Neurology, University Medical Center Göttingen, 37073 Göttingen, Germany; mbaehr@gwdg.de (M.B.); ilko.maier@med.uni-goettingen.de (I.M.); jliman@gwdg.de (J.L.)
2. Department of Geriatrics, University Medical Center Göttingen, 37073 Göttingen, Germany; mareike.kirsch@med.uni-goettingen.de (M.K.); christine.arnim@med.uni-goettingen.de (C.A.F.v.A.)
3. Department of Neuroradiology, University Hospital of Magdeburg, 39120 Magdeburg, Germany; daniel.behme@med.uni-goettingen.de
4. Department of Neuroradiology, University Medical Center Göttingen, 37073 Göttingen, Germany; christian.riedel@med.uni-goettingen.de
5. Department of Interventional and Diagnostical Neuroradiology, Clinic for Radiology and Nuclearmedicine, University Hospital Basel, 4031 Basel, Switzerland; marios.psychogios@usb.ch (M.-N.P.); alex.brehm@usb.ch (A.B.)
* Correspondence: marlena.schnieder@med.uni-goettingen.de; Tel.: +49-551-39-66356
† Contributed equally.

Abstract: Frailty is associated with an increased risk of adverse health-care outcomes in elderly patients. The Hospital Frailty Risk Score (HFRS) has been developed and proven to be capable of identifying patients which are at high risk of adverse outcomes. We aimed to investigate whether frail patients also face adverse outcomes after experiencing an endovascular treated large vessel occlusion stroke (LVOS). In this retrospective observational cohort study, we analyzed patients ≥ 65 years that were admitted during 2015–2019 with LVOS and endovascular treatment. Primary outcomes were mortality and the modified Rankin Scale (mRS) after three months. Regression models were used to determine the impact of frailty. A total of 318 patients were included in the cohort. The median HFRS was 1.6 (IQR 4.8). A total of 238 (75.1%) patients fulfilled the criteria for a low-frailty risk with a HFRS < 5.72 (22.7%) for moderate-frailty risk with an HFRS from 5–15 and 7 (2.2%) patients for a high-frailty risk. Multivariate regression analyses revealed that the HFRS was associated with an increased mortality after 90 days (CI (95%) 1.001 to 1.236; OR 1.112) and a worse mRS (CI (95%) 1.004 to 1.270; OR 1.129). We identified frailty as an impact factor on functional outcome and mortality in patients undergoing thrombectomy in LVOS.

Keywords: stroke; frailty; elderly patients; hospital frailty risk score; mechanical thrombectomy

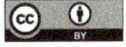

1. Introduction

Treatment of older people can be a challenge for health care systems. An aging population leads to a higher frequency of age related diseases such as dementia, cancer or stroke, often in patients with multimorbidity [1]. But hospital admission and even therapies can be a cause of harm for some older people [2]. Analyses of frailty can help to identify those patients. Frailty is described as a decline of function in multiple organ systems linked to aging and an increased risk of poor outcome [3]. Recently, a novel frailty score based on Tenth Revision of the international classification of disease (ICD-10) diagnostic codes was developed and proven to be capable of identifying patients which are at high risk of adverse outcomes [4]. In total, the score consists of 109 ICD-codes. The authors created a points system, where a certain number of points are awarded for each ICD-10 code and added together to create the final frailty risk score. ICD-10 codes with the highest impact are Dementia in Alzheimer's disease, Hemiplegia, Alzheimer's disease followed by sequelae of cerebrovascular disease and other signs involving the nervous and musculoskeletal systems, including a tendency to fall. The score has several advantages since it is easy to calculate based on the medical history of the patients with a low interrater variability [4]. Frailty, analyzed via the Hospital Frailty Risk Score (HFRS) has been shown to be correlated with poor outcomes, for example after transcatheter valve therapies [5], catheter ablation of atrial fibrillation [6], heart failure [7,8] as well as acute myocardial infarction [7]. In stroke patients, pre-stroke frailty seems to be associated with a shorter survival [9] and patients with stroke are more likely to be classified as frail [10]. Furthermore, pre-existing comorbidities in stroke are associated with a higher short-term and long-term mortality [11] and it is associated with an attenuated improvement following stroke thrombolysis [12]. But to date, there are no data regarding the impact of frailty on the efficacy of mechanical thrombectomy. Since mechanical thrombectomy has become the standard of care for large vessel occlusion stroke (LVOS) patients after publication of the first five randomized trials in 2015 [13], understanding the mechanisms influencing the outcome has been a challenge. Time from onset of stroke to treatment as well as high Alberta Stroke Program Early CT scores (ASPECTS) is crucial for a favorable outcome [14–16].

It is known that increasing age is associated with poor outcomes [13]. Octagenarians and Nonagenarians treated by mechanical thrombectomy have a higher mortality and morbidity than younger patients. Still, successful recanalization leads to a better neurological outcome and a lower mortality in these patients [17–19].

Thus, it would be helpful to implement indicators or scores which are of prognostic value in patients undergoing thrombectomy. The aim of this study was to examine the outcome of elderly patients suffering from LVO with regard to frailty.

2. Materials and Methods

2.1. Study Design, Setting and Study Population

We conducted a retrospective observational cohort study at the University Medical Center in Göttingen by using linked clinical and health administrative databases from 2015 to 2019. This included the stroke database, which we analyzed for elderly patients ≥ 65 years being admitted with LVOS and endovascular treatment. LVOS was defined as a stroke due to an occlusion of the carotid artery, middle cerebral artery in the M1 segment or proximal M2 segment, anterior cerebral artery, posterior cerebral artery or basilar artery. The trial was registered and approved prior to inclusion by the ethics committee of the University of Medicine Göttingen (Ethikkommission der Universitätsmedizin Göttingen (No: 13/7/15An)). Written consent was obtained by all participants or their legally authorized representatives.

2.2. Study Outcomes

Primary outcomes of patients were measured by the three months mortality rate as well as the modified Rankin Scale (mRS) after three months. A good outcome was defined as a mRS from 0–2 and a poor outcome as mRS from 3–6.

2.3. Data Sources

The prospectively derived stroke database contains data of patients with LVOS undergoing mechanical thrombectomy in the University Medical Center in Göttingen during 2015–2019. The collected data of the stroke database included neurological features such as the National Institute of Health Stroke Scale (NHISS), mRS at discharge and after three months, as well as neuroradiological characteristics such as the Alberta stroke program early CT score (ASPECTS) and the modified thrombolysis in cerebral infarction scale (mTICI). NHISS and mRS were assessed by an experienced neurologist, ASPECTS and mTICI by a senior neuroradiologist. Δ-NIHSS was calculated for each patient as the difference between NIHSS at admission and NIHSS at discharge. For the three-month follow up, patients were examined in person. A telephone interview was made in case the patient was not able to come to the hospital. Furthermore, baseline characteristics such as age and gender of the patients were collected, as well as the average length of stay, rate of pneumonia, rehospitalization rate and mortality after three months. To analyze frailty, the Hospital Frailty Risk Score (HFRS) was calculated for each patient of the database based on the International classification of disease (ICD)-10 codes at time of admission of the patients using the pre-morbid condition of the patients including all data available at the timepoint of stroke admission, including previous admissions. The acute stroke symptoms were not included into the score. The HFRS is a recently developed and validated score to measure frailty [4]. Moreover, individuals were categorized as low (<5), intermediate (5–15) or high risk (>15) for frailty based on previously published cut-off points [4]. Patients in the intermediate-risk and high-risk categories were defined as frail. Apart from HFRS, Elixhauser and Charlson comorbidity indices were calculated for each patient based upon diagnoses of the patients at discharge. Both indices have been reported to be a predictor for mortality [20,21].

2.4. Statistical Analysis

For descriptive statistics, continuous variables are presented in means with a standard deviation or a median with an interquartile range. Categorial variables are demonstrated as counts and percentages. Outcomes and the influence of different HFRS risk-categories on hospital stay and pneumonia were assessed using a chi-squared or Kruskal-Wallis-Test as appropriate. To analyze outcomes and mortality of patients after three months, a logistic regression analysis was performed. Univariable logistic regression models were used to identify factors associated with a statistical probability ($p < 0.001$) on the outcome and mortality of the patients and then were included into the multivariable logistic regression model. HFRS, TICI-Scale, the Elixhauser- as well as the Charlston-Comorbitity Index, age, hours ventilation, rate of pneumonia, NHISS at admission and discharge, delta-NIHSS, iv-rtPA, gender, hemicraniectomy, mRS at discharge, ASPECTS, intracranial hemorrhage and time from onset to recanalization were run as univariate models. Results were considered statistically significant when $p < 0.05$. Since there was evidence of a threshold phenomenon, the association of HFRS and mortality was assessed using a segmented linear regression model, as implemented in the R package "segmented" [22]. All statistical analysis was performed using IBM SPSS Statistics vs. 26 (IBM, Armonk, NY, USA), except from regression analysis and c-statistics, which were performed in R.

3. Results

Of the 655 patients of our stroke database, 410 patients had complete follow-up data and 318 fulfilled the inclusion criteria (LVOS with mechanical thrombectomy) with an age ≥65 years. The median age of the patients was 80.1 years (IQR 9.58), the majority of patients were female (60.4%) and 40 (12.6%) suffered from pneumonia. The clinical characteristics are presented in Table 1.

The median HFRS was 1.6 (IQR 4.8). When we calculated the HFRS risk categories, 238 (75.1%) patients met the criteria for low-risk with a HFRS < 5, while 73 (22.7%) fulfilled the criteria for moderate-risk with a HFRS from 5–15 and 7 (2.2%) patients for high-risk. Regarding the neurological characteristics, the median NIHSS on admission was 15 (IQR 10) and 8 (IQR 19) at discharge. The median mRS after 90 days was 4 (IQR 5) and 120 patients (37.7%) had died after 90 days. A total of 109 (34.3%) patients had a favorable outcome with a mRS from 0–2, whereas 209 (65.7%) of the patients had an unfavorable outcome with an mRS 4–6. The neuroradiological characteristics of the patients are listed in Table 2.

Table 1. Clinical characteristics.

Clinical Characteristics	Total n = 318
Age [median (IQR)]	80.1 (IQR 9.58)
Female [n (%)]	192 (60.4%)
Pneumonia [n (%)]	40 (12.6%)
NIHSS at admission [median (IQR)]	15.0 (IQR 10)
NIHSS at discharge [median (IQR)]	8 (IQR 19)
mRS at discharge [median (IQR)]	4 (IQR 3.75)
mRS at 90 days [median (IQR)]	4 (IQR 5)
good outcome (mRS 0–2) [n (%)]	109 (34.3%)
HFRS [median (IQR)]	1.6 (IQR 4.8)
low frailty risk (<5) [n (%)]	238 (75.1%)
moderate frailty risk (5–15) [n (%)]	73 (22.7%)
high frailty risk (>15) [n (%)]	7 (2.2%)
Charlson comorbidity index [median (IQR)]	4 (IQR 6)
Elixhauser comorbidity index [median (IQR)]	9 (IQR 13)
Hemicraniectomy [n (%)]	11 (3.5%)
intravenous thrombolysis [n (%)]	187 (58.8%)
in hospital death [n (%)]	63 (19.8%)
mortality rate after 90 days [n (%)]	120 (37.7%)

NIHSS: National Institute of Health Stroke Score, mRS: modified Rankin Scale, HFRS: Hospital Frailty Risk Score.

Table 2. Neuroradiological characteristics.

Neuroradiological Characteristics	n = 318
door-to-groin time [min (IQR)]	50 (31)
Time from onset to treatment [min (IQR)]	110 (70)
Time from onset to recanalization [min (IQR)]	231 (210)
periprocedural subarachoid hemorrhage [n (%)]	32 (10.1%)
intracerebral hemorrhage [n (%)]	39 (12.4%)
mTICI scale	
0	24 (7.6%)
1	6 (1.9%)
2a	29 (9.2%)
2b	75 (23.7%)
2c	50 (15.8%)
3	132 (41.8%)
Occlusion side	
Proximal internal carotid artery	11 (3.5%)
Carotid-T	56 (17.6%)
M1-branch of MCA	152 (47.8%)
M2-branch of MCA	54 (17%)
Basilar artery	32 (10.1%)
ACA	4 (1.3%)
PCA	7 (2.2%)
ASPECTS [median (IQR)]	8 (2)

mTICI scale: modified thrombolysis in cerebral infarction scale, MCA: middle cerebral artery, ACA: anterior cerebral artery, PCA: posterior cerebral artery, ASPECTS: Alberta stroke program early CT score, IQR: interquartile range. a,b,c: a part of the scale.

Frail patients, defined by a HFRS $\geq$ 5, were older than non-frail patients (83.8 (IQR 9.6) vs. 78.9 (IQR 9.6); p < 0.001) but there was no significant difference in age between patients with a moderate or high frailty risk (83.8 (IQR 9.9) vs. 84.2 (IQR 7.2); p = 0.753). Detailed information about the differences in the frailty groups are listed in Tables 3 and 4.

Table 3. Clinical characteristics of the different frailty groups.

Clinical Characteristics	HFRS < 5	HFRS 5–15	HFRS > 15	p-Value
age [median (IQR)]	78.9 (9.6)	83.8 (9.6)	84.2 (7.2)	$p < 0.001$
Female [n (%)]	137 (57.6%)	50 (68.5%)	5 (71.4%)	$p = 0.206$
Pneumonia [n (%)]	27 (11.3%)	11 (15.3%)	1 (14.3%)	$p = 0.664$
NIHSS at admission [median (IQR)]	15 (9)	14 (8)	17 (6)	$p = 0.254$
NIHSS at discharge [median (IQR)]	7 (16)	12 (35)	15 (37)	$p = 0.052$
mRS at discharge [median (IQR)]	3 (4)	4 (4)	5 (3)	$p = 0.027$
mRS at 90 days [median (IQR)]	4 (2)	5 (2)	6 (5)	$p < 0.001$
good outcome (mRS 0–2) [n (%)]	95 (39.9%)	14 (19.4%)	0 (0%)	$p < 0.001$
Charlson comorbidity index [median (IQR)]	4 (2)	5 (3.5)	5 (2)	$p < 0.001$
Elixhauser comorbidity index [median (IQR)]	9 (10.5)	15 (14)	13 (10)	$p = 0.005$
Hemicraniectomy [n (%)]	9 (3.8%)	2 (2.7%)	0 (0%)	$p = 0.811$
intravenous thrombolysis [n (%)]	137 (57.6%)	45 (51.6%)	5 (71.4%)	$p = 0.652$
in hospital death [n (%)]	44 (18.5%)	18 (25.0%)	1 (14.3%)	$p = 0.448$
mortality rate after 90 days [n (%)]	79 (33.2%)	36 (50.0%)	5 (71.4%)	$p = 0.005$

IQR: interquartile range, NIHSS: National Institute of Health stroke score, mRS: modified Rankin Scale.

Table 4. Neuroradiological characteristics of the different frailty groups.

Neuroradiological Characteristics	HFRS < 5	HFRS 5–15	HFRS > 15	p-Value
Door-to-groin time [min (IQR)]	50 (31)	47 (40)	54 (50)	$p = 0.572$
Onset to recanalization time [min (IQR)]	228 (198)	241.5 (293)	219.5 (103)	$p = 0.697$
onset to treatment time [min (IQR)]	107.5 (66)	115 (86)	140	$p = 0.798$
periprocedural subarachoid hemorrhage [n (%)]	23 (10.1%)	8 (11.1%)	1 (16.7%)	$p = 0.855$
intracerebral hemorrhage [n (%)]	32 (13.6%)	7 (9.7%)	0 (0%)	$p = 0.410$
TICI [n (%)]				$p = 0.676$
0	18 (7.6%)	5 (6.8%)	1 (14.3%)	
1	5 (2.1%)	1 (1.4%)	0 (0%)	
2a	17 (7.2%)	11 (15.1%)	1 (14.3%)	
2b	57 (24.2%)	15 (20.5%)	3 (42.9%)	
2c	38 (16.1%)	11 (15.1%)	1 (14.3%)	
3	101 (42.8%)	30 (41.1%)	1 (14.3%)	
Occlusion site				$p = 0.039$
Proximal ACI	10 (4.2%)	1 (1.4%)	0 (0%)	
Carotid-T	46 (19.3%)	8 (11%)	2 (28.6%)	
M1-branch of MCA	114 (47.9%)	38 (52.1%)	0 (0%)	
M2-branch of MCA	31 (13%)	18 (24.7%)	5 (71.4%)	
Basilar artery	26 (10.9%)	6 (8.2%)	0 (0%)	
ACA	3 (1.3%)	1 (1.4%)	0 (0%)	
PCA	6 (2.5%)	1 (1.4%)	0 (0%)	
ASPECTS	8 (2)	9 (1)	9 (3)	$p = 0.165$

IQR: interquartile range, mTICI: modified thrombolysis in cerebral infarction scale, ACI: internal carotid artery, ACA: anterior cerebral artery, PCA: posterior cerebral artery, ASPECTS: Alberta stroke program early CT score. a,b,c: a part of the scale.

There was no significant difference in mortality at discharge, but there was a significant association between mortality and frailty after 90 days in the logistic regression analysis. In the univariate models, we found that the likelihood of mortality after 90 days significantly increased with HFRS ($p < 0.001$; CI (95%) 1.053 to 1.1183; OR 1.16) as well as the likelihood of an unfavorable neurological outcome ($p < 0.001$; CI (95%) 1.069 to 1.248; OR 1.155). The C-statistics of the model on mortality after 90 days were 0.6293. Multivariate analyses revealed that along with age, the mTICI scale, Δ-NIHSS, ASPECTS and HFRS ($p = 0.020$; CI (95%) 1.018 to 1.240; OR 1.24) showed a significant relationship with the likelihood of mortality after 90 days, as shown in Table 5.

Table 5. Multivariate logistic regression analysis of Influence on mortality after 90 days; HFRS: Hospital Frailty Risk Score, mTICI scale: modified thrombolysis in cerebral infarction scale, ASPECTS: Alberta Stroke Program Early CT Score, NIHSS: National Institute of Health Stroke Score, Δ-NIHSS: difference between the NIHSS at admission and discharge.

Mortality after 90 Days	Odds Ratio	95% Confidence	Interval	p-Value
HFRS	1.124	1.018	1.240	0.020
Age (years)	1.159	1.090	1.232	<0.001
mTICI scale	0.760	0.581	0.993	0.044
ASPECTS	0.740	0.576	0.951	0.019
Δ-NIHSS	0.868	0.835	0.903	<0.001

Plotting the relationship between HFRS and the rate of mortality after 90 days suggested a threshold phenomenon, as seen in Figure 1.

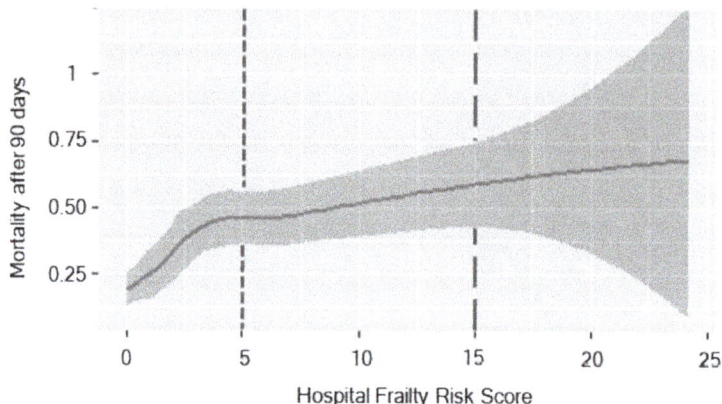

Figure 1. Association of HFRS over mortality after 90 days. The different HFRS risk categories are divided by the grey lines. The first line is the boundary between the low- and moderate-frailty risk category, the second line between moderate- and high-frailty risk. The grey shade is indicating the standard deviation.

There was a steep increase in mortality up to a frailty score of three, afterwards the gradient flattened out until it reached a plateau at about a frailty score of 15. No significant difference was detectable in the gradient of the curve.

When dividing into the three frailty-risk categories, in-hospital death in the low-risk group was 18.5% (44), in the moderate-risk group 25.0% (18) and in the high-risk group 14.3% (1) (p = 0.448). After 90 days, the mortality rate was 33.2% (79) in the low-risk group, 50.0% (36) in the moderate-risk group and 71.4% in the high-risk group (5); (p = 0.005).

Furthermore, there was a significant influence of the HFRS (p = 0.029; CI (95%) 1.012 to 1.254; OR 1.127) along with age, mTICI, ASPECTS, age, the Elixhauser Comorbidity Index and Δ-NIHSS in the multivariate analysis on neurological outcomes of the patients, as shown in Table 6.

Table 6. Multivariate logistic regression analysis of neurological outcome after 90 days measured by mRS.

Poor Neurological Outcome (mRS 3–6)	Odds Ratio	95% Confidence	Interval	p-Value
HFRS	1.127	1.012	1.254	0.029
Age	1.077	1.023	1.135	0.005
ASPECTS	0.584	0.450	0.758	<0.001
mTICI scale	0.696	0.526	0.921	0.011
Elixhauser Comorbidity Index	1.074	1.028	1.122	0.001
Δ-NIHSS	0.897	0.857	0.939	<0.001

HFRS: Hospital Frailty Risk Score, ASPECTS: Alberta Stroke Program Early CT Score, mTICI scale: modified thrombolysis in cerebral infarction scale, mRS: modified Rankin Scale, NIHSS: National Institute of Health Stroke Score.

After dividing into the three frailty categories, patients in a low frailty risk category were more likely to have a favorable outcome than those in a moderate or high frailty risk category; this reached statistical significance (95 (39.9%) vs. 14 (19.4%) vs. 0 (0%); $p < 0.001$) and can be seen in Figure 2.

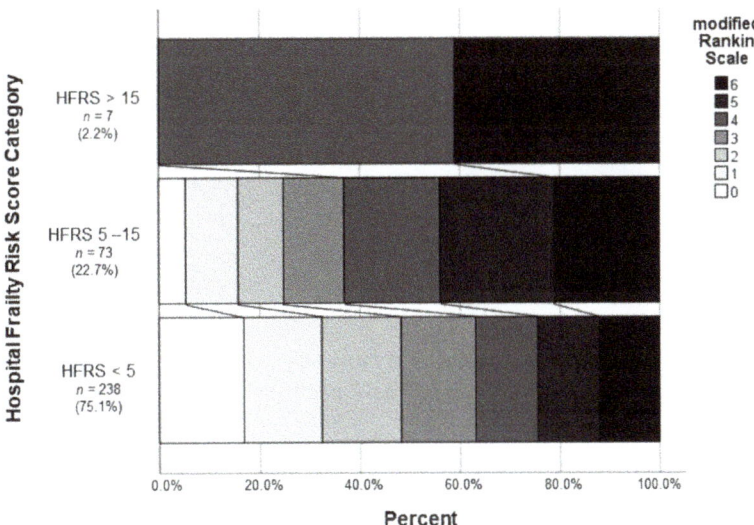

Figure 2. Proportion of the modified Rankin Scale after mechanical thrombectomy as a percentage of the different HFRS categories.

Frail patients, with a HFRS ≥ 5, did not secondary complications suffer significantly more often such as pneumonia (27 (11.3%) vs. 11 (15.3%) vs. 1 (14.3%); $p = 0.664$) and their rate of mechanical ventilation was similar to patients with a low frailty score (130 (54.6%) vs. 36 (50.0%) vs. 4 (57.1%); $p = 0.776$). The length of stay in the hospital did not differ between patients with a low, moderate or high frailty risk (10 (IQR 11) vs. 10.5 (IQR 8) vs. 9 (IQR 5) days; $p = 0.656$). No patient in the high-risk frailty group exceeded the maximum length of stay (0.29 ($\pm$2.413) vs. 0.1 ($\pm$0.118) vs. 0 ($\pm$0); $p = 0.776$). With respect to all three frailty groups, the total number of patients exceeding the g-DRG calculated maximum of stay was rather small, as can be seen in Figure 3.

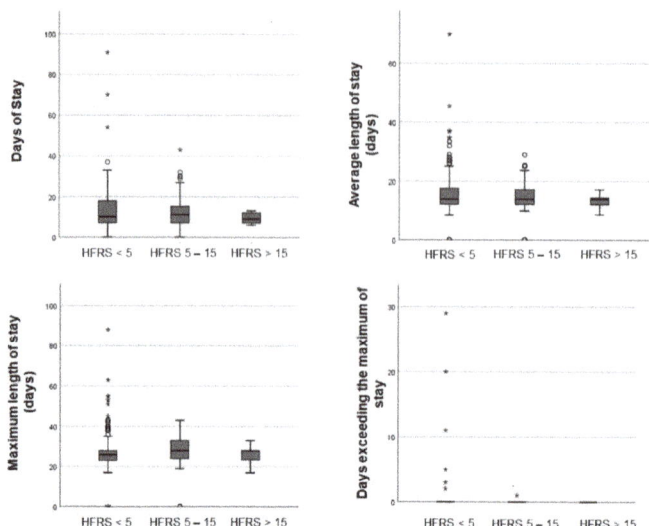

Figure 3. Boxplots of the influence of the HFRS on the length of stay in hospital. A white dot is indicating an outlier (3rd quartile + 1.5 interquartile range or 1st quartile − 1.5 interquartile range) and a * an extreme outlier (3rd quartile + 3 interquartile range or 1st quartile − 3 interquartile range).

A similar length of stay is also reflected in the renumeration for the patients. Renumeration was similar without a significant difference in the three different risk groups (low-risk 18525.83 EUR (IQR 7900.15 EUR) vs. moderate-risk 22418.75 EUR (IQR 7285.41 EUR) vs. high-risk 19903.06 EUR (IQR 10070.45 EUR); $p = 0.401$).

4. Discussion

In this monocentric cohort, more than 75% of all endovascular treated strokes were older than 65 years and our study could demonstrate that frailty, as assessed by the HFRS, has an impact on mortality after mechanical thrombectomy in large vessel occlusion stroke. Frail patients have a significantly higher mortality rate after three months than nonfrail patients. Compared to previous studies on frail patients with stroke [18], our study provides a very distinct and highly relevant subgroup of strokes, namely LVO induced strokes treated with thrombectomy. We applied the HFRS as a well evaluated frailty score, and were able to correct for multiple confounders due to our comprehensive data set.

In an aging population, frailty and the associated treatment risk is of emerging interest. Multiple scores been developed to predict mortality in patients, such as the Charlson Comorbidity Index and Elixhauser Comorbidity Index [20,21]. However, in our study, the Elixhauser Comorbidity Index and Charlson Comorbidity Index were not able to predict mortality in thrombectomized patients.

The ICD-10 based hospital frailty risk score is based on administrative data and therefore is an easy and accessible score to measure frailty, possibly enabling the physician to calculate the risk for adverse events prior to hospital admission and enabling consultation of patients or relatives.

Previously this score has been used to evaluate outcome after transcatheter valve therapies [5]. In contrast to TAVI procedures, the magnitude of the effect in thrombectomized patients is lower than those undergoing TAVI (HR TAVI 3.1, OR thrombectomy: 1.2).

Moreover, frailty is not only a predictor of mortality in patients, additional to age [13], ASPECTS [15] and other parameters such as time [14]; frailty is another parameter to predict a neurological outcome of mechanical thrombectomy in large vessel occlusion stroke. Frail patients have a worse neurological outcome after 90 days compared to non-frail patients. Only 20% of the medium risk group achieve a favorable outcome after

3 months (mRs 0–2; Figure 1). The effect on neurological outcome might be influenced by premorbid disabilities, since frail patients suffer more often from dementia and premorbid stroke [23] than non-frail patients. Although more detailed analyses are warranted to better understand the possible influence of distinct premorbid diseases on disability and, hence on outcome, further data on premorbid disability beyond specific diseases might also help to address this in future studies.

Apart from mortality and neurological outcomes, we did not find a significant difference in secondary complications or prolonged stays in hospital between different frailty groups. This is in contrast to previous data of a general hospital population [24] and a population after degenerative spine operations [25], in which an association between frailty and prolonged hospitalization had been shown. But medical interventions in stroke patients, leading to a prolonged hospital stay such as hemicraniectomy are rarely performed in frail patients. Moreover, it may be possible that other secondary complications like acute renal failure and septicemia are not treated extensively in high-risk frailty patients, as it is more likely that frail patients were sent back to care facilities in a palliative regime after disabling stroke. Another possibility is that the cut-offs differentiating between low, moderate and high-risk groups may not be accurate for stroke patients. This is indicated by the different curves of the association between mortality and HFRS in our study comparing to the original work [4]. Since HFRS was not intended to describe adverse outcomes in a specific stroke population, future studies are needed to validate the cut-offs in stroke patients.

One strength of our study is the complete data set without missing data, which minimizes a bias.

Another advantage of the HFRS is that it can be implemented automatically in hospital information systems. This refers to patients for whom the necessary administrative data are already available at the time of a new stroke admission. Because the ICD-10 code is routinely recorded electronically, determination of the HFRS can be automatically embedded in the hospital's electronic medical record and even has the potential to be programmed into frailty-attuned clinical decision support systems. Having the HFRS be automatically available at hospital admission may avoid the challenges of implementing manual scores such as the Clinical Frailty Scale and improve standardization of frailty assessment. This may have additional potential, particularly in stroke patients, where every second counts and acute disability (e.g., hemiplegia, aphasia) may complicate clinical judgement of premorbid frailty status on admission.

Whether the HFRS, a purely clinical frailty assessment or a combination of both is better suited to predict outcome in frail stroke patients needs to be clarified in further studies. In addition, further studies are needed to determine whether a frailty assessment can guide and optimize clinical care at the individual patient level.

Our study has several limitations. One limitation, not only of our study but also the HFRS, is the lack of complete administrative patient data at admission, which may lead to a misclassification bias. Several diagnoses, for example unspecified fall or care diagnoses involving the use of rehabilitation procedures which are part of the HFRS, are not always documented in patients' medical history, leading to an incomplete and therefore lower score. This is not only a shortcoming of our study but a general problem for the HFRS, in particular when used in a clinical setting. In addition, not all ICD-scores used to calculate the HFRS are used in the German reimbursement system.

Another limitation, leading to a possible selection bias, is that we only included patients who underwent mechanical thrombectomy and not those with LVOS without treatment. This was because frail patients are more likely to be excluded from mechanical thrombectomy compared to non-frail patients due their premorbid disabilities. Therefore, the rather positive clinical outcome results of the frail group may be overestimated. Especially in the high-risk frailty group, the number of patients is rather low. Therefore, it may be possible that our study underpowered this patient subgroup. This problem could be addressed by applying larger patient cohorts, e.g., from multicentric registries, to further explore the effects of strokes on high-risk frailty.

5. Conclusions

Frailty leads to a higher mortality and morbidity in patients with large vessel occlusion, even in medium frail patients, only 20% reach a favorable outcome. Therefore, identifying frail patients and stratifying risk categories using the HFRS may help to communicate with patients and families about the incidence of potential outcomes.

Author Contributions: Conceptualization, J.L. and C.A.F.v.A.; methodology, M.S., J.L., C.A.F.v.A. and M.K.; validation, J.L., C.A.F.v.A.; formal analysis, M.S.; investigation, D.B., I.M., M.-N.P. and A.B.; resources, M.B., C.H.R. and J.L.; data curation, M.S.; writing—original draft preparation, M.S.; writing—review and editing, A.B., J.L. and C.A.F.v.A.; visualization, M.S.; supervision, M.B., J.L. and C.A.F.v.A.; project administration, M.B. and C.H.R.; All authors have read and agreed to the published version of the manuscript.

Funding: This research received no external funding.

Institutional Review Board Statement: The trial was registered and approved prior to inclusion by the ethics committee of the University Medicine Göttingen (Ethikkommission der Universitätsmedizin Göttingen (No: 13/7/15An)). All methods were carried out in accordance with the declaration of Helsinki.

Informed Consent Statement: Informed consent was obtained from all subjects involved in the study.

Data Availability Statement: The data presented in this study are available on request from the corresponding author due to the need to respect the privacy of the patients.

Conflicts of Interest: The authors declare no conflict of interest.

References

1. Rechel, B.; Grundy, E.; Robine, J.-M.; Cylus, J.; Mackenbach, J.P.; Knai, C.; McKee, M. Ageing in the European Union. *Lancet* **2013**, *381*, 1312–1322. [CrossRef]
2. Hubbard, R.E.; Peel, N.M.; Samanta, M.; Gray, L.C.; Mitnitski, A.; Rockwood, K. Frailty Status at Admission to Hospital Predicts Multiple Adverse Outcomes. *Age Ageing* **2017**, *46*, 801–806. [CrossRef] [PubMed]
3. Clegg, A.; Young, J.; Iliffe, S.; Rikkert, M.O.; Rockwood, K. Frailty in Elderly People. *Lancet* **2013**, *381*, 752–762. [CrossRef]
4. Gilbert, T.; Neuburger, J.; Kraindler, J.; Keeble, E.; Smith, P.; Ariti, C.; Arora, S.; Street, A.; Parker, S.; Roberts, H.C.; et al. Development and Validation of a Hospital Frailty Risk Score Focusing on Older People in Acute Care Settings Using Electronic Hospital Records: An Observational Study. *Lancet* **2018**, *391*, 1775–1782. [CrossRef]
5. Kundi, H.; Popma, J.J.; Reynolds, M.R.; Strom, J.B.; Pinto, D.S.; Valsdottir, L.R.; Shen, C.; Choi, E.; Yeh, R.W. Frailty and Related Outcomes in Patients Undergoing Transcatheter Valve Therapies in a Nationwide Cohort. *Eur. Heart J.* **2019**, *40*, 2231–2239. [CrossRef] [PubMed]
6. Kundi, H.; Noseworthy, P.A.; Valsdottir, L.R.; Shen, C.; Yao, X.; Yeh, R.W.; Kramer, D.B. Relation of Frailty to Outcomes After Catheter Ablation of Atrial Fibrillation. *Am. J. Cardiol.* **2020**, *125*, 1317–1323. [CrossRef]
7. Kundi, H.; Wadhera, R.K.; Strom, J.B.; Valsdottir, L.R.; Shen, C.; Kazi, D.S.; Yeh, R.W. Association of Frailty With 30-Day Outcomes for Acute Myocardial Infarction, Heart Failure, and Pneumonia Among Elderly Adults. *JAMA Cardiol.* **2019**, *4*, 1084–1091. [CrossRef]
8. Kwok, C.S.; Zieroth, S.; Spall, H.G.C.V.; Helliwell, T.; Clarson, L.; Mohamed, M.; Mallen, C.; Duckett, S.; Mamas, M.A. The Hospital Frailty Risk Score and Its Association with In-Hospital Mortality, Cost, Length of Stay and Discharge Location in Patients with Heart Failure Short Running Title: Frailty and Outcomes in Heart Failure. *Int. J. Cardiol.* **2020**, *300*, 184–190. [CrossRef]
9. Winovich, D.T.; Longstreth, W.T.; Arnold, A.M.; Varadhan, R.; Zeki Al Hazzouri, A.; Cushman, M.; Newman, A.B.; Odden, M.C. Factors Associated with Ischemic Stroke Survival and Recovery in Older Adults. *Stroke* **2017**, *48*, 1818–1826. [CrossRef]
10. Palmer, K.; Vetrano, D.L.; Padua, L.; Romano, V.; Rivoiro, C.; Scelfo, B.; Marengoni, A.; Bernabei, R.; Onder, G. Frailty Syndromes in Persons with Cerebrovascular Disease: A Systematic Review and Meta-Analysis. *Front. Neurol.* **2019**, *10*. [CrossRef]
11. Schmidt, M.; Jacobsen, J.B.; Johnsen, S.P.; Bøtker, H.E.; Sørensen, H.T. Eighteen-Year Trends in Stroke Mortality and the Prognostic Influence of Comorbidity. *Neurology* **2014**, *82*, 340–350. [CrossRef]
12. Evans, N.R.; Wall, J.; To, B.; Wallis, S.J.; Romero-Ortuno, R.; Warburton, E.A. Clinical Frailty Independently Predicts Early Mortality after Ischaemic Stroke. *Age Ageing* **2020**, *49*, 588–591. [CrossRef]
13. Goyal, M.; Menon, B.K.; van Zwam, W.H.; Dippel, D.W.J.; Mitchell, P.J.; Demchuk, A.M.; Dávalos, A.; Majoie, C.B.L.M.; van der Lugt, A.; de Miquel, M.A.; et al. Endovascular Thrombectomy after Large-Vessel Ischaemic Stroke: A Meta-Analysis of Individual Patient Data from Five Randomised Trials. *Lancet* **2016**, *387*, 1723–1731. [CrossRef]
14. Saver, J.L.; Goyal, M.; van der Lugt, A.; Menon, B.K.; Majoie, C.B.L.M.; Dippel, D.W.; Campbell, B.C.; Nogueira, R.G.; Demchuk, A.M.; Tomasello, A.; et al. Time to Treatment with Endovascular Thrombectomy and Outcomes from Ischemic Stroke: A Meta-Analysis. *JAMA* **2016**, *316*, 1279–1289. [CrossRef]

15. Hill, M.D.; Rowley, H.A.; Adler, F.; Eliasziw, M.; Furlan, A.; Higashida, R.T.; Wechsler, L.R.; Roberts, H.C.; Dillon, W.P.; Fischbein, N.J.; et al. Selection of Acute Ischemic Stroke Patients for Intra-Arterial Thrombolysis with Pro-Urokinase by Using ASPECTS. *Stroke* **2003**, *34*, 1925–1931. [CrossRef]
16. Tsogkas, I.; Knauth, M.; Schregel, K.; Behme, D.; Wasser, K.; Maier, I.; Liman, J.; Psychogios, M.N. Added Value of CT Perfusion Compared to CT Angiography in Predicting Clinical Outcomes of Stroke Patients Treated with Mechanical Thrombectomy. *Eur. Radiol.* **2016**, *26*, 4213–4219. [CrossRef]
17. Meyer, L.; Alexandrou, M.; Flottmann, F.; Deb-Chatterji, M.; Abdullayev, N.; Maus, V.; Politi, M.; Bernkopf, K.; Roth, C.; Kastrup, A.; et al. Endovascular Treatment of Very Elderly Patients Aged ≥90 with Acute Ischemic Stroke. *J. Am. Heart Assoc.* **2020**, *9*, e014377. [CrossRef]
18. Drouard-de Rousiers, E.; Ludovic, L.; Sébastien, R.; Consoli, A.; Mazighi, M.; Labreuche, J.; Kyheng, M.; Gory, B.; Dargazanli, C.; Arquizan, C.; et al. Impact of Reperfusion for Nonagenarians Treated by Mechanical Thrombectomy. *Stroke* **2019**, *50*, 3164–3169. [CrossRef]
19. Derex, L.; Haesebaert, J.; Odier, C.; Alesefir, W.; Berthezène, Y.; Buisson, M.; Daneault, N.; Deschaintre, Y.; Eker, O.F.; Gioia, L.; et al. Predictors of Outcome After Mechanical Thrombectomy in Stroke Patients Aged ≥85 Years. *Can. J. Neurol. Sci. J. Can. Sci. Neurol.* **2021**, 1–6. [CrossRef]
20. Moore, B.J.; White, S.; Washington, R.; Coenen, N.; Elixhauser, A. Identifying Increased Risk of Readmission and In-Hospital Mortality Using Hospital Administrative Data: The AHRQ Elixhauser Comorbidity Index. *Med. Care* **2017**, *55*, 698–705. [CrossRef]
21. Bannay, A.; Chaignot, C.; Blotière, P.-O.; Basson, M.; Weill, A.; Ricordeau, P.; Alla, F. The Best Use of the Charlson Comorbidity Index with Electronic Health Care Database to Predict Mortality. *Med. Care* **2016**, *54*, 188–194. [CrossRef]
22. Muggeo, V.M.R. Segmented: An R Package to Fit Regression Models with Broken-Line Relationships. *R News* **2008**, *8*, 20–25.
23. Eckart, A.; Hauser, S.I.; Haubitz, S.; Struja, T.; Kutz, A.; Koch, D.; Neeser, O.; Meier, M.A.; Mueller, B.; Schuetz, P. Validation of the Hospital Frailty Risk Score in a Tertiary Care Hospital in Switzerland: Results of a Prospective, Observational Study. *BMJ Open* **2019**, *9*, e026923. [CrossRef]
24. McAlister, F.; van Walraven, C. External Validation of the Hospital Frailty Risk Score and Comparison with the Hospital-Patient One-Year Mortality Risk Score to Predict Outcomes in Elderly Hospitalised Patients: A Retrospective Cohort Study. *BMJ Qual. Saf.* **2019**, *28*, 284–288. [CrossRef] [PubMed]
25. Hannah, T.C.; Neifert, S.N.; Caridi, J.M.; Martini, M.L.; Lamb, C.; Rothrock, R.J.; Yuk, F.J.; Gilligan, J.; Genadry, L.; Gal, J.S. Utility of the Hospital Frailty Risk Score for Predicting Adverse Outcomes in Degenerative Spine Surgery Cohorts. *Neurosurgery* **2020**. [CrossRef] [PubMed]

Article

Acute Recanalization of Large Vessel Occlusion in the Anterior Circulation Stroke: Is Mechanical Thrombectomy Alone Better in Patients over 80 Years of Age? Findings from a Retrospective Observational Study

Dagmar Krajíčková [1], Antonín Krajina [2], Roman Herzig [1,*], Oldřich Vyšata [1,3], Libor Šimůnek [1] and Martin Vališ [1]

1. Department of Neurology, Comprehensive Stroke Center, Charles University Faculty of Medicine and University Hospital, Sokolská 581, CZ-500 05 Hradec Králové, Czech Republic; dagmar.krajickova@fnhk.cz (D.K.); vysatao@gmail.com (O.V.); libor.simunek@email.cz (L.Š.); valismar@seznam.cz (M.V.)
2. Department of Radiology, Comprehensive Stroke Center, Charles University Faculty of Medicine and University Hospital, CZ-500 05 Hradec Králové, Czech Republic; antonin.krajina@fnhk.cz
3. Department of Computing and Control Engineering, University of Chemistry and Technology in Prague, Czech Republic, CZ-166 28 Prague 6, Czech Republic
* Correspondence: herzig.roman@seznam.cz

Abstract: Real-world data report worse 3-month clinical outcomes in elderly patients with acute ischemic stroke (AIS) treated with mechanical thrombectomy (MT). The aim was to identify factors influencing clinical outcome in elderly patients with anterior circulation AIS treated with MT (±intravenous thrombolysis (IVT)). In a retrospective, monocentric study, analysis of prospectively collected data of 138 patients (≥80 years) was performed. IVT was an independent negative predictor (OR 0.356; 95% CI: 0.134–0.942) and female sex an independent positive predictor (OR 4.179, 95% CI: 1.300–13.438) of 3-month good clinical outcome (modified Rankin scale 0–2). Female sex was also an independent negative predictor of 3-month mortality (OR 0.244, 95% CI: 0.100–0.599). Other independent negative predictors of 3-month good clinical outcome were older age, lower pre-stroke self-sufficiency, more severe neurological deficit and longer procedural intervals. Mortality was also independently predicted by longer procedural interval and by the occurrence of symptomatic intracerebral hemorrhage ($p < 0.05$ in all cases). Our results demonstrated, that in patients aged ≥80 years with anterior circulation AIS undergoing MT (±IVT), IVT reduced the chance of 3-month good clinical outcome and female sex was associated with a greater likelihood of 3-month good clinical outcome and lower probability of 3-month mortality.

Keywords: anterior circulation; acute ischemic stroke; large vessel occlusion; elderly patients; mechanical thrombectomy; intravenous thrombolysis; bridging therapy; recanalization; clinical outcome

1. Introduction

Mechanical thrombectomy (MT) is currently the standard treatment for acute ischemic stroke (AIS) in the anterior circulation due to the emergent large vessel occlusion (ELVO). MT has been shown to lead to higher recanalization rates and better clinical outcomes in selected patients compared to intravenous thrombolysis (IVT) alone [1–5]. Although the guidelines recommend, unless there is a contraindication, treatment with intravenous recombinant tissue plasminogen activator (rtPA) before MT (bridging therapy) [6,7], there are doubts about the benefit of IVT preceding MT [8–16]. Real-world data consistently report worse 3-month clinical outcomes in elderly patients compared to younger patients [17–24]. Nevertheless, the factors influencing the clinical outcome in elderly patients have not been fully elucidated.

The aim was to identify factors influencing the recanalization rate, the occurrence of symptomatic intracerebral hemorrhage (sICH) and the clinical outcome in elderly patients

(≥80 years) with anterior circulation AIS due to ELVO undergoing MT (±IVT) in routine clinical practice.

2. Materials and Methods

2.1. Data Source and Study Population

All relevant data used for this retrospective analysis were manually extracted from hospital information systems and available individual patient medical charts, including documentation from the referring hospital (in the case of patients with secondary transport), emergency physician notes, neurology notes, and medication administration records.

In a retrospective, monocentric study, a set of 138 consecutive elderly patients (≥80 years) with anterior circulation AIS due to ELVO treated with MT using second generation stent-retrievers (±IVT) from January 2013 to June 2019 in the Comprehensive Stroke Center (CSC), University Hospital in Hradec Králové, Czech Republic, was analyzed. Some patients were transported to the CSC directly, others were transported to the CSC for MT from primary stroke centers (PSC). The indication for MT was determined in accordance with the valid guidelines [6,25–28].

2.2. Computed Tomography Imaging

Non-enhanced computed tomography (NECT) of the brain with the assessment of the Alberta Stroke Program Early CT Score (ASPECTS) and CT angiography (CTA) of the cervical and intracranial arteries including the evaluation of the collateral system was performed in all patients. For CTA, a non-ionic contrast iomeprol (Iomeron 400, Bracco, Torviscosa, Italy) was administered intravenously (total volume of 60 mL, speed 4 mL/s). Patients treated more than 6 h from symptoms onset and patients with unknown AIS onset time also underwent perfusion CT (PCT) examination using 40 mL of the same contrast medium infused intravenously at 5 mL/s. The time to maximum (Tmax) delay > 6 s was used for the display of ischemic penumbra and, the relative cerebral blood flow < 30% of that in normal tissue for a diagnosis of ischemic core (irreversibly injured brain tissue) [29]. In patients with IVT administered in the PSC, a control brain NECT was performed in the CSC prior to MT initiation to exclude bleeding complications and the development of extensive cerebral infarction. A Somatom Definition AS + (Siemens, Forchheim, Germany) scanner was used for CT examinations.

2.3. Intravenous Thrombolysis

Intravenous thrombolysis with a standard dose of 0.9 mg/kg (maximum dose 90 mg) of recombinant tissue plasminogen activator (Actilyse, Boehringer Ingelheim, Ingelheim am Rhein, Germany) was applied in all patients with known stroke onset time fulfilling the inclusion and exclusion criteria according to the valid guidelines. Furthermore, 10% of the rtPA dose was administered as intravenous bolus, followed by a 60-min infusion of the remaining 90% of the dose [30].

2.4. Digital Subtraction Angiography and Mechanical Thrombectomy

Within a 6-h time window from AIS symptoms onset, MT was performed in patients with ASPECTS ≥ 6 on NECT. The result of PCT was crucial in patients treated more than 6 h from AIS symptoms onset and in patients with unknown AIS onset time—MT was performed in patients with a small ischemic core (≤70 mL; based of the results of previous studies [31]) and with the presence of ischemic penumbra. Patients without mismatch were excluded from therapy. A poor condition of the collateral system, if representing the only unfavorable prognostic factor, was not a reason for the exclusion from the MT. MT was started as soon as possible, not waiting for the IVT effect, if applied.

A biplane angio machine (Philips Allura FD 20/20, Best, The Netherlands) was used for DSA examination. Non-ionic contrast iodixanol (Visipaque 320, GE Healthcare AS, Oslo, Norway) was administered intra-arterially using a Seldinger technique (total volume of 6 mL, speed 7 mL/s). For MT, second-generation stent-retrievers were used—Trevo (Trevo

ProVue, Concentric Medical, Mountain View, CA, USA), Solitaire (Solitaire, Covidien, Dublin, Ireland), Eric 4 (ERIC 4 Retrieval Device, MicroVention Terumo, Saint-Germain-en-Laye, France), and Preset (pREset, Phenox GmbH, Bochum, Germany). The choice of stent-retriever depended on the decision of the radiologist. In the majority of procedures, the balloon guiding catheter (Merci 8F, Concentric Medical, Mountain View, CA, USA) was placed within the internal carotid artery (ICA). In the presence of a loop, the catheter was placed below it. A microcatheter (0.021 inch) with stent-retriever was subsequently introduced. The stent-retriever was deployed across the occlusion and after 4 min the stent was slowly retrieved, while flow arrest in the accessing artery was applied by balloon inflation. Manual aspiration was applied through the guiding catheter via sidearm using a 20-cc syringe. In most cases, the procedure was performed under conscious sedation, without general anesthesia. Blood pressure was kept above 140 mm Hg.

2.5. Observed Parameters

The following data were collected: demographic data (age, sex, occurrence of vascular risk factors—arterial hypertension, diabetes mellitus, dyslipidemia, coronary artery disease, atrial fibrillation, prior stroke/transient ischemic attack), pre-intervention data (pre-stroke modified Rankin scale (mRS) value [32], direct/interhospital transfer, neurologic deficit—assessed using the National Institutes of Health Stroke Scale (NIHSS) [33], initial ASPECTS values, presence of leukoaraiosis (defined as CT signs of hypodense lesions around the anterior and posterior horns of the lateral ventricles [34]), location of vessel occlusion), and procedural characteristics (time intervals—the time when the patient was last seen normal was used in patients with an unknown AIS onset time, number of stent-retriever passes (SRPs), recanalization rate assessed using TICI score with successful recanalization defined as TICI 2b/3 [35], occurrence of sICH defined according to the Safe Implementation of Thrombolysis in Stroke-Monitoring Study (SITS-MOST) criteria [36] and 3-month clinical outcome assessed using mRS—with good clinical outcome defined as 0–2 points). Clinical outcome was assessed by a certified treating neurologist not blinded for the result of the MT. In patients, who were unable to attend a follow-up visit at the CSC, a telephone interview with another treating physician or the family members was used.

2.6. Statistical Analysis

The normality of the distributions was confirmed using the Kolmogorov–Smirnov test. Fisher's exact test was used to assess the relationship between categorical variables. The Mann–Whitney U-test or unpaired *t*-test was used, depending on data normality, to evaluate the impact of quantitative parameters.

A multivariate linear logistic regression model was used for the prediction of successful recanalization, sICH occurrence, 3-month good clinical outcome, and 3-month mortality. Bonferroni test was used for multiple comparison. Multiple colinear time predictors have been reduced to "onset-to-groin puncture" and "groin puncture-to-end of intervention" independent predictors.

Standard multivariate logistic regression was separately used for each binary output variable of interest. In the initial model, 28 predictors were used. First, we examined possible hidden relationships between output variables and explanatory ones as they could cause difficulty to the estimation process on one hand, but on the other, could also provide direct implications between these two groups of variables.

Explanatory variables involved in such relationship with an output variable were excluded from the data set when estimating the corresponding model for this output variable. Then complete models were estimated using all input variables without hidden relationships with the dependent variable. As not all estimated coefficients in the complete models were significant at the level of 0.95, we examined the justification of their inclusion into the model with the likelihood ratio (LR) test. Due to the large number of explanatory insignificant variables and their possible mutual dependency in many cases, the testing was proceeded as follows. First, we removed all statistically insignificant variables from the complete model and used the LR test to verify whether such exclusion was statistically justifiable. If not, we returned the previously eliminated variables into the model in a piecewise mode according their p values in the full model until the null hypothesis of excluding the rest of them was not rejected by the LR test. For all explanatory variables included in final models we calculated their odds ratio and its corresponding confidence intervals.

The MATLAB Statistical Toolbox (MathWorks, Natick, MA, USA) was used for statistical analysis.

2.7. Ethics

The entire study was conducted in accordance with the Declaration of Helsinki of 1964 and its later amendments (including the last in 2013). All procedures were performed in accordance with institutional guidelines. The study was approved by the Ethics Committee of the University Hospital Hradec Králové (approval No. 201912 S16R). All conscious patients signed informed consent forms for the eligible and available diagnostics and treatment. Independent witnesses verified the signatures in cases in which there were technical problems.

3. Results

The set consisted of 138 elderly patients ($\geq$80 years) (98 females; mean age 84.6 $\pm$ 3.5 years), out of whom 57 (41.3%) patients were treated with MT alone (MT-A) and 81 (58.7%) patients with MT + IVT. Baseline characteristics are presented in Table 1.

Table 1. Baseline characteristics.

Characteristic	MT-A (n = 57)	IVT + MT (n = 81)	p
Age, (years) [†]	84.6 ± 3.7 (83) (82–87)	84.2 ± 3.4 (84) (81.75–87)	0.51
Female sex	43 (75.4)	55 (67.9)	0.79
Medical history			
Arterial hypertension	50 (87.7)	72 (88.9)	1.00
Diabetes mellitus	19 (33.3)	25 (30.9)	0.86
Dyslipidemia	21 (36.8)	30 (37.0)	1.00
Coronary artery disease	22 (38.6)	27 (33.3)	0.74
Atrial fibrillation	22 (38.6)	34 (42.0)	0.87
Prior stroke/TIA	15 (26.3)	17 (21.0)	0.69
Pre-stroke mRS			
0–2	32 (56.1)	56 (69.1)	0.49
3–5	15 (26.3)	13 (16.0)	0.30
Uncertain	10 (17.5)	12 (14.8)	0.82
Unknown symptom onset	22 (38.6)	13 (16.0)	0.04
Direct transfer to the CSC	45 (78.9)	55 (67.9)	0.18
Initial qualifying NIHSS [†]	14.9 ± 4.6 (15) (12–18)	15.0 ± 4.9 (15) (13–17)	0.87
Initial CT characteristics			
ASPECTS—all patients [†]	8.7 ± 1.0 (9) (8–9)	8.1 ± 1.4 (8) (7–9)	0.002
ASPECTS—direct transfer to the CSC [†]	8.8 ± 1.1 (9) (9–10)	8.1 ± 1.4 (8) (7–9)	0.008
ASPECTS—interhospital transfer [†]	8.4 ± 0.8 (9) (8–9)	7.9 ± 1.3 (8) (7–9)	0.24
Leukoaraiosis	21 (36.8)	33 (40.7)	0.87
Occluded vessel			
M1	35 (61.4)	47 (58.0)	0.89
M2	10 (17.5)	11 (13.6)	0.64
Distal ICA + M1 (L occlusion)	9 (15.8)	11 (13.6)	0.63
Distal ICA + M1 + A1 (T occlusion)	1 (1.8)	4 (4.9)	0.65
ICA + M1 (tandem occlusion)	2 (3.5)	8 (9.9)	0.09
IVT	0 (0)	81 (100.0)	
IVT ≤ 3 h	0 (0)	75 (92.6)	

Data are n (%) for categorical variables or mean ± SD (median) (IQR) for numerical variables [†]. ASPECTS, Alberta Stroke Program Early CT Score; CSC, Comprehensive Stroke Center; CT, computed tomography; ICA, internal carotid artery; IQR, interquartile range; IVT, intravenous thrombolysis; M1, middle cerebral artery—segment 1; M2, middle cerebral artery—segment 2; mRS, modified Rankin scale; MT, mechanical thrombectomy; MT-A, MT alone; n, number of patients; NIHSS, National Institutes of Health Stroke Scale; SD, standard deviation; TIA, transient ischemic attack.

In patients treated with MT-A versus MT + IVT, there was significantly more frequent unknown symptom onset (38.6% versus 16.0%, $p = 0.04$) and ASPECTS values were significantly higher—both in the whole sets (mean 8.7 versus 8.1, $p = 0.002$) and in the subgroups of patients with direct transfer to the CSC (8.8 versus 8.1, $p = 0.008$).

As the first stent-retriever, Trevo was used 104 times (75.4%), Solitaire 32 times (23.2%), and both Eric 4 and Preset were used once. Two types of stent-retrievers were used twice during one procedure. One SRP was sufficient in 49.3% of patients, more than three SRPs were needed in 10.1% of patients. Furthermore, 26 out of 38 patients with secondary transport to the CSC were treated with IVT in the PSC. This represents only 32.1% out of 81 patients treated with IVT and this small proportion does not allow evaluation of the benefit and risk of this treatment prior to patients' transfer to the CSC. As presented in Table 2, IVT administration did not delay the start of MT, the interval from the known time of onset-to-groin puncture was even slightly shorter in the IVT + MT group than in the MT-A group. Door intervention center-to-groin puncture time was shorter by about half in patients with secondary transport to the CSC than in patients with direct transfer, because the emergency department and intervention team were pre-activated by the PSC. In the whole group, sICH occurred in 6.5% of patients—more frequently in patients with unknown time of symptoms onset (8.6%), with interhospital transfer (7.9%), with leukoaraiosis (11.1%), and with IVT (8.6%). The same factors reduced the chances of the achievement of a good clinical outcome (30.4% in the whole group) and increased the mortality (36.2% in the whole group)—28.6% and 40.0% in patients with unknown time of symptoms onset, 26.3% and 42.1% with interhospital transfer, 22.2% and 42.6% with leukoaraiosis and, 25.9% and 40.7% with IVT. By day 10, only 26% of patients had died, with the largest number (40%) dying between days 31 and 90. Pre-stroke mRS affected both the achievement of good clinical outcome (45.5% in patients with pre-stroke mRS ≤ 2) and mortality (29.5% in patients with pre-stroke mRS ≤ 2 and 46.4% with pre-stroke mRS 3–5). Procedural characteristics and outcomes in particular groups are presented in Table 2.

Table 2. Procedural characteristics and outcomes.

	Characteristic	MT-A (n = 57)	IVT + MT (n = 81)	p
	Onset-to-needle †		117.7 ± 38.6 (120.0) (98.5–140.0)	
Time intervals (min)	Onset-to-groin puncture †	209.0 ± 93.4 (184.0) (141–265)	197.0 ± 63.3 (178.5) (145–229.5)	0.42
	Door intervention center-to-groin puncture †	78.6 ± 32.9 (79.5) (56–106)	72.8 ± 27.8 (74) (51.75–91.25)	0.31
	Direct transfer to the CSC †	89.5 ± 27.7 (85.5) (70.5–105)	85.5 ± 22.0 (83.0) (72.5–101)	0.42
	Interhospital transfer †	40.8 ± 22.2 (30.0) (27–50.5)	47.5 ± 19.2 (40.5) (32.5–56)	0.35
	Groin puncture-to-end of intervention †	46.8 ± 27.2 (40.0) (28–58)	46.2 ± 27.3 (38.5) (25–56)	0.91
	Onset-to-end of intervention †	257.7 ± 98.2 (255) (173–313)	242.8 ± 67.3 (228.5) (191.5–286)	0.37
Stent-retriever passes	All patients †	2.1 ± 1.6 (2) (1–3)	1.9 ± 1.0 (2) (1–3)	
	1	27 (47.4)	41 (50.6)	0.88
	2	14 (24.6)	19 (23.5)	1.00
	≥3	7 (12.3)	7 (8.7)	0.58
Recanalization grade	TICI 0	6 (10.5)	2 (2.5)	0.08
	TICI 1	0 (0)	2 (2.5)	0.51
	TICI 2a	9 (15.8)	14 (17.3)	1.00
	TICI 2b	14 (24.6)	25 (30.9)	0.58
	TICI 3	28 (49.1)	38 (46.9)	0.88
	TICI ≥2b	42 (73.7)	63 (77.8)	0.90

Table 2. Cont.

	Characteristic	MT-A (n = 57)	IVT + MT (n = 81)	p
sICH occurrence	All patients	2 (3.5)	7 (8.6)	0.32
	Pre-stroke mRS ≤ 2	1/32 (3.1)	5/56 (8.9)	0.41
	Unknown symptom onset	1/22 (4.5)	2/13 (15.4)	0.55
	Direct transfer to the CSC	2/45 (4.4)	4/55 (7.3)	0.69
	Interhospital transfer	0 (0)	3/26 (11.5)	
	Leukoaraiosis	1/21 (4.8)	5/33 (15.2)	0.40
	IVT		7 (8.6)	
3-month good clinical outcome (mRS 0–2)	All patients	21 (36.8)	21 (25.9)	0.38
	Pre-stroke mRS ≤ 2	21/32 (65.7)	19/56 (33.9)	0.12
	Unknown symptom onset	8/22 (36.4)	2/13 (15.4)	0.46
	Direct transfer to the CSC	17/45 (37.8)	15/55 (27.3)	0.54
	Interhospital transfer	4/12 (33.3)	6/26 (23.1)	0.71
	Leukoaraiosis	5/21 (23.8)	7/33 (21.2)	1.00
	IVT		21 (25.9)	
3-month mortality (mRS 6)	All patients	17 (29.8)	33 (40.7)	0.21
	Day 1–10	5/17 (29.4)	8/33 (24.2)	0.76
	Day 11–30	6/17 (35.3)	11/33 (33.3)	1.00
	Day 31–90	6/17 (35.3)	14/33 (42.4)	1.00
	Pre-stroke mRS ≤ 2	7 (21.9)	19 (33.9)	0.48
	Unknown symptom onset	8/22 (36.4)	6/13 (46.2)	0.75
	Direct transfer to the CSC	12/45 (26.7)	22/55 (40.0)	0.42
	Interhospital transfer	5/12 (41.7)	11/26 (42.3)	1.00
	Leukoaraiosis	8/21 (38.1)	15/33 (45.5)	0.80
	IVT		33 (40.7)	

Data are n (%) for categorical variables or mean ± SD (median) (IQR) for numerical variables †. CSC, Comprehensive Stroke Center; IQR, interquartile range; IVT, intravenous thrombolysis; mRS, modified Rankin scale; MT, mechanical thrombectomy; MT-A, MT alone; n, number of patients; SD, standard deviation; sICH, symptomatic intracerebral hemorrhage; TICI, Thrombolysis in Cerebral Infarction.

As presented in Table 3, higher number of stent-retriever passes was identified as an independent negative predictor of the achievement of successful recanalization. Higher ASPECTS value was identified as an independent negative predictor and the presence of leukoaraiosis as an independent positive predictor of the sICH occurrence. IVT was identified as an independent negative predictor of the achievement of 3-month good clinical outcome. Female sex was identified as an independent positive predictor of the achievement of 3-month good clinical outcome and as an independent negative predictor of 3-month mortality. Other independent negative predictors of the achievement of 3-month good clinical outcome were, as expected, older age, lower pre-stroke self-sufficiency, more severe neurological deficit and longer time intervals (onset-to-groin, groin puncture-to-end of intervention). In addition to older age, mortality was independently predicted by the longer groin puncture-to-end of intervention interval and by the sICH occurrence (Table 3).

Table 3. Significant independent predictors of the observed parameters—results of multivariate logistic regression analysis.

Observed Parameter	Predictor	OR (95% CI)	p
Successful recanalization (TICI 2b/3)	Number of stent-retriever passes	0.537 (0.376–0.766)	6×10^{-4}
sICH	ASPECTS	0.559 (0.320–0.977)	0.041
	Leukoaraiosis	4.947 (1.036–23.619)	0.045
3-month good clinical outcome (mRS 0–2)	Age	0.803 (0.689–0.937)	0.005
	Female sex	4.179 (1.300–13.438)	0.016
	Pre-stroke mRS	0.052 (0.006–0.477)	0.009
	NIHSS value	0.856 (0.756–0.968)	0.013
	IVT	0.356 (0.134–0.942)	0.038
	Onset-to-groin interval	0.991 (0.984–0.999)	0.023
	Groin puncture-to-end of intervention	0.964 (0.941–0.987)	0.002

Table 3. *Cont.*

Observed Parameter	Predictor	OR (95% CI)	p
3-month mortality (mRS 6)	Age	1.250 (1.106–1.413)	3×10^{-4}
	Female sex	0.244 (0.100–0.599)	0.002
	Groin puncture-to-end of intervention	1.015 (1.001–1.030)	0.040
	sICH	6.681 (1.171–38.105)	0.032

ASPECTS, Alberta Stroke Program Early CT Score; CI, confidence interval; IVT, intravenous thrombolysis; mRS, modified Rankin scale; NIHSS, National Institutes of Health Stroke Scale; OR, odds ratio; sICH, symptomatic intracerebral hemorrhage; TICI, Thrombolysis in Cerebral Infarction.

4. Discussion

About 30% of patients with AIS are aged 80 and over, 17% are even older than 85 years, and the proportion of elderly patients will continue to increase as the population ages [37,38]. The fact that AIS due to ELVO in elderly patients has a poor prognosis without MT (in the medical arm/IVT group of HERMES meta-analysis only 13.9% of these patients achieved mRS 0–2 and their mortality was 45.2% [18]) supports the legitimacy of the use of MT in this age group, although its results are significantly worse compared to younger patients despite similar successful recanalization rates [17–24]. In the HERMES meta-analysis, in patients treated with MT, mRS ≤ 2 was achieved in 46% of patients aged 57–77 years and only in 29.8% of patients aged ≥80 years, and, mortality was 15.3% and 28% in particular groups [1,3,5]. In the STRATIS registry of patients treated with MT, rates of good clinical outcomes significantly decreased for each 5-year increment of age from <65 to >90 years, from 64.3% to 26.5%, while mortality significantly increased from 7.9% to 35.1% [19]. In the TREVO registry, 33.7% of patients aged ≥80 years reached mRS ≤ 2 and their mortality was 27.2%, while the same values for younger patients were 62.2 and 9.6%, respectively [20]. Out of 560 patients treated with MT in seven US centers, 108 patients aged ≥80 years also had significantly worse clinical outcomes when compared with younger patients—mRS ≤ 2 was achieved in 20.5% versus 44.4% and mortality was 34.3% versus 20% in particular groups [21]. Our results are comparable to those published—3-month good clinical outcome (mRS ≤ 2) was achieved in 30.4% of our patients aged ≥80 years and their 3-month mortality was 36.2%.

Older patients have poor clinical outcome at 3 months despite high rates of the achieved recanalization. In our group, successful recanalization (TICI 2b/3) was achieved in 76.1% of patients aged ≥80 years. In the work published in 2016, early neurological improvement depended on successful recanalization, not on the age of MT-treated patients. However, older patients exhibited poor mid-term functional outcome due to post-stroke complications and other factors that were not, or only indirectly, related to the brain tissue damage induced by the incident stroke [39]. Corresponding to our finding is that a larger proportion of patients aged ≥80 years died later—40% of them between days 31 and 90, when a direct association with brain tissue damage due to stroke is unlikely. Factors that adversely affect the prognosis in older patients may be pre-existing neuronal loss and reduced neuronal plasticity, leukoaraiosis, higher rate of comorbidities, and post-stroke complications (e.g., infections or injuries due to falls) [40,41]. In our patients with leukoaraiosis, when compared to the whole group, we recorded a higher occurrence of sICHs (11.1% versus 6.5%) and higher 3-month mortality (42.6% versus 36.2%) and a less frequent 3-month good clinical outcome (22.2% versus 30.4%). Due to pre-existing changes, the brain of elderly patients has depleted or borderline functional capacity, and is therefore able to tolerate only a small volume of infarction [42,43].

Whether treatment with IVT before MT in patients with anterior circulation stroke due to ELVO is of any benefit is currently one of the most important unanswered questions in acute stroke management [16]. To date, the results of randomized control trials (RCTs), as well as several registries and multicenter and single-center studies, suggest that MT-A is equally effective and not inferior to MT + IVT, if patients are immediately treated in stroke centers with rapid access to endovascular procedures. This was recently confirmed by multicenter RCTs from China and Japan (DIRECT-MT [44], DEVT [45], and SKIP [46]), which did not show a statistically significant difference between patients treated with MT-A versus MT + IVT in self-sufficiency at 3 months (36.4%, 54.3%, and 59.4% versus 36.8%, 46.6%, and 57.3%, resp.) or in mortality (17.7%, 17.2%, and 7.9% versus 18.8%, 17.8%, and 8.7%, resp.). In the DIRECT-MT trial, even a 5% higher successful recanalization rate achieved in patients treated with MT + IVT did not lead to a better functional outcome, and a relatively lower achievement of independence in both treatment groups was probably due to remarkably low rates of favorable collaterals [44]. Meta-analysis of six older RCTs with 940 patients treated with IVT and endovascular treatment and 107 patients treated with endovascular treatment alone showed that endovascular treatment was associated with a higher likelihood of the achievement of better outcome at 3 months—both in the group with IVT (OR 1.83) and without IVT (OR 2.47) [10]. The results of the meta-analysis of eight RCTs were similar [13]. No statistically significant differences were also confirmed by the pooled analysis of SWIFT and STAR studies [11]. Similar clinical outcomes at 90 days (either good clinical outcome, mortality, or both) in patients treated with MT-A and MT + IVT were also found in the Catalan SONIIA registry from 2011 to 2015 [12], Bernese Stroke Registry (with the exception of a lower mortality in the MT-A group) [9] (even after adding patients from the Essen registry, despite the fact that MT was delayed by 1 h in patients with MT + IVT [14]), and in other studies [8,15]. However, there are also works reporting better outcomes in patients treated with MT + IVT than with MT-A. In the German REVASK registry from 2012 to 2013, comparing patients with MT + IVT and MT-A, good 3-month clinical outcome was achieved in 47.5% versus 38.1% and mortality was 17.8% versus 27.8% in particular groups. As well as in our patient set, patients with MT + IVT had shorter times to groin puncture [47]. IVT was a predictor of the achievement of good outcome in another German registry from 2015 to 2018 (OR 1.49) [23], and better functional outcome (adjusted OR (aOR) 1.47 and 1.4, resp.) and lower mortality (aOR 0.58 and 0.74, resp.) were found in patients treated with IVT + MT versus MT-A in the Dutch MR CLEAN registry from 2014 to 2016 [48] and in the international SITS-ISTR registry from 2014 to 2016 [49]. Data regarding the effect of IVT preceding MT on ICH frequency vary. In the SONIIA registry [12], MR CLEAN registry [48], and SITS-ISTR registry [49], the occurrence of sICH in both treatment groups was similar—3.4%, 5.9%, and 3.5%, respectively, in the IVT + MT group versus 2.7%, 5.3%, and 3.0%, respectively, in the MT-A group. On the other hand, the German registries showed a significantly higher incidence of sICH in patients with MT + IVT (4.5%, 5.3%, and 3.5%, resp.) versus patients with MT-A (2.5%, 2.7%, and 1.6%, resp.) [9,14,47] and also of ICH according to the ECASS II definition [50] irrespective of the new clinical symptoms (15% versus 11% in particular groups) [23]. In the Bernese Stroke Registry, lower rate of asymptomatic ICH was observed in the MT-A versus MT + IVT group (12.5% versus 20%) [9]. Some authors [51,52] state that extensive leukoaraiosis may increase the risk of sICH in addition to IVT, and our results correspond with this.

We found the evaluation of the effect of IVT adjusted for age only in the study from Australia from 2016 to 2018 performed by Sharobeam et al. [22]. In older ($\geq$80 years) versus younger patients, treated for anterior circulation stroke with MT using second generation stent-retrievers, IVT was used in 34% versus 45%, procedure duration was 35 versus 31 min, the occurrence of sICH according to the SITS-MOST definition was 4% versus 5%, mRS 0–2 at 90 days was achieved in 28% versus 55%, and mortality rate was 27% versus 16% in particular groups. IVT was significantly associated with a favorable outcome in younger patients (OR 2.90), but not in elderly patients. In our study, IVT was identified as an independent negative predictor of the achievement of 3-month good clinical outcome (OR 0.356).

Females, representing 71% of our patients, achieved a better outcome—female sex was identified as an independent positive predictor of the achievement of 3-month good clinical outcome (OR 4.179) and as an independent negative predictor of 3-month mortality (OR 0.244). The conclusions of recent studies that reported sex differences in clinical outcome after MT are inconsistent. Studies analyzing large groups of younger patients (median age of females 69–70 years) from RCTs conclude that despite the fact that females were older and had a higher comorbidity compared to males, their clinical outcome after MT was comparable and according to the study performed by Sheth et al., females had significantly more years of optimal life (disability-adjusted life year) when compared to males (10.6 versus 8.5 years) [53,54]. In contrast, in the Japanese RESCUE registry, females (mean age 79.7 years), when compared to males (mean age 72.8 years), were less likely to achieve a good clinical outcome (27.3% versus 44.2%; aOR 0.80) and had higher mortality (12.3% versus 9.9%; aOR 0.78) [55]. The most similar to our cohort is the cohort of 279 patients treated with MT in a single, large, academic CSC in the USA between 2015 and 2017. Females, representing 52% of patients, were older than males (median age 81 versus 71.5 years). Although at discharge both males and females had a similar probability of functional independence (aOR 0.71), at 90 days the probability of functional independence was apparently lower in females (aOR 0.37). Post hoc multivariate logistic regression analysis in subgroups by age indicated a greater sex difference for independence in females under 75 years (OR 0.24), while OR for females older than 75 years compared to males was 0.54. However, the authors point out that the results of the subanalysis may not be reliable and are likely underpowered. The fact that both rates of successful recanalization and clinical outcome at discharge were similar between females and males, suggests that a worse long-term clinical outcome may reflect a less favorable situation of females not directly related to MT, such as their more frequent social isolation or lower social level. Females in this group were less likely to be married (38.2% versus 67.5%) and were more likely to have government-sponsored insurance (86.8% versus 73.1%) when compared to males [56]. The absence of greater social disparities and the general availability of outpatient or inpatient social services for the elderly in our country may have contributed to better long-term clinical outcomes after MT in females in our cohort, but do not explain the difference in outcome between the sexes.

Other independent negative predictors of the achievement of 3-month good clinical outcome were, as expected, older age, lower pre-stroke self-sufficiency, more severe neurological deficit, and longer time intervals (onset-to-groin, groin puncture-to-end of intervention). In addition to older age, mortality was independently predicted by the longer groin puncture-to-end of intervention interval and by the sICH occurrence.

Several limitations of the present study should be mentioned. First, it has a retrospective character with a sample extracted from a single stroke center database; therefore, the results may not be generalizable. Second, the data collection methods among databases may be the source of selection bias. Third, a relatively small number of patients in particular treatment subgroups limits the power for comparative analysis.

5. Conclusions

Our results demonstrated, that in patients with anterior circulation AIS due to ELVO aged ≥ 80 years and undergoing MT ($\pm$IVT), IVT reduced the chance of the achievement of 3-month good clinical outcome and female sex was associated with a greater likelihood of the achievement of 3-month good clinical outcome and lower probability of 3-month mortality. However, these results require verification on a larger set of patients.

Author Contributions: Conceptualization, D.K. and R.H.; data curation, D.K., A.K. and L.Š.; formal analysis, R.H. and O.V.; funding acquisition, M.V.; investigation, D.K., A.K. and L.Š.; methodology, D.K. and R.H.; project administration, D.K., R.H. and L.Š.; resources, D.K., A.K., R.H. and L.Š.; software, O.V.; supervision, R.H.; validation, R.H.; writing—original draft, D.K., R.H. and O.V.; writing—review and editing, D.K., A.K., R.H., O.V., L.Š. and M.V. All authors have read and agreed to the published version of the manuscript.

Funding: This work was supported in part by the Ministry of Health of the Czech Republic (grant number DRO—UHHK 00179906) and Charles University, Czech Republic (grant number PROGRES Q40).

Institutional Review Board Statement: The study was conducted according to the guidelines of the Declaration of Helsinki, and approved by the Ethics Committee of the University Hospital Hradec Králové, Czech Republic (approval No. 201912 S16R) on 5 December 2019.

Informed Consent Statement: Given the retrospective nature of the study, the individual consent to participate was not required after the approval from the local Ethics Committee.

Data Availability Statement: The datasets analyzed during the current study are available from the corresponding author on reasonable request.

Conflicts of Interest: The authors declare no conflict of interest. The funders had no role in the design of the study; in the collection, analyses, or interpretation of data; in the writing of the manuscript, or in the decision to publish the results.

References

1. Berkhemer, O.A.; Fransen, P.S.S.; Beumer, D.; Van den Berg, L.A.; Lingsma, H.F.; Yoo, A.J.; Schonewille, W.J.; Vos, J.A.; Nederkoorn, P.J.; Wermer, M.J.H.; et al. A randomized trial of intraarterial treatment for acute ischemic stroke. *N. Engl. J. Med.* **2015**, *372*, 11–20. [CrossRef]
2. Campbell, B.C.; Mitchell, P.J.; Kleinig, T.; Dewey, H.M.; Churilov, L.; Yassi, N.; Yan, B.; Dowling, R.J.; Parsons, M.W.; Oxley, T.J.; et al. Endovascular therapy for ischemic stroke with perfusion-imaging selection. *N. Engl. J. Med.* **2015**, *372*, 1009–1018. [CrossRef]
3. Goyal, M.; Demchuk, A.M.; Menon, B.K.; Eesa, M.; Rempel, J.L.; Thornton, J.; Roy, D.; Jovin, T.G.; Willinsky, R.A.; Sapkota, B.L.; et al. Randomized assessment of rapid endovascular treatment of ischemic stroke. *N. Engl. J. Med.* **2015**, *372*, 1019–1030. [CrossRef] [PubMed]
4. Saver, J.L.; Goyal, M.; Bonafe, A.; Diener, H.-C.; Levy, E.I.; Pereira, V.M.; Albers, G.W.; Cognard, C.; Cohen, D.J.; Hacke, W.; et al. Stent-retriever thrombectomy after intravenous t-PA vs. t-PA alone in stroke. *N. Engl. J. Med.* **2015**, *372*, 2285–2295. [CrossRef] [PubMed]
5. Jovin, T.G.; Chamorro, A.; Cobo, E.; De Miquel, M.A.; Molina, C.A.; Rovira, A.; Román, L.S.; Serena, J.; Abilleira, S.; Ribo, M.; et al. Thrombectomy within 8 h after symptom onset in ischemic stroke. *N. Engl. J. Med.* **2015**, *372*, 2296–2306. [CrossRef] [PubMed]
6. Powers, W.J.; Rabinstein, A.A.; Ackerson, T.; Adeoye, O.M.; Bambakidis, N.C.; Becker, K.; Biller, J.; Brown, M.; Demaerschalk, B.M.; Hoh, B.; et al. Guidelines for the early management of patients with acute ischemic stroke: A guideline for healthcare professionals from the American Heart Association/American Stroke Association. *Stroke* **2018**, *49*, e46–e110. [CrossRef]
7. Šaňák, D.; Mikulík, R.; Tomek, A.; Bar, M.; Herzig, R.; Neumann, J.; Škoda, O.; Školoudík, D.; Václavík, D.; Roček, M.; et al. Doporučení pro mechanickou trombektomii akutního mozkového infarktu—Verze 2019. *Cesk. Slov. Neurol. N.* **2019**, *82/115*, 700–705. [CrossRef]
8. Leker, R.R.; Pikis, S.; Gomori, J.M.; Cohen, J.E. Is bridging necessary? A pilot study of bridging versus primary stentretriever-based endovascular reperfusion in large anterior circulation strokes. *J. Stroke Cerebrovasc. Dis.* **2015**, *24*, 1163–1167. [CrossRef]
9. Broeg-Morvay, A.; Mordasini, P.; Bernasconi, C.; Bühlmann, M.; Pult, F.; Arnold, M.; Schroth, G.; Jung, S.; Mattle, H.P.; Gralla, J.; et al. Direct mechanical intervention versus combined intravenous and mechanical intervention in large anterior circulation stroke: A matched-pairs analysis. *Stroke* **2016**, *47*, 1037–1044. [CrossRef]
10. Tsivgoulis, G.; Katsanos, A.H.; Mavridis, D.; Magoufis, G.; Arthur, A.; Alexandrov, A.V. Mechanical thrombectomy improves functional outcomes independent of pretreatment with intravenous thrombolysis. *Stroke* **2016**, *47*, 1661–1664. [CrossRef]
11. Coutinho, J.M.; Liebeskind, D.S.; Slater, L.A.; Nogueira, R.G.; Clark, W.; Dávalos, A.; Bonafé, A.; Jahan, R.; Fischer, U.; Gralla, J.; et al. Combined intravenous thrombolysis and thrombectomy vs. thrombectomy alone for acute ischemic stroke: A pooled analysis of the SWIFT and STAR studies. *JAMA Neurol.* **2017**, *74*, 268–274. [CrossRef]
12. 12. Abilleira, S.; Ribera, A.; Cardona, P.; Rubiera, M.; López-Cancio, E.; Amaro, S.; Rodríguez-Campello, A.; Camps-Renom, P.; Cánovas, D.; De Miquel, M.A.; et al. Outcomes after direct thrombectomy or combined intravenous and endovascular treatment are not different. *Stroke* **2017**, *48*, 375–378. [CrossRef] [PubMed]
13. Fischer, U.; Kaesmacher, J.; Pereira, V.M.; Chapot, R.; Siddiqui, A.H.; Froehler, M.T.; Cognard, C.; Furlan, A.J.; Saver, J.L.; Gralla, J. Direct mechanical thrombectomy versus combined intravenous and mechanical thrombectomy in large-artery anterior circulation stroke: A topical review. *Stroke* **2017**, *48*, 2912–2918. [CrossRef] [PubMed]
14. Bellwald, S.; Weber, R.; Dobrocky, T.; Nordmeyer, H.; Jung, S.; Hadisurya, J.; Mordasini, P.; Mono, M.L.; Stracke, C.P.; Sarikaya, H.; et al. Direct mechanical intervention versus bridging therapy in stroke patients eligible for intravenous thrombolysis: A pooled analysis of 2 registries. *Stroke* **2017**, *48*, 3282–3288. [CrossRef] [PubMed]
15. Rai, A.T.; Boo, S.; Buseman, C.; Adcock, A.K.; Tarabishy, A.R.; Miller, M.M.; Roberts, T.D.; Domico, J.R.; Carpenter, J.S. Intravenous thrombolysis before endovascular therapy for large vessel strokes can lead to significantly higher hospital costs without improving outcomes. *J. Neurointerv. Surg.* **2018**, *10*, 17–21. [CrossRef]
16. Malhotra, A.; Wu, X.; Payabvash, S.; Matouk, C.C.; Forman, H.P.; Gandhi, D.; Sanelli, P.; Schindler, J. Comparative effectiveness of endovascular thrombectomy in elderly stroke patients. *Stroke* **2019**, *50*, 963–969. [CrossRef]

17. Chandra, R.V.; Leslie-Mazwi, T.M.; Oh, D.C.; Chaudhry, Z.A.; Mehta, B.P.; Rost, N.S.; Rabinov, J.D.; Hirsch, J.A.; González, R.G.; Schwamm, L.H.; et al. Elderly patients are at higher risk for poor outcomes after intra-arterial therapy. *Stroke* **2012**, *43*, 2356–2361. [CrossRef]
18. Goyal, M.; Menon, B.K.; Van Zwam, W.H.; Dippel, D.W.; Mitchell, P.J.; Demchuk, A.M.; Dávalos, A.; Majoie, C.B.; Van der Lugt, A.; De Miquel, M.A.; et al. Endovascular thrombectomy after large-vessel ischaemic stroke: A meta-analysis of individual patient data from five randomised trials. *Lancet* **2016**, *387*, 1723–1731. [CrossRef]
19. Mueller-Kronast, B.K.; Zaidat, O.O.; Froehler, M.T.; Jahan, R.; Aziz-Sultan, M.A.; Klucznik, R.P.; Saver, J.L.; Hellinger, F.R.; Yavagal, D.R.; Yao, T.L.; et al. Systematic evaluation of patients treated with neurothrombectomy devices for acute ischemic stroke: Primary results of the STRATIS registry. *Stroke* **2017**, *48*, 2760–2768. [CrossRef]
20. Binning, M.J.; Bartolini, B.; Baxter, B.; Budzik, R.; English, J.; Gupta, R.; Hedayat, H.; Krajina, A.; Liebeskind, D.; Nogueira, R.G.; et al. Trevo 2000: Results of a large real-world registry for stent retriever for acute ischemic stroke. *J. Am. Heart Assoc.* **2018**, *7*, e010867. [CrossRef]
21. Alawieh, A.; Chatterjee, A.; Feng, W.; Porto, G.; Vargas, J.; Kellogg, R.; Turk, A.S.; Turner, R.D.; Chaudry, M.I.; Spiotta, A.M. Thrombectomy for acute ischemic stroke in the elderly: A 'real world' experience. *J. Neurointerv. Surg.* **2018**, *10*, 1209–1217. [CrossRef]
22. Sharobeam, A.; Cordato, D.J.; Manning, N.; Cheung, A.; Wenderoth, J.; Cappelen-Smith, C. Functional outcomes at 90 days in octogerians undergoing thrombectomy for acute ischemic stroke: A prospective cohort study and meta-analysis. *Front. Neurol.* **2019**, *10*, 254. [CrossRef]
23. Wollenweber, F.A.; Tiedt, S.; Alegiani, A.; Alber, B.; Bangard, C.; Berrouschot, J.; Bode, F.J.; Boeckh-Behrens, T.; Bohner, G.; Bormann, A.; et al. Functional outcome following stroke thrombectomy in clinical practice. *Stroke* **2019**, *50*, 2500–2506. [CrossRef] [PubMed]
24. Martini, M.; Mocco, J.; Turk, A.; Siddiqui, A.H.; Fiorella, D.; Hanel, R.; Woodward, K.; Rai, A.; Frei, D.; Almandoz, J.E.D.; et al. An international multicenter retrospective study to survey the landscape of thrombectomy in the treatment of anterior circulaton acute ischemic stroke: Outcomes with respect to age. *J. Neurointerv. Surg.* **2020**, *12*, 115–121. [CrossRef]
25. Adams, H.P.; Del Zoppo, G.; Alberts, M.J.; Bhatt, D.L.; Brass, L.; Furlan, A.; Grubb, R.L.; Higashida, R.T.; Jauch, E.C.; Kidwell, C.; et al. Guidelines for the early management of adults with ischemic stroke: A guideline from the American Heart Association/American Stroke Association Stroke Council, Clinical Cardiology Council, Cardiovascular Radiology and Intervention Council, and the Atherosclerotic Peripheral Vascular Disease and Quality of Care Outcomes in Research Interdisciplinary Working Groups: The American Academy of Neurology affirms the value of this guideline as an educational tool for neurologists. *Stroke* **2007**, *38*, 1655–1711. [CrossRef]
26. Jauch, E.C.; Saver, J.L.; Adams, H.P.; Bruno, A.; Connors, J.J.; Demaerschalk, B.M.; Khatri, P.; McMullan, P.W.; Qureshi, A.I.; Rosenfield, K.; et al. Guidelines for the early management of patients with acute ischemic stroke: A guideline for healthcare professionals from the American Heart Association/American Stroke Association. *Stroke* **2013**, *44*, 870–947. [CrossRef]
27. Šaňák, D.; Neumann, J.; Tomek, A.; Školoudík, D.; Škoda, O.; Mikulík, R.; Herzig, R.; Václavík, D.; Bar, M.; Roček, M.; et al. Doporučení pro rekanalizační léčbu akutního mozkového infarktu—Verze 2016. *Cesk. Slov. Neurol. N.* **2016**, *79/112*, 231–234. [CrossRef]
28. Wahlgren, N.; Moreira, T.; Michel, P.; Steiner, T.; Jansen, O.; Cognard, C.; Mattle, H.P.; Van Zwam, W.; Holmin, S.; Tatlisumak, T.; et al. Mechanical thrombectomy in acute ischemic stroke: Consensus statement by ESO-Karolinska Stroke Update 2014/2015, supported by ESO, ESMINT, ESNR and EAN. *Int. J. Stroke* **2016**, *11*, 134–147. [CrossRef] [PubMed]
29. Campbell, B.C.; Christensen, S.; Levi, C.R.; Desmond, P.M.; Donnan, G.A.; Davis, S.M.; Parsons, M.W. Cerebral blood flow is the optimal CT perfusion parameter for assessing infarct core. *Stroke* **2011**, *42*, 3435–3440. [CrossRef] [PubMed]
30. Neumann, J.; Tomek, A.; Školoudík, D.; Škoda, O.; Mikulík, R.; Herzig, R.; Václavík, D.; Bar, M.; Šaňák, D. Doporučený postup pro intravenózní trombolýzu v léčbě akutního mozkového infarktu—Verze 2014. *Cesk. Slov. Neurol. N.* **2014**, *77/110*, 381–385.
31. Šaňák, D.; Nosál', V.; Horák, D.; Bártková, A.; Zeleňák, K.; Herzig, R.; Bučil, J.; Školoudík, D.; Burval, S.; Cisariková, V.; et al. Impact of diffusion-weighted MRI-measured initial cerebral infarction volume on clinical outcome in acute stroke patients with middle cerebral artery occlusion treated by thrombolysis. *Neuroradiology* **2006**, *48*, 632–639. [CrossRef]
32. Van Swieten, J.C.; Koudstaal, P.J.; Visser, M.C.; Schouten, H.J.; Van Gijn, J. Interobserver agreement for the assessment of handicap in stroke patients. *Stroke* **1988**, *19*, 604–607. [CrossRef] [PubMed]
33. Goldstein, L.B.; Samsa, G.P. Reliability of the National Institute of Health Stroke Scale. Extension to non-neurologists in the context of a clinical trial. *Stroke* **1997**, *28*, 307–310. [CrossRef]
34. Marek, M.; Horyniecki, M.; Fraczek, M.; Kluczewska, E. Leukoaraiosis—New concepts and modern imaging. *Pol. J. Radiol.* **2018**, *83*, e76–e81. [CrossRef]
35. Yoo, A.J.; Simonsen, C.Z.; Prabhakaran, S.; Chaudhry, Z.A.; Issa, M.A.; Fugate, J.E.; Linfante, I.; Liebeskind, D.S.; Khatri, P.; Jovin, T.G.; et al. Refining angiographic biomarkers of revascularization: Improving outcome prediction after intra-arterial therapy. *Stroke* **2013**, *44*, 2509–2512. [CrossRef]
36. Wahlgren, N.; Ahmed, N.; Dávalos, A.; Ford, G.A.; Grond, M.; Hacke, W.; Hennerici, M.G.; Kaste, M.; Kuelkens, S.; Larrue, V.; et al. Thrombolysis with alteplase for acute ischaemic stroke in the Safe Implementation of Thrombolysis in Stroke-Monitoring Study (SITS-MOST): An observational study. *Lancet* **2007**, *369*, 275–282. [CrossRef]

37. Marini, C.; Baldassarre, M.; Russo, T.; De Santis, F.; Sacco, S.; Ciancarelli, I.; Carolei, A. Burden of first-ever ischemic stroke in the oldest old: Evidence from a population-based study. *Neurology* **2004**, *62*, 77–81. [CrossRef] [PubMed]
38. Russo, T.; Felzani, G.; Marini, C. Stroke in the very old: A systematic review of studies on incidence, outcome, and resource use. *J. Aging Res.* **2011**, *2011*, 108785. [CrossRef] [PubMed]
39. Kleine, J.F.; Boeckh-Behrens, T.; Prothmann, S.; Zimmer, C.; Liebig, T. Discrepancy between early neurological course and mid-term outcome in older stroke patients after mechanical thrombectomy. *J. Neurointerv. Surg.* **2016**, *8*, 671–676. [CrossRef]
40. Arsava, E.M.; Rahman, R.; Rosand, J.; Lu, J.; Smith, E.E.; Rost, N.S.; Singhal, A.B.; Lev, M.H.; Furie, K.L.; Koroshetz, W.J.; et al. Severity of leukoaraiosis correlates with clinical outcome after ischemic stroke. *Neurology* **2009**, *72*, 1403–1410. [CrossRef]
41. Henninger, H.; Lin, E.; Baker, S.P.; Wakhloo, A.K.; Takhtani, D.; Moonis, M. Leukoaraiosis predicts poor 90-day outcome after acute large cerebral artery occlusion. *Cerebrovasc. Dis.* **2012**, *33*, 525–531. [CrossRef] [PubMed]
42. Ribo, M.; Flores, A.; Mansilla, E.; Rubiera, M.; Tomasello, A.; Coscojuela, P.; Pagola, J.; Rodriguez-Luna, D.; Muchada, M.; Alvarez-Sabín, J.; et al. Age-adjusted infarct volume threshold for good outcome after endovascular treatment. *J. Neurointerv. Surg.* **2014**, *6*, 418–422. [CrossRef]
43. Lima, A.; Haussen, D.C.; Rebello, L.C.; Dehkharghani, S.; Grossberg, J.; Grigoryan, M.; Frankel, M.; Nogueira, R.G. Endovascular therapy for large vessel stroke in the elderly: Hope in the new stroke era. *Cerebrovasc. Dis.* **2016**, *42*, 421–427. [CrossRef]
44. Yang, P.; Zhang, Y.; Zhang, L.; Zhang, Y.; Treurniet, K.M..; Chen, W.; Peng, Y.; Han, H.; Wang, J.; Wang, S.; et al. Endovascular thrombectomy with or without intravenous alteplase in acute stroke. *J. Clin. Med.* **2020**, *382*, 1981–1993. [CrossRef]
45. Zi, W.; Qiu, Z.; Li, F.; Sang, H.; Wu, D.; Luo, W.; Liu, S.; Yuan, J.; Song, J.; Shi, Z.; et al. Effect of endovascular treatment alone vs. intravenous alteplase plus endovascular treatment on functional independence in patients with acute ischemic stroke. The DEVT randomised clinical trial. *JAMA* **2021**, *325*, 234–243. [CrossRef] [PubMed]
46. Suzuki, K.; Matsumaru, Y.; Takeuchi, M.; Morimoto, M.; Kanazawa, R.; Takayama, Y.; Kamila, Y.; Shigeta, K.; Okubo, S.; Haykawa, M.; et al. Effect of mechanical thrombectomy without vs. with intravenous thrombolysis on functional outcome among patients with acute ischemic stroke. The SKIP randomised clinical trial. *JAMA* **2021**, *325*, 244–253. [CrossRef] [PubMed]
47. Minnerup, J.; Wersching, H.; Teuber, A.; Wellmann, J.; Eyding, J.; Weber, R.; Reimann, G.; Weber, W.; Krause, L.U.; Kurth, T.; et al. Outcome after thrombectomy and intravenous thrombolysis in patients with acute ischemic stroke: A prospective observational study. *Stroke* **2016**, *47*, 1584–1592. [CrossRef]
48. Chalos, V.; LeCouffe, N.E.; Uyttenboogaart, M.; Lingsma, H.F.; Mulder, M.J.H.L.; Venema, E.; Treurniet, K.M.; Eshghi, O.; Van der Worp, H.B.; Van der Lugt, A.; et al. Endovascular treatment with or without prior intravenous alteplase for acute ischemic stroke. *J. Am. Heart Assoc.* **2019**, *8*, e011592. [CrossRef] [PubMed]
49. Ahmed, N.; Mazya, M.; Nunes, A.P.; Moreira, T.; Ollikainen, J.P.; Escudero-Martinez, I.; Bigliardi, G.; Dorado, L.; Dávalos, A.; Egido, J.A.; et al. Safety and outcomes of thrombectomy in ischemic stroke with vs. without intravenous thrombolysis. *Neurology* **2021**, *97*, e765–e776. [CrossRef]
50. Hacke, W.; Kaste, M.; Fieschi, C.; Von Kummer, R.; Davalos, A.; Meier, D.; Larrue, V.; Bluhmki, E.; Davis, S.; Donnan, G.; et al. Randomised double-blind placebo-controlled trial of thrombolytic therapy with intravenous alteplase in acute ischaemic stroke (ECASS II). *Lancet* **1998**, *352*, 1245–1251. [CrossRef]
51. Kidwell, C.S.; Latour, L.; Saver, J.L.; Alger, J.R.; Starkman, S.; Duckwiler, G.; Jahan, R.; Vinuela, F.; Kang, D.W.; Warach, S. Thrombolytic toxicity: Blood brain barrier disruption in human ischemic stroke. *Cerebrovasc. Dis.* **2008**, *25*, 338–343. [CrossRef] [PubMed]
52. Strbian, D.; Engelter, S.; Michel, P.; Meretoja, A.; Sekoranja, L.; Ahlhelm, F.J.; Mustanoja, S.; Kuzmanovic, I.; Sairanen, T.; Forss, N.; et al. Symptomatic intracranial hemorrhage after stroke thrombolysis: The SEDAN score. *Ann. Neurol.* **2012**, *71*, 634–641. [CrossRef] [PubMed]
53. Chalos, V.; De Ridder, I.R.; Lingsma, H.F.; Brown, S.; Van Oostenbrugge, R.J.; Goyal, M.; Campbell, B.C.V.; Muir, K.W.; Guillemin, F.; Bracard, S.; et al. Does sex modify the effect of endovascular treatment for ischemic stroke? *Stroke* **2019**, *50*, 2413–2419. [CrossRef]
54. Sheth, S.A.; Lee, S.; Warach, S.J.; Gralla, J.; Jahan, R.; Goayl, M.; Nogueira, R.G.; Zaidat, O.O.; Pereira, V.M.; Siddiqui, A.; et al. Sex differences in outcome after endovascular stroke therapy for acute ischemic stroke. *Stroke* **2019**, *50*, 2420–2427. [CrossRef]
55. Uchida, K.; Yoshimura, S.; Sakai, N.; Yamagami, H.; Morimoto, T. Sex differences in management and outcomes of acute ischemic stroke with large vessel occlusion. *Stroke* **2019**, *50*, 1915–1918. [CrossRef]
56. Madsen, T.E.; DeCroce-Movson, E.; Hemendinger, M.; McTaggart, R.A.; Yaghi, S.; Cutting, S.; Furie, K.L.; Saad, A.; Siket, M.S.; Jayaraman, M.V. Sex differences in 90-day outcomes after mechanical thrombectomy for acute ischemic stroke. *J. Neurointerv. Surg.* **2019**, *11*, 221–225. [CrossRef] [PubMed]

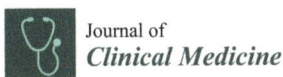

Article

C-Reactive Protein and White Blood Cell Count in Non-Infective Acute Ischemic Stroke Patients Treated with Intravenous Thrombolysis

Marcin Wnuk [1,2,*], Justyna Derbisz [1,2], Leszek Drabik [3,4] and Agnieszka Slowik [1,2]

1. Department of Neurology, Jagiellonian University Medical College, 31-688 Krakow, Poland; justyna.derbisz@gmail.com (J.D.); slowik@neuro.cm-uj.krakow.pl (A.S.)
2. University Hospital in Krakow, 30-688 Krakow, Poland
3. Department of Pharmacology, Jagiellonian University Medical College, 31-531 Krakow, Poland; leszek.drabik@uj.edu.pl
4. John Paul II Hospital, Krakow, 31-202 Krakow, Poland
* Correspondence: marcin.wnuk@uj.edu.pl

Citation: Wnuk, M.; Derbisz, J.; Drabik, L.; Slowik, A. C-Reactive Protein and White Blood Cell Count in Non-Infective Acute Ischemic Stroke Patients Treated with Intravenous Thrombolysis. *J. Clin. Med.* **2021**, *10*, 1610. https://doi.org/10.3390/jcm10081610

Academic Editor: Hyo Suk Nam

Received: 12 March 2021
Accepted: 7 April 2021
Published: 10 April 2021

Publisher's Note: MDPI stays neutral with regard to jurisdictional claims in published maps and institutional affiliations.

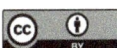

Copyright: © 2021 by the authors. Licensee MDPI, Basel, Switzerland. This article is an open access article distributed under the terms and conditions of the Creative Commons Attribution (CC BY) license (https://creativecommons.org/licenses/by/4.0/).

Abstract: Background: Previous studies on inflammatory biomarkers in acute ischemic stroke (AIS) produced divergent results. We evaluated whether C-reactive protein (CRP) and white blood cell count (WBC) measured fasting 12–24 h after intravenous thrombolysis (IVT) were associated with outcome in AIS patients without concomitant infection. **Methods:** The study included 352 AIS patients treated with IVT. Excluded were patients with community-acquired or nosocomial infection. Outcome was measured on discharge and 90 days after stroke onset with the modified Rankin scale (mRS) and defined as poor outcome (mRS 3–6) or death (mRS = 6). **Results:** Final analysis included 158 patients (median age 72 years (interquartile range 63-82), 53.2% (*n* = 84) women). Poor outcome on discharge and at day 90 was 3.8-fold and 5.8-fold higher for patients with CRP ≥ 8.65 mg/L (fifth quintile of CRP), respectively, compared with first quintile (<1.71 mg/L). These results remained significant after adjustment for potential confounders (odds ratio (OR) on discharge = 10.68, 95% CI: 2.54–44.83, OR at day 90 after stroke = 7.21, 95% CI: 1.44–36.00). In-hospital death was 6.3-fold higher for patients with fifth quintile of CRP as compared with first quintile and remained independent from other variables (OR = 4.79, 95% CI: 1.29–17.88). Independent predictors of 90-day mortality were WBC < 6.4×10^9 /L (OR = 5.00, 95% CI: 1.49–16.78), baseline National Institute of Health Stroke Scale (NIHSS) score (OR = 1.13 per point, 95% CI: 1.01–1.25) and bleeding brain complications (OR = 5.53, 95% CI: 1.59–19.25) but not CRP ≥ 8.65 mg/L. **Conclusions:** Non-infective CRP levels are an independent risk factor for poor short- and long-term outcomes and in-hospital mortality in AIS patients treated with IVT. Decreased WBC but not CRP is a predictor for 90-day mortality.

Keywords: stroke; thrombolysis; C-reactive protein; white blood cell count; prognosis; outcome

1. Introduction

Numerous biomarkers [1,2], including inflammatory ones, were found to be associated with atherosclerosis and cardiovascular events [3]. This applied to the levels of C-reactive protein (CRP) which increase during the first 24 h after hospital admission was independently associated with an increased risk of 30-day mortality in patients with acute myocardial infarction [4]. Increased white blood cell count (WBC) was instead an independent risk factor for long-term mortality in patients with coronary artery disease [5].

In patients with acute ischemic stroke (AIS) treated with intravenous thrombolysis (IVT), CRP within 24 h from symptom onset [6] and WBC within 24 h after IVT [7] were associated with a poor long-term functional outcome. However, there were also numerous studies which produced divergent results concerning the prognostic role of CRP in patients with AIS, likely due to a high proportion of patients with an infection. The negative prognostic influence of CRP was not ameliorated by IVT [8], whereas in several studies other prognostic factors were found to be more important in long-term prognosis [9–11]. It was shown that from 18.2 [12] to 23.6% [13] of AIS patients developed an infection during hospitalization, with pneumonia and urinary tract infection being the most common [14]. Although the elevation of inflammatory markers is usually observed in infections, a CRP increase in AIS may reflect non-infective ischemia-induced inflammation contributing to a hypercoagulable state and extensive tissue damage [15]. There is no widely accepted cut-off point in the literature for infective CRP in the AIS studies [9,16]. Although the specific cut-off value (>6 mg/dL) was used to exclude possible concomitant infection in a study by Montaner et al. [8], the clinical assessment plays a more important role in the exclusion of infection. Therefore, previous studies might have produced inconsistent findings of the prognostic role of CRP in AIS patients due to the variable and inadequate threshold of a biomarker used. CRP level and WBC may also be affected by measurements which took place in different clinical conditions, such as different time of the day, after previous food intake and under the influence of non-steroidal anti-inflammatory drugs [17–19]. For example, fasting is associated with a significant decrease in the CRP level [17], whereas WBC increases by nearly 10% two hours after meal consumption [19].

Many factors, including age, comorbidities and severity as measured with the National Institute of Health Stroke Scale (NIHSS) affect long-term prognosis after AIS treated with IVT [20]. There is still a need for other markers which could help predict long-term prognosis among AIS patients.

Therefore, the aim of the current study was to evaluate whether CRP levels and WBC measured fasting 12–24 h after IVT were associated with short- and long-term outcome in AIS patients without concomitant infection.

2. Materials and Methods

2.1. Patient Recruitment, CRP and WBC Measurements

The study was performed as a retrospective analysis of the prospectively collected data of 352 AIS patients from the Krakow Stroke Data Bank, a single-center stroke registry established in the University Hospital in Krakow in 2007. All patients were of Caucasian origin and were treated with IVT between June 2014 and December 2018. Excluded were patients with infection (n = 83) as described previously [13]. The lack of infection was determined by the exclusion of patients with fever, signs of infection in the physical examination, or those who needed antibiotics during subsequent hospitalization. Moreover, all patients underwent a routine chest x-ray, urine test and internal medicine consultation during the first 3 days since admission. Additionally, follow-up internal medicine consultation was performed in case of CRP elevation and before discharge. As the presence of malignant tumor was the exclusion criteria for IVT in AIS, there were no patients with this condition enrolled in our study.

After further exclusion of patients without available information regarding CRP and WBC levels measured fasting between 12 and 24 h after IVT, there were 158 remaining patients included in the final analysis. Our institutional protocol for fasting blood measurements requires overnight fasting for at least 6 h [21] and blood withdrawal before breakfast between 7 and 8 a.m. [22].

We collected the data about demographics, vascular risk factors, stroke etiology and NIHSS on admission and after IVT. Patients were followed-up according to the previously described protocol [13]. Outcome was measured with the modified Rankin scale (mRS). We obtained information about prognosis on discharge and 90 days after stroke onset and defined as poor outcome (mRS 3–6) or death (mRS = 6). Bleeding brain complications secondary to IVT were defined according to the ECASS-1 classification [23,24].

The study was approved by the Jagiellonian University Ethical Committee (KBET 54/B/2007). We obtained informed consent from all patients which was either written or verbal in the presence of at least two physicians in case of the inability to use the dominant hand due to stroke.

2.2. Statistics

The study was powered to have an 80% chance to detect a 50% difference in CRP between the group with mRS 0–2 and 3–6 at the 0.05 significance level. In order to demonstrate such a difference or greater, 26 subjects or more were required in each group based on the values from a published article [16].

The baseline clinical characteristics according to the quintiles of CRP and quartiles of WBC were compared using the univariate analysis of variance, Kruskal–Wallis rank ANOVA and chi-squared test, as appropriate. Values were presented as counts and percentages, means and standard deviations or medians (interquartile ranges), as appropriate. The multivariate models included age, sex and body mass index (BMI) (model 1); age, sex, BMI, hypertension, mRS score before stroke > 0, baseline NIHSS score, hemorrhagic brain complications and fasting hyperglycemia (model 2A); and age, sex, BMI, hypertension, maximal systolic blood pressure within 24 h after IVT, mRS score before stroke > 0, baseline NIHSS score, hemorrhagic brain complications and mechanical thrombectomy (model 2B). The Hosmer–Lemeshow test and ROC (Receiver Operating Characteristic) scores were used to evaluate the goodness of fit. Models with the lowest Akaike information criterion and highest Nagelkerke pseudo R2 were presented. The level of significance was set at a p-value ≤ 0.05. The data were processed using STATISTICA version 13.0 (Statsoft Inc., Tulsa, OK, USA).

3. Results

3.1. Patient Characteristics, Serum CRP Levels and WBC 12–24 h after IVT

The cohort of 158 patients with AIS treated with IVT is presented in Table 1 according to the CRP quintiles. The median age was 72 years (interquartile range 63–82), and 53.2% (n = 84) of patients were women. Mechanical thrombectomy was performed in 47 (29.7%) patients.

Table 1. Baseline clinical characteristics of the patients based on C-reactive protein (CRP) quintiles.

	Q1 CRP < 1.71 (n = 32)	Q2 CRP 1.71–3.11 (n = 32)	Q3 CRP 3.12–5.09 (n = 31)	Q4 CRP 5.10–8.64 (n = 32)	Q5 CRP $\geq$ 8.65 (n = 31)	p-Value
Age (years)	68 (58–76)	73 (68–80)	73 (69–80)	72 (64–83)	77 (62–86)	0.246
Women, n (%)	15 (46.9)	15 (46.9)	14 (45.2)	19 (59.4)	21 (67.8)	0.292
BMI (kg/m^2)	24.7 (22.8–27.7)	24.8 (23.3–27.7)	27.5 (24.2–29.3)	27.1 (25.2–29.9)	26.8 (25.0–29.7)	0.006
Hypertension, n (%)	22 (68.8)	23 (71.2)	27 (87.1)	26 (81.2)	30 (96.8)	0.031
Hypercholesterolemia, n (%)	12 (37.5)	8 (25.0)	11 (35.5)	11 34.4)	6 (19.4)	0.461
Diabetes mellitus, n (%)	9 (28.1)	8 (25.0)	7 (22.6)	7 (21.9)	11 (35.5)	0.744
Smoking, n (%)	6 (18.8)	2 (6.3)	2 (6.5)	8 (25.8)	5 (16.1)	0.151
Ischemic heart disease, n (%)	7 (21.9)	3 (9.4)	7 (22.6)	10 (31.2)	8 (25.8)	0.307
Atrial fibrillation, n (%)	6 (18.8)	10 (31.3)	11 (35.5)	8 (25.0)	9 (29.0)	0.635
Previous stroke, n (%)	7 (21.9)	3 (9.4)	8 (25.8)	6 (18.8)	4 (12.9)	0.432
mRS score before stroke >0	3 (9.4)	1 (3.1)	1 (3.2)	4 (12.5)	2 (6.4)	0.523
Stroke etiology, n (%)						
-large-vessel disease	5 (15.6)	5 (15.6)	5 (16.1)	3 (9.4)	5 (16.1)	
-small-vessel disease	1 (3.1)	1 (3.1)	0 (0.0)	0 (0.0)	0 (0.0)	
-cardioembolic	6 (18.8)	11 (34.4)	12 (38.7)	11 (34.4)	10 (32.3)	0.932
-other	19 (59.4)	14 (43.8)	13 (41.9)	18 (56.3)	15 (48.4)	
- undetermined	1 (3.1)	1 (3.1)	1 (3.2)	0 (0.0)	1 (3.2)	

Table 1. Cont.

	Q1 CRP < 1.71 (n = 32)	Q2 CRP 1.71–3.11 (n = 32)	Q3 CRP 3.12–5.09 (n = 31)	Q4 CRP 5.10–8.64 (n = 32)	Q5 CRP ≥ 8.65 (n = 31)	p-Value
Mechanical thrombectomy, n (%)	5 (15.60)	8 (25.0)	10 (32.3)	11 (34.4)	13 (41.9)	0.198
Time from stroke onset to thrombolysis (min)	119 (94–175)	145 (93–174)	117 (85–174)	90 (76–176)	121 (83–160)	0.556
NIHSS score on admission	9.7 ± 6.3	9.2 ± 6.7	12.5 ± 6.9	11.6 ± 6.3	14.6 ± 6.4	0.013
NIHSS score after r-tPA	4.4 ± 4.6	5.3 ± 5.5	8.1 ± 9.7	5.7 ± 6.9	11.9 ± 8.7	<0.001
Post-IVT hemorrhagic brain complications, n (%)						
-no complication	29 (90.6)	27 (84.4)	25 (80.7)	27 (84.4)	22 (71.0)	
-HI type 1	1 (3.1)	3 (9.4)	2 (6.5)	2 (6.3)	3 (9.7)	
-HI type 2	1 (3.1)	1 (3.1)	1 (3.2)	2 (6.3)	3 (9.7)	0.874
-PH type 1	1 (3.1)	1 93.1)	2 (6.5)	0 (0.0)	1 (3.2)	
-PH type 2	0 (0.0)	0 (0.0)	1 (3.2)	1 (3.1)	2 96.5)	
Maximal SBP within 24 h after r-tPA (mmHg)	144 (123–156)	145 (125–160)	145 (134–166)	151 (139–169)	143 (134–160)	0.536
Maximal DBP within 24 h after r-tPA (mmHg)	80 (72–90)	80 (72–89)	80 (70–90)	80 (70–85)	77 (70–80)	0.694
Fasting glucose (mmol/L)	6.5 (5.5–7.3)	6.2 (5.4–7.0)	6.1 (5.4–8.2)	6.8 (5.5–7.9)	6.9 (5.9–8.2)	0.491
Creatinine (μmol/L)	82 (65–94)	74 (63–100)	77 (69–97)	82 (71–91)	76 (65–93)	0.892
WBC (×10^9/L)	7.1 (6.0–8.7)	7.8 (6.6–8.8)	7.5 (5.4–9.2)	8.2 (6.9–10.9)	8.9 (6.4–11.5)	0.145

Values are presented as n (%), mean ± standard deviation, median and interquartile range. Abbreviations: BMI—body mass index, DBP—diastolic blood pressure, IVT—intravenous thrombolysis, HI—hemorrhagic infarction, mRS—modified Rankin scale, MT—mechanical thrombectomy, NIHSS—National Institutes of Health Stroke Scale, PH—parenchymal hematoma, r-tPA—recombinant tissue plasminogen activator, SBP—systolic blood pressure, and WBC—white blood cells count. Q1–Q5 denotes five groups according to the quintile of CRP (mg/L).

The median CRP 12–24 h after IVT was 3.94 (2.01–5.12 mg/L) and 15.2% (n = 24) of patients had CRP > 10 mg/L. The BMI, NIHSS score on admission and after IVT and prevalence of hypertension increased with the increase in CRP. The median WBC was 7.76 (6.40–9.61 × 10^9/L). Large-vessel disease stroke was associated with a higher WBC (Supplemental Table S1). There was no correlation between CRP and fasting glucose levels (r = 0.11, p = 0.167).

3.2. Serum CRP Levels and WBC 12–24 h after IVT and Poor Functional Outcome on Discharge and at Day 90 after Stroke

Patients with poor functional outcome on discharge (n = 52, 32.9%) and at day 90 after stroke (n = 39, 25.3%) had higher CRP measured fasting between 12 and 24 h after IVT compared with the remainder (5.92 (3.31–12.10) vs. 3.16 (1.76–5.73) mg/L, p < 0.001 and 5.91 (2.87–11.27) vs. 3.43 (1.71–5.96) mg/L, p < 0.001, respectively). The area under the receiver operating characteristic curve (AUC) of CRP for predicting poor functional outcome at day 90 was 0.667 (95% CI, 0.559–0.773, p = 0.002). With a cut-off point of 8.65 mg/L, the sensitivity, specificity and accuracy were 43.6%, 89.6% and 77.9%, respectively. The frequency of poor functional outcome on discharge and at day 90 was 3.8-fold and 5.8-fold higher for patients with CRP ≥ 8.65 mg/L (the fifth quintile of CRP), respectively, compared with the first quintile (<1.71 mg/L) (Figure 1). The odds ratio of poor functional outcome for patients in the highest quintile of CRP on discharge remained significant after adjustment for age, sex, BMI, hypertension, mRS score before stroke >0, baseline NIHSS score, hemorrhagic brain complications and fasting hyperglycemia (Table 2). The association between CRP and poor functional outcome at day 90 after stroke was significant in the multivariable model adjusted for multiple confounders including age, sex, baseline

NIHSS score, bleeding brain complications and mechanical thrombectomy (Table 2). The CRP ≥ 8.65 mg/L was predicted by the NIHSS score on admission and hypertension (Supplemental Table S2).

There was no significant association between the quartiles of WBC and the frequency of poor functional outcome on discharge and at day 90 (Figure 1).

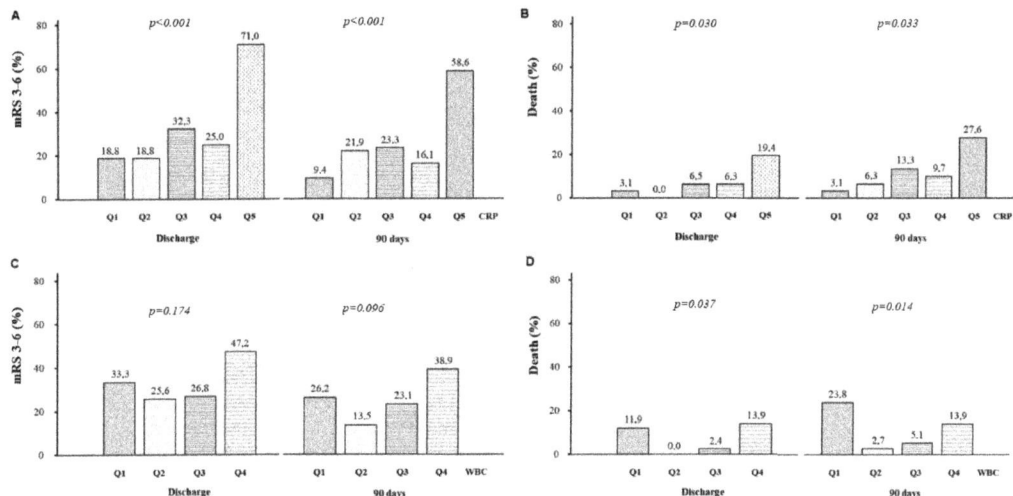

Figure 1. Panel (**A**,**B**). The proportion of patients with disability (modified Rankin Scale, mRS 3–6) or death (mRS = 6) on discharge and at day 90 after stroke onset, according to the quintile (quintile 1–quintile 5, Q1–Q5) of C-reactive protein (CRP) values. Panel (**C**,**D**). The proportion of patients with disability or death on discharge and at day 90 after stroke onset, according to the quartile (quartile 1–quartile 4, Q1–Q4) of white blood cell count (WBC).

Table 2. C-reactive protein and poor functional outcome (mRS 3–6) on discharge and at day 90 after stroke.

On Discharge		Model 1		Model 2A	
	Events n, (%)	OR (95% CI)	p-value	OR (95% CI)	p-value
Q1 (<1.71, n = 32)	6 (18.8)	1.00 (reference)	-	1.00 (reference)	-
Q2 (1.71–3.11, n = 32)	6 (18.8)	1.00 (0.28–3.56)	1.00	1.28 (0.27–5.96)	0.756
Q3 (3.12–5.09, n = 31)	10 (32.3)	2.13 (0.66–6.94)	0.209	1.65 (0.40–6.86)	0.493
Q4 (5.10–8.64, n = 32)	8 (25.0)	1.33 (0.40–4.45)	0.647	1.02 (0.24–4.29)	0.982
Q5 (≥8.65, n = 31)	22 (71.0)	9.70 (2.94–31.98)	<0.001	10.68 (2.54–44.83)	0.001
P for trend			<0.001		0.004
AIC			182.19		132.89
AUC			0.744 ± 0.05		0.895 ± 0.03
R2 Nagelkerke			0.241		0.560
Hosmer–Lemeshow test p-value			0.369		0.057
At day 90 after stroke		Model 1		Model 2B	
	Events n, (%)	OR (95% CI)	p-value	OR (95% CI)	p-value
Q1 (<1.71, n = 32)	3 (9.4)	1.00 (reference)	-	1.00 (reference)	-
Q2 (1.71–3.11, n = 32)	7 (21.9)	2.90 (0.65–13.0)	0.165	4.11 (0.73–23.7)	0.109
Q3 (3.12–5.09, n = 31)	7 (22.5)	3.18 (0.71–14.4)	0.132	1.86 (0.33–10.63)	0.484
Q4 (5.10–8.64, n = 32)	5 (15.7)	1.64 (0.34–7.83)	0.535	0.75 (0.12–4.53)	0.754
Q5 (≥ 8.65, n = 31)	17 (54.8)	12.56 (2.95–53.5)	0.001	7.21 (1.44–36.0)	0.016

Table 2. Cont.

On Discharge	Model 1	Model 2A
P for trend	0.022	0.021
AIC	152.42	125.16
AUC	0.776 ± 0.04	0.887 ± 0.03
R2 Nagelkerke	0.291	0.521
Hosmer–Lemeshow test p-value	0.169	0.569

Model 1 included age, sex and BMI. Model 2A included age, sex, BMI, hypertension, mRS score before stroke >0, baseline NIHSS score, hemorrhagic brain complications and fasting hyperglycemia. Model 2B included age, sex, BMI, hypertension, maximal SBP within 24 h after r-tPA, mRS score before stroke >0, baseline NIHSS score, hemorrhagic brain complications and mechanical thrombectomy. Abbreviations, see Table 1. AIC denotes Akaike information criterion, AUC—the area under the curve, CI—confidence interval, OR—odds ratio, Q1–Q5 five groups according to the quintile of CRP (mg/L).

3.3. Serum CRP Levels and WBC 12–24 h after IVT and Early Neurological Deterioration and Bleeding

Neurological deterioration after IVT, defined as an increase of two or more points in the NIHSS scale [25] between admission and 12–24 h after IVT, was observed in seven (4.43%) patients. The CRP and WBC values did not differ between groups with and without neurological deterioration (5.77 (3.45–9.31) vs. 3.79 (1.03–7.36) mg/L, $p = 0.22$ and 10.42 (4.95–13.95) vs. 7.77 (6.44–9.77) $\times 10^9$/L, $p = 0.29$, respectively). Intracranial bleeding (ECASS class 1–4) was observed in 28 (17.72%) patients (6.96%, 5.06%, 3.16% and 2.53% for classes 1–4, respectively). We observed a trend toward higher CRP (5.18 (2.99–9.44) vs. 3.56 (1.84–7.34) mg/L), $p = 0.09$, and no difference in WBC (7.12 (6.11–10.38) vs. 7.86 (6.51–9.45) $\times 10^9$/L, $p = 0.43$), in patients with and without bleeding, ECASS class 1–4.

3.4. Serum CRP Levels and WBC 12–24 h after IVT and In-Hospital and 90-Day Mortality

Patients who died in hospital ($n = 11$, 7.0%) and within 90 days after stroke ($n = 18$, 11.4%) had higher CRP levels compared with the survivors (8.99 (4.39–15.42) vs. 3.67 (1.93–6.93) mg/L, $p = 0.01$ and 6.51 (4.39–10.67) vs. 3.49 (1.83–6.23) mg/L, $p = 0.006$, respectively). The frequency of in-hospital death was 6.3-fold higher for patients with the fifth quintile of CRP as compared with the first quintile (Figure 1). In-hospital mortality was independently predicted by CRP $\geq$ 8.65 mg/L and hemorrhagic brain complications (Table 3). The independent predictors of 90-day mortality were WBC $< 6.4 \times 10^9$/L, baseline NIHSS score and hemorrhagic brain complications, but not CRP $\geq$ 8.65 mg/L (Table 3).

Table 3. Predictors of death on discharge and at day 90 after stroke.

On Discharge	OR	95% CI	p-Value	OR	95% CI	p-Value
Age (per 1 year)	1.00	0.96–10.5	0.861	-	-	-
Sex (female)	4.32	0.90–20.68	0.067	-	-	-
BMI (per 1 unit)	1.05	0.92–1.21	0.441	-	-	-
Baseline NIHSS score (per 1 point)	1.15	1.03–1.28	0.012	-	-	-
Mechanical thrombectomy	3.10	0.90–10.73	0.074	-	-	-
Hemorrhagic brain complications (ECASS 1–3 score)	6.82	1.91–24.28	0.003	5.66	1.52–21.11	0.010
CRP $\geq$ 8.65 mg/L	5.86	1.66–20.70	0.006	4.79	1.29–17.88	0.020
WBC $< 6.4 \times 10^9$/L	2.48	0.71–8.59	0.152	-	-	-
AIC						72.21
AUC						0.794 ± 0.07
R2 Nagelkerke						0.208
Hosmer–Lemeshow test p-value						0.689
At day 90 after stroke	OR	95% CI	p-value	OR	95% CI	p-value
Age (per 1 year)	1.03	0.99–1.08	0.161	-	-	-
Sex (female)	3.50	1.10–11.18	0.034	-	-	-
BMI (per 1 unit)	1.04	0.93–1.16	0.523	-	-	-

Table 3. Cont.

On Discharge	OR	95% CI	p-Value	OR	95% CI	p-Value
Baseline NIHSS score (per 1 point)	1.17	1.07–1.28	<0.001	1.13	1.01–1.25	0.036
Hemorrhagic brain complications (ECASS 1–3 score)	8.19	2.86–23.50	<0.001	5.53	1.59–19.25	0.007
CRP $\geq$ 8.65 mg/L	4.38	1.55–12.39	0.005	-	-	-
WBC < 6.4 $\times 10^9$/L	4.06	1.48–11.16	0.007	5.00	1.49–16.78	0.009
AIC						87.03
AUC						0.877 $\pm$ 0.04
R2 Nagelkerke						0.406
Hosmer–Lemeshow test p-value						0.420

Abbreviations, see Tables 1 and 2.

The AUC of WBC for 90-day mortality was 0.660 (95% CI, 0.518–0.802, $p = 0.027$). The WBC value of 6.4 × 10^9/L offered the best overall sensitivity, specificity and accuracy of 76.5, 23.5 and 74.0%, respectively. The WBC < 6.4 × 10^9/L was associated with a 4.7-fold and 8.8-fold higher rate of deaths compared with the WBC 6.40–7.75 × 10^9/L and 7.76–9.60 × 10^9/L (Figure 1). The WBC < 6.4 × 10^9/L was predicted by large vessel stroke etiology (Supplemental Table S3).

4. Discussion

The current study supported an association between fasting CRP levels measured 12–24 h after IVT and analyzed in quintiles and long-term functional outcome after AIS in patients without concomitant infection. Previous prospective study performed on a large cohort of more than 3000 patients confirmed the prognostic significance of CRP measured within 24 h from symptom onset in the whole group of patients assessed with mRS three months after AIS, and, admittedly, after adjustment for IVT, this association was still maintained [6]. A similar conclusion came from the study evaluating 436 AIS patients without infection in China, in which elevated CRP levels within 24 h after IVT were found to increase nearly 5-fold the risk of 3-month poor functional outcome [7]. On the other hand, in the study of Karlinski et al., also evaluating AIS patients without infection, CRP assessed within 24 h from symptom onset was not associated with 3-month outcome, however, patients were dichotomized according to the abnormal level of CRP, that is, lower than or above 5 ng/mL [16]. In another study, the change in CRP between admission and the seventh day of hospitalization did not affect long-term outcome either [11]. However, the long-term prognostic role of CRP in AIS patients without infection treated with IVT seemed to be also supported by the studies in patients undergoing another reperfusion therapy of AIS, that is, mechanical thrombectomy. In a recent study, a similar to our research cut-off level of CRP was found to be associated with long-term outcome in AIS patients who underwent endovascular therapy independent of other variables [26].

In our study, no association between CRP levels and 3-month mortality after AIS treated with IVT was found. Our conclusions stayed in line with the previous results coming from the Chinese study which also did not support a correlation of CRP with all-cause mortality at 3 months [7]. Interestingly, in the same study, high WBC increased 2-fold the risk of death at 3 months [7]. Increased WBC the next day after mechanical thrombectomy was found to significantly correlate with the NIHSS score at day 90 after stroke onset [27]. We found instead that the lowest WBC quartile was an independent risk factor for increased long-term mortality at 3 months in AIS patients without infection. Together with the observed trend for higher mortality in the quartile of the highest WBC, it seemed that the association between WBC and the risk of death might resemble the U-curve.

In our specific group of patients, the association of CRP with short-term outcome was also revealed. Our observation resembled the results from another Chinese study which searched for the predictors of poor response to IVT [28]. The authors proposed even the ACBS scale, as there were four parameters which remained significant in the multivariate analysis, with CRP apart from age, glucose levels and systolic blood pressure at baseline [28]. Elevated CRP levels were also found to correlate negatively with the reduction in neurological deficit measured with the NIHSS 12–24 h after IVT [29]. Thus, it seems that assessment of CRP within the first 24 h after admission in AIS patients without infection treated with IVT could be helpful in the evaluation of their short-term clinical outcome. However, uncertainty exists concerning the appropriate time point for CRP measurement in AIS patients. Most previous studies assessed CRP levels within 24 h after admission [16], whereas in others measurements took place within 24 h from AIS onset [6] or upon arrival to the emergency department [28]. In our study, we used the specific time frame for CRP assessment, that is, between 12 and 24 h after IVT, which was previously used in another study evaluating the prognostic role of trends in CRP levels [29]. Another study on a group of more than a thousand AIS patients receiving IVT showed that CRP levels assessed within 24 h from admission or in the following days better predicted long-term functional outcome that the admission values [30]. It is worth mentioning that in reference to another blood parameter such as glucose, its values measured fasting the next morning after admission had more potent long-term prognostic significance than the admission values [22]. Therefore, as levels of CRP might be biased by food intake [17], we measured CRP levels in our AIS patients after at least 6 h overnight fasting [21], according to our institutional protocol [22]

There were no associations between CRP levels and neurological worsening or bleeding brain complications in our study. Previous studies showed that patients with elevated CRP more often suffered from bleeding brain complications, however, this association was not confirmed after adjustment for other clinical parameters, including age, stroke severity and recent infection [16], which resembles the results of our study. As to neurological deterioration, higher CRP levels were found to be associated with its increased risk in another study after adjustment for multiple confounders [6] that was not confirmed in our study, probably due to the smaller sample size. In another study, the association between CRP and neurological deterioration was supported only for AIS patients who did not receive IVT [31].

The role of CRP in the pathophysiology of stroke is complicated, however, during AIS, systemic inflammation is induced, which may result in increased body temperature, WBC and CRP levels [32]. In a rabbit model of stroke, CRP levels after a cerebrovascular event correlated with the size of the infarct, and were perceived by the authors as a good marker of prognosis during AIS assessment [33]. Early treatment with IVT may result in the reduction in inflammatory response due to inhibition of the brain tissue necrosis [32].

In our study, CRP after adjustment for numerous variables including hypertension predicted poor functional outcomes. Interestingly, we observed that hypertension was the strongest predictor of the highest levels of CRP in the multivariate analysis (Supplemental Table S2). We hypothesize that elevated CRP may reflect the risk of an unfavorable outcome that was attributed to hypertension in other studies [34]. Future studies are needed to evaluate those mechanisms. Although there was no statistically significant correlation between CRP and fasting glucose levels, we cannot exclude the true correlation with the increase in the sample size.

Non-infective CRP in patients with AIS may deliver prognostic information distinct from that carried by CRP measured during the acute phase of infection. Non-infective CRP elevation may reflect stroke-induced inflammation and endothelial dysfunction contributing to a hypercoagulable state and extensive tissue damage. High levels of CRP are an independent marker of cardiovascular risk, which may be reduced by a statin therapy independently to a lipid-lowering drug action [35]. Aimed anti-inflammatory treatment targeting interleukin-1, endothelial selectins and leukocyte infiltration shows promising results in preclinical and small clinical studies in AIS [36]. Therefore, we view the results of our study as hypothesis-generating, whereas future studies are needed to evaluate whether such treatment could be effective in diminishing inflammatory processes induced by AIS and manifested by non-infective CRP increase. Finally, the unique timing of sample collections that takes into consideration the CRP-kinetics may contribute to our observations.

Our study has important limitations. First, the sample of patients was relatively small and therefore subgroup analyses, especially related to WBC, should be interpreted with caution. Second, we did not analyze the influence of change in CRP levels during hospitalization on long-term functional outcome. Third, we also did not take into account the differential of WBC which was recently shown to be an important prognostic factor in AIS patients [37]. Fourth, the reported statistical associations do not necessarily mean a cause-effect relationship.

5. Conclusions

In conclusion, CRP levels measured fasting between 12 and 24 h after IVT are an independent risk factor for poor short- and long-term outcomes in AIS patients without infection, as well as for in-hospital mortality. The lowest quartile of WBC predicts 3-month mortality; however, this finding needs further investigation. Future studies are also expected to create a prognostic scale for short- and long-term prognosis after AIS with CRP as one of the reasonable parameters.

Supplementary Materials: The following are available online at https://www.mdpi.com/article/10.3390/jcm10081610/s1. Supplementary Table S1. Baseline clinical characteristics of the patients based on white blood cell count (WBC) quartiles; Supplementary Table S2. Predictors of the CRP $\geq$ 8.65 mg/L (fifth quintile); Supplementary Table S3. Predictors of white blood cells count < 6.4×10^9/L (first quartile).

Author Contributions: M.W. (conceptualization, methodology, draft writing and editing), J.D. (data acquisition), L.D. (formal analysis, methodology, draft writing and editing) and A.S. (supervision and draft review). All authors have read and agreed to the published version of the manuscript.

Funding: This research was funded by the grant from The National Centre for Research and Development, Poland under the ERA-NET NEURON program, contract no.: ERA-NET-NEURON/21/2020 and from the Jagiellonian University grant N41/DBS/000464.

Institutional Review Board Statement: The study was conducted according to the guidelines of the Declaration of Helsinki, and approved by the Jagiellonian University Ethical Committee (KBET/54/B/2007).

Informed Consent Statement: We obtained informed consent from all patients which was either written or verbal in the presence of at least two physicians in case of the inability to use the dominant hand due to stroke.

Data Availability Statement: The data supporting the findings of the present study will be made available for any qualified investigator from the corresponding author upon reasonable request.

Conflicts of Interest: The authors declare no conflict of interest.

References

1. Wnuk, M.; Pera, J.; Jagiełła, J.; Szczygieł, E.; Ferens, A.; Spisak, K.; Wołkow, P.; Kmieć, M.; Burkot, J.; Chrzanowska-Waśko, J.; et al. The rs2200733 variant on chromosome 4q25 is a risk factor for cardioembolic stroke related to atrial fibrillation in Polish patients. *Neurol. Neurochir. Pol.* **2011**, *45*, 148–152. [CrossRef]
2. Drabik, L.; Konieczyńska, M.; Undas, A. Clot Lysis Time Predicts Stroke During Anticoagulant Therapy in Patients with Atrial Fibrillation. *Can. J. Cardiol.* **2020**, *36*, 119–126. [CrossRef]
3. Soeki, T.; Sata, M. Inflammatory Biomarkers and Atherosclerosis. *Int. Heart J.* **2016**, *57*, 134–139. [CrossRef] [PubMed]
4. Milwidsky, A.; Ziv-Baran, T.; Letourneau-Shesaf, S.; Keren, G.; Taieb, P.; Berliner, S.; Shacham, Y. CRP velocity and short-term mortality in ST segment elevation myocardial infarction. *Biomarkers* **2017**, *22*, 383–386. [CrossRef]
5. Zhao, X.; Jiang, L.; Xu, L.; Tian, J.; Xu, Y.; Zhao, Y.; Feng, X.; Wu, Y.; Zhang, Y.; Wang, D.; et al. Predictive value of in-hospital white blood cell count in Chinese patients with triple-vessel coronary disease. *Eur. J. Prev. Cardiol.* **2019**, *26*, 872–882. [CrossRef] [PubMed]
6. Matsuo, R.; Ago, T.; Hata, J.; Wakisaka, Y.; Kuroda, J.; Kuwashiro, T.; Kitazono, T.; Kamouchi, M.; on behalf of the Fukuoka Stroke Registry Investigators. Plasma C-Reactive Protein and Clinical Outcomes after Acute Ischemic Stroke: A Prospective Observational Study. *PLoS ONE* **2016**, *11*, e0156790. [CrossRef]

7. Qu, X.; Shi, J.; Cao, Y.; Zhang, M.; Xu, J. Prognostic Value of White Blood Cell Counts and C-reactive Protein in Acute Ischemic Stroke Patients After Intravenous Thrombolysis. *Curr. Neurovasc. Res.* **2018**, *15*, 10–17. [CrossRef]
8. Montaner, J.; Fernandez-Cadenas, I.; Molina, C.A.; Ribó, M.; Huertas, R.; Rosell, A.; Penalba, A.; Ortega, L.; Chacón, P.; Alvarez-Sabín, J. Poststroke C-Reactive Protein Is a Powerful Prognostic Tool Among Candidates for Thrombolysis. *Stroke* **2006**, *37*, 1205–1210. [CrossRef] [PubMed]
9. Topakian, R.; Strasak, A.M.; Nussbaumer, K.; Haring, H.-P.; Aichner, F.T. Prognostic value of admission C-reactive protein in stroke patients undergoing IV thrombolysis. *J. Neurol.* **2008**, *255*, 1190–1196. [CrossRef] [PubMed]
10. Winbeck, K.; Poppert, H.; Etgen, T.; Conrad, B.; Sander, D. Prognostic Relevance of Early Serial C-Reactive Protein Measurements After First Ischemic Stroke. *Stroke* **2002**, *33*, 2459–2464. [CrossRef]
11. Lee, S.; Song, I.-U.; Na, S.-H.; Jeong, D.-S.; Chung, S.-W. Association Between Long-term Functional Outcome and Change in hs-CRP Level in Patients With Acute Ischemic Stroke. *Neurologist* **2020**, *25*, 122–125. [CrossRef]
12. Mendes de Sá, F.; Mendes Bertoncello Fontes, C.; Lia Mondelli, A. Major infections in hospitalized patients with stroke: A pro-spective study. *Int. Arch. Med.* **2016**, *9*, 1–8.
13. Derbisz, J.; Nowak, K.; Wnuk, M.; Pulyk, R.; Jagiella, J.; Slowik, J.; Dziedzic, T.; Slowik, A. Prognostic Significance of Stroke-Associated Infection and other Readily Available Parameters in Acute Ischemic Stroke Treated by Intravenous Thrombolysis. *J. Stroke Cerebrovasc. Dis.* **2021**, *30*, 105525. [CrossRef]
14. Weimar, C.; Roth, M.P.; Zillessen, G.; Glahn, J.; Wimmer, M.L.; Busse, O.; Haberl, R.L.; Diener, H.-C.; on behalf of the German Stroke Date Bank Collaborators. Complications following Acute Ischemic Stroke. *Eur. Neurol.* **2002**, *48*, 133–140. [CrossRef]
15. Sproston, N.R.; Ashworth, J.J. Role of C-Reactive Protein at Sites of Inflammation and Infection. *Front. Immunol.* **2018**, *9*, 754. [CrossRef]
16. Karlinski, M.; Bembenek, J.; Grabska, K.; Kobayashi, A.; Baranowska, A.; Litwin, T.; Czlonkowska, A. Routine serum C-reactive protein and stroke outcome after intravenous thrombolysis. *Acta Neurol. Scand.* **2014**, *130*, 305–311. [CrossRef] [PubMed]
17. Alam, I.; Gul, R.; Chong, J.; Tan, C.T.Y.; Chin, H.X.; Wong, G.; Doggui, R.; Larbi, A. Recurrent circadian fasting (RCF) improves blood pressure, bi-omarkers of cardiometabolic risk and regulates inflammation in men. *J. Transl. Med.* **2019**, *17*, 272. [CrossRef] [PubMed]
18. Tarp, S.; Bartels, E.M.; Bliddal, H.; Furst, D.E.; Boers, M.; Danneskiold-Samsøe, B.; Rasmussen, M.; Christensen, R. Effect of nonsteroidal antiinflammatory drugs on the C-reactive protein level in rheumatoid arthritis: A meta-analysis of randomized controlled trials. *Arthritis Rheum.* **2012**, *64*, 3511–3521. [CrossRef]
19. Kościelniak, M.B.K.; Charchut, M.A.; Wójcik, M.M.; Sztefko, K.; Tomasik, P.J. Impact of Fasting on Complete Blood Count Assayed in Capillary Blood Samples. *Lab. Med.* **2017**, *48*, 357–361. [CrossRef] [PubMed]
20. Clua-Espuny, J.L.; Abilleira, S.; Queralt-Tomas, L.; Gonzalez-Henares, A.; Gil-Guillen, V.; Muria-Subirats, E.; Ballesta-Ors, J. Long-Term Survival After Stroke According to Reperfusion Therapy, Cardiovascular Therapy and Gender. *Cardiol. Res.* **2019**, *10*, 89–97. [CrossRef]
21. Nordestgaard, B.G.; Langsted, A.; Mora, S.; Kolovou, G.; Baum, H.; Bruckert, E.; Watts, G.F.; Sypniewska, G.; Wiklund, O.; Boren, J.; et al. Fasting is not routinely required for determination of a lipid profile: Clinical and laboratory implications including flagging at desirable concentration cut-points—A joint con-sensus statement from the European Atherosclerosis Society and European Fede. *Eur. Heart J.* **2016**, *37*, 1944–1958. [CrossRef] [PubMed]
22. Wnuk, M.; Popiela, T.; Drabik, L.; Brzegowy, P.; Lasocha, B.; Wloch-Kopec, D.; Pulyk, R.; Jagiella, J.; Wiacek, M.; Kaczorowski, R.; et al. Fasting Hyperglycemia and Long-term Outcome in Patients with Acute Ischemic Stroke Treated with Mechanical Thrombectomy. *J. Stroke Cerebrovasc. Dis.* **2020**, *29*, 104774. [CrossRef] [PubMed]
23. Trouillas, P.; Von Kummer, R. Classification and Pathogenesis of Cerebral Hemorrhages After Thrombolysis in Ischemic Stroke. *Stroke* **2006**, *37*, 556–561. [CrossRef]
24. Undas, A.; Drabik, L.; Potpara, T. Bleeding in anticoagulated patients with atrial fibrillation: Practical considerations. *Pol. Arch. Intern. Med.* **2020**, *130*, 47–58. [CrossRef] [PubMed]
25. Kwan, J.; Hand, P. Early neurological deterioration in acute stroke: Clinical characteristics and impact on outcome. *QJM* **2006**, *99*, 625–633. [CrossRef] [PubMed]
26. Wang, L.; Wu, L.; Lang, Y.; Wu, D.; Chen, J.; Zhao, W.; Li, C.; Ji, X. Association between high-sensitivity C-reactive protein levels and clinical outcomes in acute ischemic stroke patients treated with endovascular therapy. *Ann. Transl. Med.* **2020**, *8*, 1379. [CrossRef]
27. Huber, T.; Kleine, J.F.; Kaesmacher, J.; Bette, S.; Poppert, H.; Zimmer, C.; Boeckh-Behrens, T. Blood Leukocytes as Prognostic Parameter in Stroke Thrombectomy. *Cerebrovasc. Dis.* **2016**, *42*, 32–40. [CrossRef]
28. Yue, Y.-H.; Li, Z.-Z.; Hu, L.; Zhu, X.-Q.; Xu, X.-S.; Sun, H.-X.; Wan, Z.-W.; Xue, J.; Yu, D.-H. Clinical characteristics and risk score for poor clinical outcome of acute ischemic stroke patients treated with intravenous thrombolysis therapy. *Brain Behav.* **2019**, *9*, e01351. [CrossRef]
29. Gill, D.; Sivakumaran, P.; Wilding, P.; Love, M.; Veltkamp, R.; Kar, A. Trends in C-Reactive Protein Levels Are Associated with Neurological Change Twenty-Four Hours after Thrombolysis for Acute Ischemic Stroke. *J. Stroke Cerebrovasc. Dis.* **2016**, *25*, 1966–1969. [CrossRef]
30. Rocco, A.; Ringleb, P.A.; Grittner, U.; Nolte, C.H.; Schneider, A.; Nagel, S. Follow-up C-reactive protein level is more strongly associ-ated with outcome in stroke patients than admission levels. *Neurol. Sci.* **2015**, *36*, 2235–2241. [CrossRef]

31. Seo, W.-K.; Seok, H.-Y.; Kim, J.H.; Park, M.-H.; Yu, S.-W.; Oh, K.; Koh, S.-B.; Park, K.-W. C-Reactive Protein is a Predictor of Early Neurologic Deterioration in Acute Ischemic Stroke. *J. Stroke Cerebrovasc. Dis.* **2012**, *21*, 181–186. [CrossRef] [PubMed]
32. Ye, L.; Cai, R.; Yang, M.; Qian, J.; Hong, Z. Reduction of the systemic inflammatory induced by acute cerebral infarction through ultra-early thrombolytic therapy. *Exp. Ther. Med.* **2015**, *10*, 1493–1498. [CrossRef]
33. Yu, Q.; Lin, Y.; Yang, P.; Wang, Y.; Zhao, S.; Yang, P.; Fan, J.; Liu, E. C-reactive protein is associated with the progression of acute embolic stroke in rabbit model. *J. Thromb. Thrombol.* **2011**, *33*, 301–307. [CrossRef] [PubMed]
34. Zhang, Q.; Qiu, D.-X.; Fu, R.-L.; Xu, T.-F.; Jing, M.-J.; Zhang, H.-S.; Geng, H.-H.; Zheng, L.-C.; Wang, P.-X. H-Type Hypertension and C Reactive Protein in Recurrence of Ischemic Stroke. *Int. J. Environ. Res. Public Health* **2016**, *13*, 477. [CrossRef]
35. Drieu, A.; Levard, D.; Vivien, D.; Rubio, M. Anti-inflammatory treatments for stroke: From bench to bedside. *Ther. Adv. Neurol. Disord.* **2018**, *11*, 1–15. [CrossRef] [PubMed]
36. Dinarello, C.A.; Simon, A.; Van Der Meer, J.W.M. Treating inflammation by blocking interleukin-1 in a broad spectrum of diseases. *Nat. Rev. Drug Discov.* **2012**, *11*, 633–652. [CrossRef]
37. Xue, J.; Huang, W.; Chen, X.; Li, Q.; Cai, Z.; Yu, T.; Shao, B. Neutrophil-to-Lymphocyte Ratio Is a Prognostic Marker in Acute Ischemic Stroke. *J. Stroke Cerebrovasc. Dis.* **2017**, *26*, 650–657. [CrossRef]

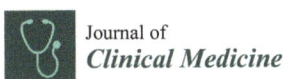

Article

Temperature-Induced Changes in Reperfused Stroke: Inflammatory and Thrombolytic Biomarkers

Paulo Ávila-Gómez [1], Pablo Hervella [1], Andrés Da Silva-Candal [1], María Pérez-Mato [2], Manuel Rodríguez-Yáñez [3], Iria López-Dequidt [3], José M. Pumar [4], José Castillo [1], Tomás Sobrino [1], Ramón Iglesias-Rey [1,*] and Francisco Campos [1,*]

[1] Clinical Neurosciences Research Laboratory (LINC), Health Research Institute of Santiago de Compostela (IDIS), E15706 Santiago de Compostela, Spain; paulo.avila.gomez@sergas.es (P.Á.-G.); pablo.hervella.lorenzo@sergas.es (P.H.); andres.alexander.da.silva.candal@sergas.es (A.D.S.-C.); jose.castillo.sanchez@sergas.es (J.C.); tomas.sobrino.moreiras@sergas.es (T.S.)

[2] Neuroscience and Cerebrovascular Research Laboratory, Department of Neurology and Stroke Center, La Paz University Hospital, Neuroscience Area of IdiPAZ Health Research Institute, Universidad Autónoma de Madrid, E28046 Madrid, Spain; mery19832005@yahoo.es

[3] Stroke Unit, Department of Neurology, Health Research Institute of Santiago de Compostela, Hospital Clínico Universitario, 15706 Santiago de Compostela, Spain; manyanez@yahoo.es (M.R.-Y.); iriaalejandralopez@googlemail.com (I.L.-D.)

[4] Department of Neuroradiology, Hospital Clínico Universitario, Health Research Institute of Santiago de Compostela (IDIS), E15706 Santiago de Compostela, Spain; josemanuel.pumar@usc.es

* Correspondence: ramon.iglesias.rey@sergas.es (R.I.-R.); francisco.campos.perez@sergas.es (F.C.); Tel./Fax: +34-981951098 (R.I.-R. & F.C.)

Received: 13 June 2020; Accepted: 2 July 2020; Published: 4 July 2020

Abstract: Although hyperthermia is associated with poor outcomes in ischaemic stroke (IS), some studies indicate that high body temperature may benefit reperfusion therapies. We assessed the association of temperature with effective reperfusion (defined as a reduction of ≥8 points in the National Institute of Health Stroke Scale (NIHSS) within the first 24 h) and poor outcome (modified Rankin Scale (mRS) > 2) in 875 retrospectively-included IS patients. We also studied the influence of temperature on thrombolytic (cellular fibronectin (cFn); matrix metalloproteinase 9 (MMP-9)) and inflammatory biomarkers (tumour necrosis factor-alpha (TNF-α), interleukin 6 (IL-6)) and their relationship with effective reperfusion. Our results showed that a higher temperature at 24 but not 6 h after stroke was associated with failed reperfusion (OR: 0.373, $p = 0.001$), poor outcome (OR: 2.190, $p = 0.005$) and higher IL-6 levels (OR: 0.958, $p < 0.0001$). Temperature at 6 h was associated with higher MMP-9 levels (R = 0.697; $p < 0.0001$) and effective reperfusion, although this last association disappeared after adjusting for confounding factors (OR: 1.178, $p = 0.166$). Our results suggest that body temperature > 37.5 °C at 24 h, but not at 6 h after stroke, is correlated with reperfusion failure, poor clinical outcome, and infarct size. Mild hyperthermia (36.5–37.5 °C) in the first 6 h window might benefit drug reperfusion therapies by promoting clot lysis.

Keywords: biomarkers; ischemic stroke; recanalization therapy; reperfusion; temperature

1. Introduction

Temperature is a long-known pivotal factor in the development and progression of neurological injuries, particularly in the field of stroke, where approximately 50% of patients develop hyperthermia (or fever) within the first 24 h [1,2]. Indeed, higher temperatures during the acute phase of ischaemic stroke (IS) have been associated with greater infarct volumes and worse functional outcomes at 3 months [2–8]. Therapeutic hypothermia helps to preserve tissue energy and halts several cell death mechanisms; thus, it is currently considered one of the most promising neuroprotective approaches in preclinical models of stroke [9,10]. Nonetheless, although therapeutic hypothermia has well-established neuroprotective effects in specific conditions, its translatability to the human clinic remains elusive [11,12].

Besides mechanical devices, reperfusion drug therapy with recombinant tissue plasminogen activator (rtPA) remains the treatment of choice during the acute phase of an ischaemic event, although its use is limited due to the risk of haemorrhage [13–15]. In this regard, body temperature also has a relevant influence on the efficacy of thrombolytic therapy. Paradoxically, although hyperthermia has been associated with poor outcomes and an increased risk of developing haemorrhagic transformation (HT) after rtPA treatment [2], some studies have shown that high body temperatures could have a beneficial effect on reperfusion therapies by enhancing the thrombolytic activity of rtPA [16–18]. For instance, previous studies have reported increased fibrinolysis using streptokinase at higher temperatures [19], while lower clot lysis was observed at lower temperatures when rtPA was added to clot suspensions [20]. In patients with acute lower limb ischaemia treated with catheter-directed thrombolysis, heating the rtPA also resulted in faster clot lysis [21]. Therefore, it is not clear if the improvement in clot lysis and efficacy of reperfusion can overcome the deleterious effect of hyperthermia on stroke outcome in rtPA-treated patients.

In this regard, it has been widely reported that, although reperfusion is associated with improved patient outcomes, it can also exacerbate temperature-dependent processes related to blood–brain barrier disruption and post-stroke inflammatory response, leading to increased brain damage [22]. For instance, rtPA upregulates matrix metalloproteinase 9 (MMP-9) expression [23], which is associated with HT and poor outcome in IS [24], and hyperthermia exacerbates the destruction of microvascular integrity by increasing MMP-9 activity [25]. Our group has also reported that circulating levels of fibronectin (cFn) predicted rtPA-associated HT after systemic thrombolysis [26]. Moreover, we have previously demonstrated that higher levels of proinflammatory markers such as interleukin 6 (IL-6) and tumour necrosis factor-alpha (TNF-α) were associated with poor outcomes and larger infarcts in IS patients with hyperthermia [27] and rtPA treatment [28].

Given the conflicting evidence on the effect of temperature on thrombolytic-reperfusion, we hypothesised that higher body temperature during the acute phase of an IS could have a beneficial effect on reperfusion therapies and patient outcomes. Thus, this work aimed to study the influence of temperature on the recanalisation effectiveness and functional outcome at 3 months in a population of IS patients receiving reperfusion therapies. To further support our analysis, we evaluated the effect of temperature on the levels of fibrinolytic and inflammatory activity biomarkers and their impact on the effectiveness of reperfusion. As a secondary objective, we analysed the influence of temperature on the percentage of patients with HT and infarct volume.

2. Materials and Methods

2.1. Study Design

This retrospective observational study was conducted on a registry of patients with IS included consecutively and prospectively from our databank. The patients were admitted to the Stroke Unit of the University Clinical Hospital of Santiago de Compostela (Spain) from January 2008 to December 2018. The study was performed in accordance with the principles of the Declaration of Helsinki of the World Medical Association and approved by the Research Ethics Committee of Santiago (project identification code 2019/616). Informed consent was obtained from each patient or their relatives after providing a full explanation of the procedures.

2.2. Inclusion Criteria

All patients included in this study met the following criteria: (1) authorisation for the anonymous use of their data for research; (2) magnetic resonance imaging (MRI) or computed tomography (CT) study at inclusion and between days four and seven; (3) hemispheric location; (4) patients undergoing reperfusion treatment with rtPA alone or in combination with thrombectomy; (5) patients with a latency time between stroke onset and inclusion of ≤6 h; and (6) a minimum follow-up (face-to-face or telephone) duration of 3 months. Patients who met any of the following criteria were not considered for the study: (1) institutionalised patients, (2) comorbidity and life expectancy <1 year, (3) without subsequent diagnostic confirmation, (4) lacunar infarctions, and (5) loss to follow-up at 3 months.

2.3. Blood Samples and Biomarker Assays

Biochemistry, haematology, and coagulation tests were performed in the central laboratory of the hospital. Measurements were made from blood samples obtained in the first 6 h after admission and the next 24 ± 6 h. Although the biomarker analysis was not performed simultaneously, it was supervised by the same researchers and carried out using the same standardised methods. For this study, we selected MMP-9 and cellular cFn as markers associated with thrombolytic activity [24,26], while IL-6 and TNF-α were selected as markers associated with inflammatory activity [27]. For these molecular assessments, venous blood samples were collected in vacutainer tubes (Becton Dickinson, San Jose, CA, USA) in the first 6 h after symptom onset (always after the administration of the thrombolytic bolus) and at 24 ± 6 h. After allowing the sample to clot for 60 min, the blood samples were centrifuged at 3000× g for 10 min and the serum was immediately aliquoted, frozen, and stored at −80 °C until analysis.

Serum levels of IL-6 were measured by enzyme-linked immunosorbent assay (ELISA) (BioLegend, San Diego, CA, USA) with a minimum assay sensitivity of 1.6 pg/mL and an intra- and inter-assay coefficient of variation (CV) of 5.0% and 6.8%, respectively, following the manufacturer's instructions. TNF-α was measured using an immunodiagnostic IMMULITE 1000 System (Siemens Healthcare Global, Los Angeles, CA, USA) with a minimum assay sensitivity of 1.7 pg/mL, an intra-assay CV of 3.5%, and an inter-assay CV of 6.5%. Finally, serum levels of active MMP-9 (GE Healthcare, Amersham, UK, Little Chalfont, Buckinghamshire, UK) and cFn (BioHit, Helsinki, Finland) were measured using commercial ELISA kits following the manufacturer's instructions. The intra- and inter-assay CVs were <8%. All biomarkers were evaluated within the first 3 months after blood sample collection.

2.4. Clinical Scale, Temperature and Therapeutic Management

All patients were admitted to the stroke unit and were treated under the Spanish Neurological Society protocol [29] by trained neurologists experienced in cerebrovascular diseases. The intensity of the neurological deficit was determined by the National Institute of Health Stroke Scale (NIHSS) upon admission to the Stroke Unit. Neurological improvement, defined as a reduction of ≥ 8 points in the NIHSS in the first 24 h, was used as a clinical marker of effective reperfusion [13]. Functional outcome was assessed at 3 months ± 15 days (face-to-face in 80.8% of the sample) using the modified Rankin Scale (mRS) (mRs categorised as poor outcome >2). Both scales were evaluated by internationally certified neurologists. Temperature was measured by the nursing staff every 6 h. For this analysis, the axillary temperature was measured at the time of admission and at 6 and 24 h. Patients with temperatures ≥37.5 °C were treated with paracetamol (500 mg p.o.) or metamizole (2 g i.v.) every 6 h.

2.5. Neuroimaging Studies

Cerebral CT or MRI studies were performed on and between days 4 and 7. All neuroimaging studies were supervised by the same neuroradiologist. Symptomatic HT was assessed at the time of recording the neurological worsening and, in any case, in the follow-up CT. HT was defined as symptomatic when it was associated with early neurological deterioration (worsening of at least 4 points in the NIHSS during the first 48 h after stroke onset). HT was classified according to the European Cooperative Acute Stroke Study (ECASS) III [30] criteria as follows: haemorrhagic infarction type 1 (HI1) was defined as small petechiae along the infarct margins, HI type 2 (HI2) was defined as more confluent petechiae within the infarct area but without space-occupying effect, parenchymal haemorrhage type 1 (PH1) was defined as blood clots not exceeding 30% of the infarct with some mild space-occupying effect, and PH type 2 (PH2) as blood clots exceeding 30% of the infarct area with significant space-occupying effect. The PH1 and PH2 groups were considered to have severe HT. The initial lesion volume was determined upon admission by diffusion-weighted imaging (DWI) through an automatic planimetric method. Lesion volume was determined in the follow-up CT using the ABC/2 method [31] until 2016, and then by automated planimetric method.

2.6. Endpoints

The main outcome variables were effective reperfusion (defined as a reduction of ≥8 points in the NIHSS in the first 24 h) and poor patient outcomes (mRS >2). Mild hyperthermia was defined as an axillary temperature between 36.5 °C and 37.5 °C. As secondary endpoints, we also analysed the association between effective reperfusion and serum levels of thrombolytic (MMP-9, cFN) and inflammatory (IL-6, TNF-α) biomarkers. Finally, we also determined the association between infarct volume and HT with temperature.

2.7. Statistical Analysis

In the descriptive analysis, categorical variables were expressed as frequencies and percentage and as means (standard deviation (SD)) or median and interquartile range (25th and 75th percentiles) for the continuous variables, depending on their adjustment to a normal distribution. The normality of the sample was determined by Kolmogorov–Smirnov tests with Lilliefors correction. Statistical inference was then performed with chi-square, Student's t, or Mann–Whitney tests according to the nature of the contrast variable and its adjustment to normality. Bivariate correlations were performed using Pearson's correlations for normally distributed variables.

The association of temperature (at admission and 6 and 24 h) with effective reperfusion, outcome at 3 months, HT, and serum levels of the studied biomarkers were assessed using logistic regression analysis models and the correlation between temperature and infarct volume was analysed by linear multivariate regression. Each model was adjusted for the independent variables in the bivariate analysis. The optimal cut-off points were calculated in the variables of interest using receiver operative curve (ROC) analysis. The results were expressed as adjusted odds ratios (ORs) or B with their respective 95% confidence intervals (CIs). p-Values < 0.05 were considered statistically significant in all tests. All analyses were conducted using IBM SPSS Statistics for Macintosh, version 20.0 (IBM Corp, Armonk, NY, USA).

3. Results

3.1. Sample Description

The sample is described in Table 1. This study included a total of 875 patients (mean age, 72.0 ± 12.5 years; 45.9% females) with acute IS. The mean temperatures at admission and 6 and 24 were 36.2 ± 0.6 °C, 36.6 ± 0.7 °C, and 36.5 ± 0.7 °C, respectively. Regarding the aetiology of the stroke, 43.5% were of cardioembolic origin, followed by atherothrombotic (23.5%) and lacunar (1.3%). Undetermined origin or other origins were reported in 31.7% of cases. Systemic fibrinolysis with rtPA was the reperfusion treatment of choice in 91.1% of cases, and intravenous or i.a. thrombolysis combined with thrombectomy in the remaining 8.9% of cases.

Table 1. Description of the 875 patients included in the study.

Characteristic	Total Sample ($n = 875$)
Age, years	72.0 ± 12.5
Women, %	45.9
Onset-treatment time, min	161.8 ± 61.2
Previous disability (modified Rankin Scale)	0 (0,0)
Hypertensive, %	63.8
Diabetics, %	22.9
Smokers, %	22.5
Alcohol consumption, %	10.3
Dyslipidaemia, %	39.3
Peripheral arterial disease, %	6.7
Atrial fibrillation, %	22.9
Ischemic heart disease, %	12.7
Temperature at admission, °C	36.2 ± 0.6
Temperature at 6 h, °C	36.6 ± 0.7
Temperature at 24 h, °C	36.5 ± 0.7
Blood glucose, mg/dL	138.6 ± 55.7
Glycosylated haemoglobin, %	6.2 ± 4.5
Leukocytes, $\times 10^3$/mL	8.3 ± 3.2
Fibrinogen, mg/dL	414.2 ± 103.2
Microalbuminuria, mg/24 h	5.7 ± 7.8
C-reactive protein, mg/L	5.5 ± 4.7
LDL-cholesterol, mg/dL	108.0 ± 40.7
HDL-cholesterol, mg/dL	41.7 ± 14.9
Triglycerides, mg/dL	114.2 ± 51.5
Sedimentation rate, mm	18.3 ± 20.4
NIHSS at admission	17 (12,22)
DWI volume at admission, mL	28.1 ± 43.5
Leukoaraiosis No, % Fazekas I, % Fazekas II, % Fazekas III, %	 41.7 36.5 15.0 6.9
Trial of ORG 10172 in acute stroke treatment (TOAST) Atherothrombotic, % Cardioembolic, % Lacunar, % Undetermined/others, %	 23.5 43.5 1.3 31.7
Type of reperfusion treatment Systemic fibrinolysis, % IV or IA thrombolysis + thrombectomy, %	 91.1 8.9
Effective reperfusion, %	44.0
Early neurological deterioration, %	9.9
Haemorrhagic transformation No, % IH1, % IH2, % PH1, % PH2, %	 68.0 21.4 5.3 3.0 2.4
Lesion volume at days 4–7, mL	51.1 ± 75.8
Modified Rankin Scale at 3 months	1 (0,3)
Good functional outcome at 3 months, %	69.3

LDL: low density lipoprotein; HDL: high density lipoprotein; NIHSS: National Institute of Health Stroke Scale; DWI: diffusion-weighted imaging; IH1: infarction type 1; IH2: infarction type 2; PH1: parenchymal haemorrhage type 1; PH2: parenchymal haemorrhage type 1; IV: intravenous; IA: intra arterial.

3.2. Analysis of the Association between Temperature and Effective Reperfusion

Among the studied population, 44% of the patients had effective reperfusion, while the remaining 56% did not (385 vs. 490 patients). The patients with effective reperfusion showed lower temperatures both at admission and at 24 h. Interestingly, a higher temperature at 6 h was associated with successful reperfusion (Figure 1).

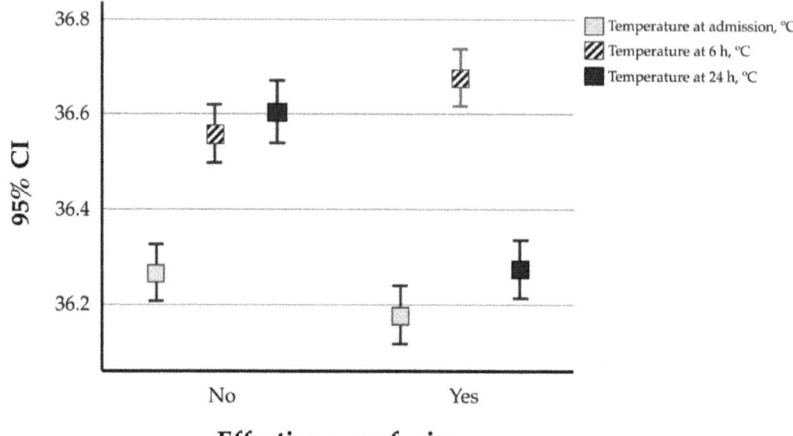

Effective reperfusion

Figure 1. Temperatures at admission and 6 h 24 h in relation to reperfusion effectiveness.

Pearson bivariate correlation analysis performed for the 3 different measurements showed a negative correlation between higher body temperature at admission ($r = -0.77$, $p = 0.022$) and at 24 h ($r = -0.266$; $p < 0.0001$) with effective reperfusion, but no association was observed for the temperature at 6 h ($r = 0.055$; $p = 0.103$). Subsequently, we performed a logistic regression analysis, adjusted for variables that showed significant differences in the bivariate analysis (age, sex, onset-treatment time, blood glucose, atrial fibrillation, NIHSS at admission, leukoaraiosis, and HT) for effective reperfusion. Logistic regression analysis showed a non-significant association between the effectiveness of reperfusion therapy and higher body temperature at 6 h (OR: 1.178; 95% CI: 0.934–1.484; $p = 0.166$). Conversely, higher body temperature at admission and 24 h was negatively associated with effective reperfusion (OR: 0.700; 95% CI: 0.552–0.887; $p = 0.003$; OR: 0.373 and 95% CI: 0.290–0.480; $p = 0.001$) (Table 2).

Table 2. Logistic regression model for temperature at three different time points associated with effective reperfusion.

	OR *	CI 95%	p
Temperature at admission	0.700	0.552–0.887	0.003
Temperature at 6 h	1.178	0.934–1.484	0.166
Temperature at 24 h	0.373	0.290–0.480	0.001

* Adjusted for age, sex, onset-treatment time, blood glucose, atrial fibrillation, National Institute of Health Stroke Scale (NIHSS) score at admission, leukoaraiosis, and haemorrhagic transformation.

3.3. Evaluation of Temperature and Functional Outcomes at 3 Months

Among the 875 patients studied, 606 (69.3%) showed good outcomes at 3 months compared to the remaining 269 (30.7%) patients. Lower temperatures at admission and 24 h were associated with better outcomes at 3 months. Conversely, a higher body temperature at 6 h was associated with good outcomes at 3 months compared to those in the poor outcome group (Figure 2).

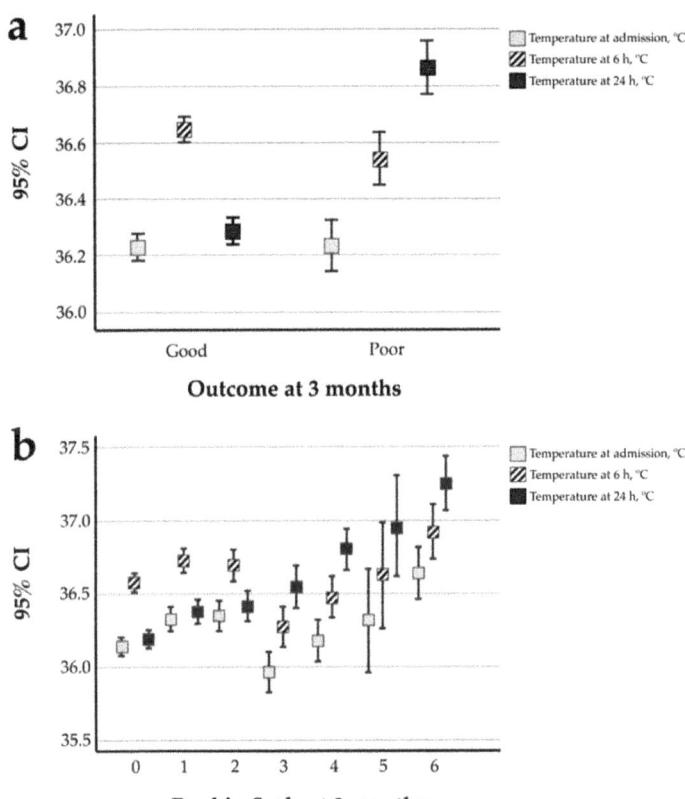

Figure 2. Evaluation of functional outcomes at 3 months. (**a**) Temperatures at admission and 6 and 24 h in relation to patient outcomes. (**b**) Temperatures at admission and 6 and 24 h in relation to modified Rankin Scale scores at 3 months.

Logistic regression models were used to evaluate poor outcome at 3 months in relation to the temperatures at the three timepoints and adjusted by the variables that showed clinical and statistical significance in the model. The analysis showed no association with basal body temperature (OR 0.817, 95% CI 0.475–1.405, p = 0.948) and temperature at 6 h (OR 0.792, 95% CI 0.465–1.350, p = 0.792). However, the temperature at 24 h was significantly associated with poor patient outcomes at 3 months (OR 2.190, 95% CI 1.264–3.793, p = 0.005) (Table 3).

Table 3. Logistic regression model for temperature at three different time points showing the relationships to poor outcomes at 3 months.

	OR *	CI 95%	p
Temperature at admission	0.817	0.475–1.405	0.465
Temperature at 6 h	0.792	0.934–1.484	0.792
Temperature at 24 h	2.190	1.264–3.793	0.005

* Adjusted for age, sex, onset-treatment time, blood glucose, atrial fibrillation, National Institute of Health Stroke Scale (NIHSS) score at admission, diffusion-weighted imaging (DWI) volume at admission, leukoaraiosis, and effective reperfusion.

3.4. Determination of Temperature-Induced Biomarkers of Thrombolytic and Inflammatory Activity and Their Associations with Effective Reperfusion

cFN and MMP-9 serum levels showed a stronger correlation with temperature at 6 h ($r = 0.701$; $p < 0.0001$; $r = 0.697$; $p < 0.0001$) compared to IL-6 and TNF-α ($r = 0.113$; $p = 0.001$; $r = 0.223$; $p < 0.0001$). Similarly, a greater association was observed between IL-6 and TNF-α levels and temperature at 24 h ($r = 0.712$; $p < 0.0001$; $r = 0.602$; $p < 0.0001$) compared to those for cFN and MMP-9 ($r = 0.195$; $p < 0.0001$; $r = 0.342$; $p < 0.0001$). Based on these findings, we performed multivariate analysis for each biomarker according to their most prominent correlation in relation to effective reperfusion. The analysis showed that MMP-9 levels at 6 h and IL-6 at 24 h were independently associated with the effectiveness of the reperfusion therapy (OR: 1.004; 95% CI: 1.002–1.006; $p < 0.0001$ and OR: 0.979; 95% CI: 0.967–0.992; $p = 0.001$). Table 4 shows the measured levels of all the studied biomarkers.

Table 4. Levers of biomarkers analysed at 6 and 24 h.

	N	Minimum	Maximum	Mean ± Standard Deviation
MMP-9 (6 h; ng/mL)	799	3.6	430.1	103.81 ± 79.16
Cellular fibronectin (6 h; ng/mL)	804	4.1	35.9	8.55 ± 4.55
TNF-α (Basal; ng/mL)	831	1.8	45.8	16.84 ± 6.65
IL-6 (Basal; ng/mL)	841	1.1	58.6	11.17 ± 10.00
MMP-9 (24 h; ng/mL)	653	3.6	339.1	87.66 ± 60.55
Cellular fibronectin (24 h; ng/mL)	662	1.7	18.3	7.11 ± 2.260
TNF-α (24 h; ng/mL)	669	7.3	65.8	27.98 ± 9.16
IL-6 (24 h; ng/mL)	666	8.4	83.6	32.45 ± 13.88

MMP-9: matrix metalloproteinase 9; TNF-α: tumour necrosis factor-alpha; IL-6: interleukin 6.

Simultaneous analysis of these two values in the logistic regression model revealed a positive association for MMP-9 levels at 6 h with effective reperfusion (OR: 1.008; 95% CI: 1.005–1.010; $p < 0.0001$). In contrast, IL-6 at 24 h was an independent factor strongly associated with reperfusion failure (OR: 0.958; 95% CI: 0.942–0.973; $p < 0.0001$) (Table 5).

Table 5. Logistic regression model for the levels of biomarkers related to effective reperfusion.

	OR *	95%CI	p
MMP-9 levels at 6 h (ng/mL)	1.008	1.005–1.010	<0.0001
IL-6 levels at 24 h (pg/mL)	0.958	0.942–0.973	<0.0001

* Adjusted for age, sex, onset-treatment time, blood glucose, atrial fibrillation, National Institute of Health Stroke Scale (NIHSS) score at admission, and leukoaraiosis. MMP-9: matrix metalloproteinase 9; IL-6: interleukin 6.

3.5. Association of Temperature with HT and Infarct Volume

In this study, 68% ($n = 595$) of patients did not have HT. Among the patients who developed HT, IH1 was the most common subtype ($n = 187$, 21.4%), followed by IH2 ($n = 46$, 5.3%), PH1 ($n = 26$, 3.0%), and PH2 ($n = 21$, 2.4%). In all groups, temperature was directly related to haemorrhagic transformation and higher temperatures were observed in the most severe cases. Patients with no HT or IH showed an increase in temperature from admission to 6 h that then declined at 24 h, while PH patients showed an increase in temperature over time. The multivariate analysis showed an association between PH and temperature (OR: 3.468; 95% CI: 1.368–8.792, $p = 0.009$), at 6 h (OR: 3.231; 95% CI: 1.254–8.326; $p = 0.015$) and at 24 h (OR: 4.588; 95% CI: 1.726–12.199, $p = 0.002$).

Regarding infarct size, the mean infarct volume at days 4–7 was 51.1 ± 75.8 mL. We observed no correlation between infarct volume and temperature at 6 h ($r = 0.066$; $p = 0.066$), although a significant correlation was observed at admission ($r = 0.110$; $p = 0.001$) and at 24 h ($r = 0.302$; $p < 0.0001$). Multivariate analysis showed no association between infarct volume and temperature at admission (B: 6.956; 95% CI: 0.620–14.531; $p = 0.072$) or at 6 h (B: 6.765; 95% CI: 0.725–14.253; $p = 0.077$). However, patients with higher temperatures at 24 h were over 20 times more likely to present greater infarct volumes between days 4 and 7 (B: 23.369; 95% CI: 16.308–30.430; $p < 0.0001$).

4. Discussion

Consistent with the findings of our previous study [2], higher body temperature at 24 h in the present study was negatively associated with effective reperfusion. This effect was also reflected by increased infarct volumes and poor outcome at 3 months in patients treated with rtPA. Higher body temperature at admission was also negatively associated with effective reperfusion but did not impair functional outcome at 3 months. Contrary to the observations at 24 h, our analysis showed that temperature at 6 h in rtPA patients was not associated with poor outcome or infarct volume. Higher body temperature at 6 h was positively associated with effective reperfusion, although this association disappeared after adjusting for confounding factors in the logistic regression analysis.

Although the positive association observed between mild temperature at 6 h and effective reperfusion was weak, previous studies support the beneficial effect of mild hyperthermia in rtPA-treated patients [16,32–35]. Indeed, the results of in vitro studies on rtPA activity are consistent with this rationale and demonstrated a direct relationship between high body temperature and clot lysis effectiveness [20]. In this regard, in the Paracetamol (Acetaminophen) In Stroke (PAIS) trial aimed to assess whether early treatment (12–24 h) with paracetamol improved functional outcome in patients with acute stroke by reducing body temperature and preventing fever, reporting that this analgesic compound did not improve functional outcomes [32]. A second sub-analysis, derived from the same PAIS trial and designed to evaluate the influence of baseline body temperature on the effect of rtPA (alteplase) and functional outcome in patients with acute IS, found that high body temperature might have a larger benefit for treatment with alteplase than that in patients with lower body temperature [33]. In brief, during the initial 6 h window after cerebral infarction when rtPA treatment was provided, the results of our analysis suggested that the effect of high body temperature on clot lysis was more relevant in terms of functional prognosis than the use of neuroprotective strategies related to hypothermia. Therefore, efforts are required to develop novel approaches to improve thrombolytic therapy [36].

Analysis of thrombolytic biomarkers showed that MMP-9 levels at 6 h were directly correlated with temperature and with the effectiveness of reperfusion therapy, which could be explained by the increase in rtPA activity, although with an increased risk of developing HT, as was observed in the analysis. These findings suggest that the threshold of the beneficial effect of body temperature is very narrow. Indeed, the beneficial effect of body temperature at 6 h was observed at an average temperature of $36.6 \pm 0.7\ °C$.

As an inflammatory biomarker, IL-6 levels at 24 h were correlated with higher body temperature and negatively associated with effective reperfusion. High serum levels of inflammatory markers in the first 24 h were previously linked with early clinical deterioration and worsened outcome in acute IS [37–39]. These findings are further supported by our recent publication, in which IL-6 levels at 24 h were associated with worsened clinical outcomes in IS patients who underwent recanalisation therapy, regardless of the reperfusion effectiveness [40]. Therefore, delayed (24 h) episodes of fever or high temperature may amplify the ischaemic lesion mediated by an inflammatory response, overcoming the benefit of rtPA treatment.

Based on these clinical findings, exhaustive monitoring of mild hyperthermia in clearly defined ranges during rtPA administration (in the first 6 h) could have a beneficial effect on reperfusion therapies when combined with hypothermia strategies in later stages of the acute phase (i.e., at 24 h).

The present study has some limitations. This single-centre study was conducted on a retrospectively enrolled patient registry. Transcranial Doppler used to determine the reperfusion rate could only be performed in 18% of the treated patients. Therefore, an 8-point or more improvement in NIHSS in the first 24 h was chosen as the endpoint as it was sensitive to the effects of early reperfusion, consistent with the results of other analyses [41,42], although the use of this clinical criterion to define effective reperfusion may lead to a bias in the classification of therapeutic response groups. The lack of imaging analysis to correlate the location of occlusions with the reperfusion effectiveness is also a critical issue that could interfere with our analysis, as patients with distal occlusions usually have higher reperfusion rates, small infarct sizes, and possibly low temperatures on admission (low inflammatory response). To overcome this critical limitation, in this study, we defined effective reperfusion as a reduction of ≥ 8 points in the NIHSS in the first 24 h, which normally involves patients with more proximal occlusions. Finally, as none of the patients included in this study reached hyperthermic values, we cannot rule out the possibility that temperatures higher than 37.5 °C at 6 h could further promote effective reperfusion, although our data seems to predict such an effect.

In conclusion, the results of our analysis support the theory that mild hyperthermia could benefit reperfusion therapies by promoting clot lysis during the first 6 h of ischaemic stroke but worsen the outcome at later stages. Thrombolytic activity at 6 h seems to be related to temperature and may improve reperfusion therapies, warranting future studies to further elucidate the therapeutic potential of controlled mild hyperthermia in combination with rtPA administration.

Author Contributions: Conceptualization, P.Á.-G., J.C. and F.C.; Data curation, P.H., J.C. and T.S.; Formal analysis, P.Á.-G. and J.C.; Funding acquisition, J.C., T.S. and R.I.-R.; Investigation, M.R.-Y., I.L.-D. and J.M.P.; Methodology, M.R.-Y., J.M.P. and J.C.; Project administration, J.C., R.I.-R. and F.C.; Resources, A.D.S.-C., M.P.-M. and I.L.-D.; Software, A.D.S.-C., M.P.-M., I.L.-D. and F.C.; Supervision, J.C., T.S. and R.I.-R.; Validation, P.H., A.D.-C. and M.P.-M.; Visualization, P.Á.-G. and P.H.; Writing—original draft, P.Á.-G. and P.H.; Writing—review & editing, J.C., T.S., R.I.-R. and F.C. All authors have read and agreed to the published version of the manuscript.

Funding: This study was partially supported by grants from the Spanish Ministry of Science and Innovation (SAF2017-84267-R), Xunta de Galicia (Consellería Educación: IN607A2018/3), Instituto de Salud Carlos III (ISCIII) (PI17/00540 and PI17/01103), Spanish Research Network on Cerebrovascular Diseases RETICS-INVICTUS PLUS (RD16/0019), and by the European Union FEDER program. Furthermore, Tomás. Sobrino (CPII17/00027) and Francisco Campos (CPII19/00020) are recipients of research contracts from the Miguel Servet Program of Instituto de Salud Carlos III. María Pérez-Mato is a Sara Borrell Researcher (CD19/00033). The sponsors did not participate in the study design, collection, analysis, or interpretation of the data, writing the report, or in the decision to submit the paper for publication.

Conflicts of Interest: The authors declare no conflicts of interest.

References

1. Castillo, J.; Davalos, A.; Marrugat, J.; Noya, M. Timing for fever-related brain damage in acute ischemic stroke. *Stroke* **1998**, *29*, 2455–2460. [CrossRef] [PubMed]
2. Millan, M.; Grau, L.; Castellanos, M.; Rodriguez-Yanez, M.; Arenillas, J.F.; Nombela, F.; Perez de la Ossa, N.; Lopez-Manzanares, L.; Serena, J.; Castillo, J.; et al. Body temperature and response to thrombolytic therapy in acute ischaemic stroke. *Eur. J. Neurol.* **2008**, *15*, 1384–1389. [CrossRef] [PubMed]
3. Saini, M.; Saqqur, M.; Kamruzzaman, A.; Lees, K.R.; Shuaib, A.; Investigators, V. Effect of hyperthermia on prognosis after acute ischemic stroke. *Stroke* **2009**, *40*, 3051–3059. [CrossRef] [PubMed]
4. Blanco, M.; Campos, F.; Rodriguez-Yanez, M.; Arias, S.; Fernandez-Ferro, J.; Gomez-Sanchez, J.C.; Castillo, J. Neuroprotection or increased brain damage mediated by temperature in stroke is time dependent. *PLoS ONE* **2012**, *7*, e30320. [CrossRef]
5. Dehkharghani, S.; Bowen, M.; Haussen, D.C.; Gleason, T.; Prater, A.; Cai, Q.; Kang, J.; Nogueira, R.G. Body Temperature Modulates Infarction Growth following Endovascular Reperfusion. *AJNR Am. J. Neuroradiol.* **2017**, *38*, 46–51. [CrossRef]
6. Forlivesi, S.; Micheletti, N.; Tomelleri, G.; Bovi, P.; Cappellari, M. Association of hyperglycemia, systolic and diastolic hypertension, and hyperthermia relative to baseline in the acute phase of stroke with poor outcome after intravenous thrombolysis. *Blood Coagul. Fibrinolysis* **2018**, *29*, 167–171. [CrossRef]
7. Greer, D.M.; Funk, S.E.; Reaven, N.L.; Ouzounelli, M.; Uman, G.C. Impact of fever on outcome in patients with stroke and neurologic injury: A comprehensive meta-analysis. *Stroke* **2008**, *39*, 3029–3035. [CrossRef]
8. De Jonge, J.C.; Wallet, J.; van der Worp, H.B. Fever worsens outcomes in animal models of ischaemic stroke: A systematic review and meta-analysis. *Eur. Stroke J.* **2019**, *4*, 29–38. [CrossRef]

9. Wang, H.; Wang, B.; Normoyle, K.P.; Jackson, K.; Spitler, K.; Sharrock, M.F.; Miller, C.M.; Best, C.; Llano, D.; Du, R. Brain temperature and its fundamental properties: A review for clinical neuroscientists. *Front. Neurosci.* **2014**, *8*, 307. [CrossRef]
10. Basto, F.M.; Lyden, P. Hypothermia in acute ischemic stroke therapy. *Handb. Clin. Neurol.* **2018**, *157*, 823–837. [CrossRef]
11. Van der Worp, H.B.; Macleod, M.R.; Bath, P.M.; Demotes, J.; Durand-Zaleski, I.; Gebhardt, B.; Gluud, C.; Kollmar, R.; Krieger, D.W.; Lees, K.R.; et al. EuroHYP-1: European multicenter, randomized, phase III clinical trial of therapeutic hypothermia plus best medical treatment vs. best medical treatment alone for acute ischemic stroke. *Int. J. Stroke* **2014**, *9*, 642–645. [CrossRef] [PubMed]
12. Vieites-Prado, A.; Iglesias-Rey, R.; Fernandez-Susavila, H.; da Silva-Candal, A.; Rodriguez-Castro, E.; Grohn, O.H.; Wellmann, S.; Sobrino, T.; Castillo, J.; Campos, F. Protective Effects and Magnetic Resonance Imaging Temperature Mapping of Systemic and Focal Hypothermia in Cerebral Ischemia. *Stroke* **2016**, *47*, 2386–2396. [CrossRef]
13. Iglesias-Rey, R.; Rodriguez-Yanez, M.; Rodriguez-Castro, E.; Pumar, J.M.; Arias, S.; Santamaria, M.; Lopez-Dequidt, I.; Hervella, P.; Correa-Paz, C.; Sobrino, T.; et al. Worse Outcome in Stroke Patients Treated with rt-PA Without Early Reperfusion: Associated Factors. *Transl. Stroke Res.* **2018**, *9*, 347–355. [CrossRef] [PubMed]
14. Xiong, Y.; Manwani, B.; Fisher, M. Management of Acute Ischemic Stroke. *Am. J. Med.* **2019**, *132*, 286–291. [CrossRef] [PubMed]
15. Kim, J.S. tPA Helpers in the Treatment of Acute Ischemic Stroke: Are They Ready for Clinical Use? *J. Stroke* **2019**, *21*, 160–174. [CrossRef]
16. Naess, H.; Idicula, T.; Lagallo, N.; Brogger, J.; Waje-Andreassen, U.; Thomassen, L. Inverse relationship of baseline body temperature and outcome between ischemic stroke patients treated and not treated with thrombolysis: The Bergen stroke study. *Acta Neurol. Scand.* **2010**, *122*, 414–417. [CrossRef] [PubMed]
17. Wrotek, S.E.; Kozak, W.E.; Hess, D.C.; Fagan, S.C. Treatment of fever after stroke: Conflicting evidence. *Pharmacotherapy* **2011**, *31*, 1085–1091. [CrossRef]
18. Khanevski, A.N.; Naess, H.; Thomassen, L.; Waje-Andreassen, U.; Nacu, A.; Kvistad, C.E. Elevated body temperature in ischemic stroke associated with neurological improvement. *Acta Neurol. Scand.* **2017**, *136*, 414–418. [CrossRef]
19. Mumme, A.; Kemen, M.; Homann, H.H.; Zumtobel, V. The temperature dependence of fibrinolysis with streptokinase. *Dtsch. Med. Wochenschr.* **1993**, *118*, 1594–1596. [CrossRef]
20. Yenari, M.A.; Palmer, J.T.; Bracci, P.M.; Steinberg, G.K. Thrombolysis with tissue plasminogen activator (tPA) is temperature dependent. *Thromb. Res.* **1995**, *77*, 475–481. [CrossRef]
21. Tsetis, D.K.; Katsamouris, A.N.; Giannoukas, A.D.; Hatzidakis, A.A.; Kostas, T.; Chamalakis, K.; Ioannou, C.; Gourtsoyiannis, N.C. Potential benefits from heating the high-dose rtPA boluses used in catheter-directed thrombolysis for acute/subacute lower limb ischemia. *J. Endovasc. Ther.* **2003**, *10*, 739–744. [CrossRef]
22. Mizuma, A.; Yenari, M.A. Anti-Inflammatory Targets for the Treatment of Reperfusion Injury in Stroke. *Front. Neurol.* **2017**, *8*, 467. [CrossRef] [PubMed]
23. Tsuji, K.; Aoki, T.; Tejima, E.; Arai, K.; Lee, S.R.; Atochin, D.N.; Huang, P.L.; Wang, X.; Montaner, J.; Lo, E.H. Tissue plasminogen activator promotes matrix metalloproteinase-9 upregulation after focal cerebral ischemia. *Stroke* **2005**, *36*, 1954–1959. [CrossRef] [PubMed]
24. Castellanos, M.; Leira, R.; Serena, J.; Pumar, J.M.; Lizasoain, I.; Castillo, J.; Davalos, A. Plasma metalloproteinase-9 concentration predicts hemorrhagic transformation in acute ischemic stroke. *Stroke* **2003**, *34*, 40–46. [CrossRef] [PubMed]
25. Meng, Q.; He, C.; Shuaib, A.; Wang, C.X. Hyperthermia worsens ischaemic brain injury through destruction of microvessels in an embolic model in rats. *Int. J. Hyperth.* **2012**, *28*, 24–32. [CrossRef] [PubMed]
26. Castellanos, M.; Leira, R.; Serena, J.; Blanco, M.; Pedraza, S.; Castillo, J.; Davalos, A. Plasma cellular-fibronectin concentration predicts hemorrhagic transformation after thrombolytic therapy in acute ischemic stroke. *Stroke* **2004**, *35*, 1671–1676. [CrossRef]
27. Leira, R.; Rodriguez-Yanez, M.; Castellanos, M.; Blanco, M.; Nombela, F.; Sobrino, T.; Lizasoain, I.; Davalos, A.; Castillo, J. Hyperthermia is a surrogate marker of inflammation-mediated cause of brain damage in acute ischaemic stroke. *J. Intern. Med.* **2006**, *260*, 343–349. [CrossRef]

28. Rodriguez, J.A.; Sobrino, T.; Orbe, J.; Purroy, A.; Martinez-Vila, E.; Castillo, J.; Paramo, J.A. proMetalloproteinase-10 is associated with brain damage and clinical outcome in acute ischemic stroke. *J. Thromb. Haemost.* **2013**, *11*, 1464–1473. [CrossRef]
29. Alonso de Lecinana, M.; Egido, J.A.; Casado, I.; Ribo, M.; Davalos, A.; Masjuan, J.; Caniego, J.L.; Martinez Vila, E.; Diez Tejedor, E.; ad hoc Committee of the SEN Study Group for Cerebrovascular Diseases; et al. Guidelines for the treatment of acute ischaemic stroke. *Neurologia* **2014**, *29*, 102–122. [CrossRef]
30. Hacke, W.; Kaste, M.; Bluhmki, E.; Brozman, M.; Davalos, A.; Guidetti, D.; Larrue, V.; Lees, K.R.; Medeghri, Z.; Machnig, T.; et al. Thrombolysis with alteplase 3 to 4.5 h after acute ischemic stroke. *N. Engl. J. Med.* **2008**, *359*, 1317–1329. [CrossRef]
31. Sims, J.R.; Gharai, L.R.; Schaefer, P.W.; Vangel, M.; Rosenthal, E.S.; Lev, M.H.; Schwamm, L.H. ABC/2 for rapid clinical estimate of infarct, perfusion, and mismatch volumes. *Neurology* **2009**, *72*, 2104–2110. [CrossRef] [PubMed]
32. Den Hertog, H.M.; van der Worp, H.B.; van Gemert, H.M.; Algra, A.; Kappelle, L.J.; van Gijn, J.; Koudstaal, P.J.; Dippel, D.W.; Investigators, P. The Paracetamol (Acetaminophen) In Stroke (PAIS) trial: A multicentre, randomised, placebo-controlled, phase III trial. *Lancet. Neurol.* **2009**, *8*, 434–440. [CrossRef]
33. De Ridder, I.; den Hertog, H.; van Gemert, M.; Dippel, D.; van der Worp, B.; PAIS investigators. Increased benefit of alteplase in patients with ischemic stroke and a high body temperature. *Cerebrovasc. Dis.* **2013**, *35*, 60–63. [CrossRef] [PubMed]
34. Kim, S.H.; Saver, J.L. Initial body temperature in ischemic stroke: Nonpotentiation of tissue-type plasminogen activator benefit and inverse association with severity. *Stroke* **2015**, *46*, 132–136. [CrossRef] [PubMed]
35. Meunier, J.M.; Chang, W.T.; Bluett, B.; Wenker, E.; Lindsell, C.J.; Shaw, G.J. Temperature affects thrombolytic efficacy using rt-PA and eptifibatide, an in vitro study. *Ther. Hypothermia Temp. Manag.* **2012**, *2*, 112–118. [CrossRef]
36. Bonnard, T.; Gauberti, M.; Martinez de Lizarrondo, S.; Campos, F.; Vivien, D. Recent Advances in Nanomedicine for Ischemic and Hemorrhagic Stroke. *Stroke* **2019**, *50*, 1318–1324. [CrossRef]
37. Vila, N.; Castillo, J.; Davalos, A.; Chamorro, A. Proinflammatory cytokines and early neurological worsening in ischemic stroke. *Stroke* **2000**, *31*, 2325–2329. [CrossRef]
38. Bustamante, A.; Sobrino, T.; Giralt, D.; Garcia-Berrocoso, T.; Llombart, V.; Ugarriza, I.; Espadaler, M.; Rodriguez, N.; Sudlow, C.; Castellanos, M.; et al. Prognostic value of blood interleukin-6 in the prediction of functional outcome after stroke: A systematic review and meta-analysis. *J. Neuroimmunol.* **2014**, *274*, 215–224. [CrossRef]
39. Vila, N.; Castillo, J.; Davalos, A.; Esteve, A.; Planas, A.M.; Chamorro, A. Levels of anti-inflammatory cytokines and neurological worsening in acute ischemic stroke. *Stroke* **2003**, *34*, 671–675. [CrossRef]
40. Hervella, P.; Rodriguez-Castro, E.; Rodriguez-Yanez, M.; Arias, S.; Santamaria-Cadavid, M.; Lopez-Dequidt, I.; Estany-Gestal, A.; Maqueda, E.; Lopez-Loureiro, I.; Sobrino, T.; et al. Intra- and extra-hospital improvement in ischemic stroke patients: Influence of reperfusion therapy and molecular mechanisms. *Sci. Rep.* **2020**, *10*, 3513. [CrossRef]
41. Kharitonova, T.; Mikulik, R.O.; Roine, R.; Soinne, L.; Ahmed, N.; Wahlgren, N. Safe Implementation of Thrombolysis in Stroke Investigators.Association of Early National Institutes of Health Stroke Scale Improvement With Vessel Recanalization and Functional Outcome After Intravenous Thrombolysis in Ischemic Stroke. *Stroke* **2011**, *42*, 1638. [CrossRef] [PubMed]
42. Lansberg, G.M.; Christensen, S.; Kemp, S.; Mlynash, M.; Mishra, N.; Federau, C.; Tsai, P.J.; Kim, S.; Nogueria, G.R.; Jovin, T.; et al. Computed Tomographic Perfusion to Predict Response to Recanalization in Ischemic Stroke. *Ann. Neurol.* **2017**, *81*, 849. [CrossRef] [PubMed]

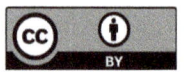

© 2020 by the authors. Licensee MDPI, Basel, Switzerland. This article is an open access article distributed under the terms and conditions of the Creative Commons Attribution (CC BY) license (http://creativecommons.org/licenses/by/4.0/).

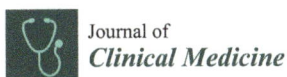

Article

Acute Kidney Injury after Endovascular Treatment in Patients with Acute Ischemic Stroke

Joonsang Yoo [1,2], Jeong-Ho Hong [1], Seong-Joon Lee [3], Yong-Won Kim [4], Ji Man Hong [3], Chang-Hyun Kim [5], Jin Wook Choi [6], Dong-Hun Kang [7], Yong-Sun Kim [8], Yang-Ha Hwang [4], Jin Soo Lee [3] and Sung-Il Sohn [1,*]

1. Department of Neurology, Keimyung University School of Medicine, Daegu 42601, Korea; quarksea@gmail.com (J.Y.); neurohong79@gmail.com (J.-H.H.)
2. Department of Neurology, National Health Insurance Service Ilsan Hospital, Goyang 10444, Korea
3. Department of Neurology, Ajou University School of Medicine, Suwon 16500, Korea; editisan@hanmail.net (S.-J.L.); dacda@hanmail.net (J.M.H.); jinsoo22@gmail.com (J.S.L.)
4. Department of Neurology, School of Medicine, Kyungpook National University, Daegu 41944, Korea; yw.kim23@gmail.com (Y.-W.K.); yangha.hwang@gmail.com (Y.-H.H.)
5. Department of Neurosurgery, Keimyung University School of Medicine, Daegu 42601, Korea; ppori2k@naver.com
6. Department of Radiology, Ajou University School of Medicine, Suwon 16500, Korea; radjwchoi@gmail.com
7. Department of Neurosurgery, School of Medicine, Kyungpook National University, Daegu 41944, Korea; kdhdock@hotmail.com
8. Department of Radiology, School of Medicine, Kyungpook National University, Daegu 41944, Korea; yongkim@knu.ac.kr
* Correspondence: sungil.sohn@gmail.com; Tel.: +82-53-258-7833; Fax: +82-53-258-4380

Received: 10 April 2020; Accepted: 11 May 2020; Published: 14 May 2020

Abstract: Acute kidney injury (AKI) is often associated with the use of contrast agents. We evaluated the frequency of AKI, factors associated with AKI after endovascular treatment (EVT), and associations with AKI and clinical outcomes. We retrospectively analyzed consecutively enrolled patients with acute ischemic stroke who underwent EVT at three stroke centers in Korea. We compared the characteristics of patients with and without AKI and independent factors associated with AKI after EVT. We also investigated the effects of AKI on functional outcomes and mortality at 3 months. Of the 601 patients analyzed, 59 patients (9.8%) developed AKI and five patients (0.8%) started renal replacement therapy after EVT. In the multivariate analysis, diabetes mellitus (odds ratio (OR), 2.341; 95% CI, 1.283–4.269; $p = 0.005$), the contrast agent dose (OR, 1.107 per 10 mL; 95% CI, 1.032–1.187; $p = 0.004$), and unsuccessful reperfusion (OR, 1.909; 95% CI, 1.019–3.520; $p = 0.040$) were independently associated with AKI. The presence of AKI was associated with a poor functional outcome (OR, 5.145; 95% CI, 2.177–13.850; $p < 0.001$) and mortality (OR, 8.164; 95% CI, 4.046–16.709; $p < 0.001$) at 3 months. AKI may also affect the outcomes of ischemic stroke patients undergoing EVT. When implementing EVT, practitioners should be aware of these risk factors.

Keywords: ischemic stroke; acute kidney injury; contrast media; endovascular treatment; outcome

1. Introduction

Acute kidney injury (AKI) is an acute worsening of renal function often associated with the use of contrast agents [1,2]. Although the understanding of contrast-associated AKI (CA-AKI) has improved, CA-AKI remains an important issue in procedures using contrast agents such as computed tomography angiography (CTA), computed tomography perfusion (CTP), and endovascular treatment (EVT). The risk of AKI is also increased by acute ischemic stroke itself [3]. AKI is not uncommon and may lead to poorer outcomes in ischemic stroke patients [4–6].

Recently, EVT has been established as a treatment for acute ischemic stroke [7–9]. Several studies of AKI in acute ischemic stroke patients have been performed, but research is still lacking on AKI in stroke patients who have undergone EVT. Prior to the popularity of EVT, there were pioneering AKI studies of patients who underwent EVT, but it was difficult to determine the characteristics of the AKI patients or the risk factors associated with AKI because of the relatively small number of included patients [10,11]. There has been recent research on the effect of baseline renal impairment on CA-AKI, but little is known about the factors associated with CA-AKI [12]. Therefore, in this study, we investigated the incidence of AKI, the risk factors associated with AKI after EVT, and the effect of AKI on the outcomes of ischemic stroke patients who underwent EVT.

2. Materials and Methods

2.1. Study Participants

This study is a retrospective analysis of data from the Acute Stroke due to Intracranial Atherosclerotic occlusion and Neurointervention Korean Retrospective (ASIAN KR) registry. Details of the registry have been previously published [13,14]. Briefly, data in the registry were collected from the patients of three university stroke centers in Korea from January 2011 to February 2016. During the study period, acute stroke patients who underwent EVT were consecutively enrolled. In this study, we included patients with an onset-to-puncture time of ≤24 h. All patient data were anonymized, and each patient was assigned an identification number. The data collection protocol was approved by the institutional review board of each hospital.

2.2. Clinical Assessment and EVT Process

Imaging and clinical analyses were performed in a core lab after the de-identification process. The initial stroke severity and serum creatinine level were assessed at the time of arrival, before images were taken. Follow-up serum creatinine results were collected from the next day to 7 days after the baseline images. Stroke severity was evaluated using the National Institutes of Health Stroke Scale (NIHSS) score. Renal function was assessed using the estimated glomerular filtration rate (eGFR) with the Modification of Diet in Renal Disease formula. Baseline renal function was classified into four groups by eGFR values of 90 mL/min/1.73 m^2 or above (Stage I), 60 to 89 mL/min/1.73 m^2 (Stage II), 30 to 59 mL/min/1.73 m^2 (Stage III), and under 30 mL/min/1.73 m^2 (Stage IV and V). The number of patients with Stage V CKD was only three; therefore, they were classified together with Stage IV CKD. AKI was evaluated using the Kidney Disease Improving Global Outcomes criteria [15,16]. Patients were considered to have AKI if they had an increment in serum creatinine of 0.3 mg/dL within 48 h or an increment in serum creatinine 1.5 times that recorded at baseline within 7 days. An increment in serum creatinine 2.0–2.9 times that recorded at baseline within 7 days indicated AKI Stage 2. An increment in serum creatinine three or more times that recorded at baseline, an increase in serum creatinine to 4.0 mg/dL or more, or the initiation of renal replacement therapy indicated AKI Stage 3. We also investigated whether CTA was performed before EVT. The device used for the EVT procedure was chosen by the treating physician. A direct aspiration device or a stent retriever was recommended as a primary reperfusion device. Balloon guide catheters, intracranial or extracranial angioplasty, and/or stenting were implemented as needed. Either Visipaque (Iodixanol, GE healthcare, Marlborough, MA, USA) or Pamiray (Iopamidol, Dongkook Pharm., Seoul, Korea) was used as the contrast medium during the EVT procedure. The contrast dose was based on the prescribed records. However, it was recalculated based on cerebral angiography imaging and procedure because a large amount of the contrast was discarded during the procedure. First, the usual dose of contrast medium used in each hospital was checked according to the artery and procedure. The total amount of contrast agent administrated to the patients was retrospectively calculated by assigning each image series and routine procedural dose. Reperfusion status was evaluated using the modified thrombolysis in cerebral infarction (mTICI) grade on the final angiogram [17]. Successful reperfusion was defined as an mTICI grade of 2b or 3. Time intervals, including onset-to-door time, door-to-puncture time, and total procedure time, were assessed. The procedure time was defined as the time from puncture to the final angiogram. Hemorrhagic transformation was evaluated using follow-up computed tomography or magnetic resonance imaging. Intracerebral hemorrhages were classified in accordance with the European Cooperative Acute Stroke Study criteria [18]. Functional status was assessed using the modified Rankin scale (mRS) score. A poor clinical outcome was defined as an mRS of 3 or more at 3 months. If a patient's preclinical mRS was 3 or more and the 3-month mRS did not worsen, the patient was not classified as having a poor clinical outcome. We also identified mortality at 3 months.

2.3. Statistical Analyses

Data are expressed as means ± standard deviations, medians (interquartile ranges (IQR)), or numbers (percentages), as statistically appropriate. We compared the imaging and clinical variables between the groups with and without AKI using chi-squared tests, independent Student's t-tests, or Wilcoxon rank-sum tests, respectively. To identify the factors associated with AKI, we performed multivariate analysis after adjusting for age, sex, the initial stroke severity, baseline renal function, the performance of CTA before EVT, and factors with $p < 0.1$ in the univariate analysis. We also assessed the factors associated with a poor clinical outcome and mortality at 3 months. To investigate these associations, we performed a multivariate analysis after adjusting for the presence or stage of AKI, age, sex, the initial NIHSS score, baseline renal function, and factors with p-value < 0.1 in the univariate analysis. All p-values were two-tailed, and variables were considered significant at p-value < 0.05. All statistical analyses were performed using R version 3.6.2 (http://www.R-project.org).

3. Results

During the study period, a total of 720 patients were enrolled in the ASIAN KR registry. After excluding 21 patients because they had undergone EVT more than 24 h after onset, because of early mortality due to malignant brain edema, or because of hemodialysis before admission, 699 patients were eligible for this study. Of these, 98 patients lacked baseline or follow-up renal function tests. Finally, 601 patients (86.0%) were included in our analysis (Figure 1). The mean age of the included patients was 68.0 ± 12.2 years, and 333 patients (55.4%) were men. CTA before EVT was performed in 510 patients (84.9%), and the mean dose for CTA was 82.6 ± 7.6 mL. The mean dose of the contrast agent was 71.2 ± 37.2 mL, and 452 of the included patients (75.2%) had successful reperfusion. Patients with successful reperfusion used smaller amounts of the contrast agent than those with unsuccessful reperfusion (68.5 ± 36.0 vs. 79.1 ± 39.5 mL, $p = 0.004$). Most of the excluded patients (95 patients, 96.9%) were excluded due to missing follow-up creatinine levels. The excluded patients tended to be younger than the included patients (68.0 ± 12.2 years vs. 63.8 ± 12.6 years, $p = 0.003$) and had better baseline renal function (eGFR: 64.6 ± 26.1 vs. 72.4 ± 24.6 mL/min/1.73 m^2, $p = 0.005$) and less severe stroke (initial NIHSS: 17 (13–21) vs. 14 (9–18), $p < 0.001$). None of the excluded patients required renal replacement therapy during their hospital stay. The excluded patients also showed better clinical outcomes at 3 months (mRS 3 (1–5) vs. 1 (0–2), $p < 0.001$) (Table S1).

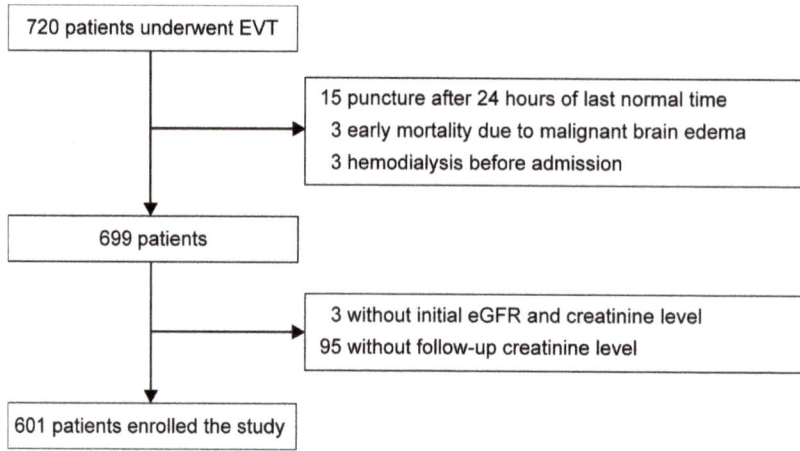

Figure 1. Patients enrollment. EVT, endovascular treatment; eGFR, estimated glomerular filtration rate.

3.1. Factors Associated with Acute Kidney Injury

Among the 601 included patients, 59 (9.8%) developed AKI within 7 days of EVT. Of these, 22 (3.7%) were classified with AKI Stage 1, 14 (2.3%) were classified with AKI Stage 2, and 23 (3.8%) were classified with AKI Stage 3. Of the patients with AKI, renal replacement therapy was initiated in five patients (0.8%). The age and sex were similar between patients with and without AKI (Table 1). The amount of contrast medium used was higher in patients with AKI (69.1 ± 36.0 vs. 89.8 ± 42.9 mL, $p = 0.001$). In the multivariate analysis, diabetes mellitus (odds ratio, 2.341; 95% CI, 1.283–4.269; $p = 0.005$), contrast dose (odds ratio, 1.107 per 10 mL; 95% CI, 1.032–1.187; $p = 0.004$), and unsuccessful reperfusion (odds ratio, 1.909; 95% CI, 1.019–3.520; $p = 0.040$) were independently associated with the presence of AKI (Table 2). The performance of CTA before EVT was associated with an increased AKI risk, but the increase was not statistically significant (odds ratio, 2.112; 95% CI, 0.786–7.406; $p = 0.181$).

3.2. Factors Associated with Functional Outcome and Mortality at 3 Months

Follow-up was conducted at 3 months for all patients to determine functional outcome and mortality. There were 330 patients (54.9%) who showed poor functional outcomes at 3 months. Of the 59 patients with AKI, 52 (88.1%) showed poor outcomes, and only seven (11.9%) showed good outcomes ($p < 0.001$) (Table S2). In the multivariate analysis, the presence of AKI was independently associated with a poor outcome (odds ratio, 5.145; 95% CI, 2.177–13.850; $p < 0.001$) (Table 3, Model 1). AKI Stage 2 (odds ratio, 13.709; 95% CI, 2.108–280.187; $p = 0.022$) and Stage 3 (odds ratio, 6.028; 95% CI, 1.452–42.593; $p = 0.030$) was also associated with a poor functional outcome at 3 months (Table 3, Model 2 and Figure 2). Baseline renal function showed an association with functional outcome (p value for trend = 0.005); however, it did not show an independent association in the multivariate analysis. The dose of contrast medium used was also associated with a poor functional outcome (odds ratio, 1.080 per 10 mL increase; 95% CI, 1.013–1.155; $p = 0.021$).

During the 3-month follow-up, 86 patients (14.3%) died. Of these, 29 (33.7%) had AKI. Of the 515 survivors, 30 (5.8%) had AKI ($p < 0.001$) (Table S3). In the multivariate analysis, the presence of AKI was significantly associated with mortality (odds ratio, 8.164; 95% CI, 4.046–16.709; $p < 0.001$) (Table 4, Model 1). AKI Stage 2 (odds ratio, 20.845; 95% CI, 5.907–82.054; $p < 0.001$) and Stage 3 (odds ratio, 13.670; 95% CI, 4.740–41.925; $p < 0.001$) were also independently associated with mortality at 3 months (Table 4, Model 2).

Table 1. Patient characteristics according to the presence of acute kidney injury.

	No Acute Kidney Injury (n = 542)	Acute Kidney Injury (n = 59)	p-Value
Age, years	67.9 ± 12.2	68.3 ± 11.8	0.827
Sex, men	307 (56.6)	26 (44.1)	0.088
Risk factors			
Hypertension	336 (62.0)	45 (76.3)	0.043
Diabetes mellitus	139 (25.6)	28 (47.5)	0.001
Atrial fibrillation	267 (49.3)	31 (52.5)	0.733
Dyslipidemia	160 (29.5)	20 (33.9)	0.584
Smoking	118 (21.8)	10 (16.9)	0.489
Previous stroke or history of TIA	96 (17.7)	11 (18.6)	>0.999
Medication prior to admission			
Antiplatelets	145 (26.8)	17 (28.8)	0.854
Anticoagulants	73 (13.5)	6 (10.2)	0.611
Statins	26 (4.8)	8 (13.6)	0.013
Baseline renal function			0.996 *
eGFR ≥90 mL/min/1.73 m^2	84 (15.5)	14 (23.7)	
eGFR 60–89 mL/min/1.73 m^2	194 (35.8)	17 (28.8)	
eGFR 30–59 mL/min/1.73 m^2	233 (43.0)	19 (32.2)	
eGFR <30 mL/min/1.73 m^2	31 (5.7)	9 (15.3)	
CTA before EVT	455 (83.9)	55 (93.2)	0.090
Contrast agent			0.807
Iodixanol	391 (72.1)	44 (74.6)	
Iopamidol	151 (27.9)	15 (25.4)	
Contrast dose, mL	69.1 ± 36.0	89.8 ± 42.9	0.001
Laboratory findings			
Hemoglobin, g/dL	13.5 ± 1.8	12.8 ± 2.1	0.025
White blood cells, ×10^9/L	8.7 ± 3.4	9.8 ± 4.2	0.063
Platelets, ×10^9/L	221 ± 69	226 ± 75	0.645
Glucose, mmol/L	7.7 ± 3.0	8.9 ± 3.8	0.029
Stroke-related factors			
NIHSS score on admission	17 (13–21)	19 (14.5–21.5)	0.022
ASPECTS †	7 (5–9)	5 (3–8)	0.004
Intravenous tPA	279 (51.5)	31 (52.5)	0.985
Onset to puncture time, min	270 (180–445)	251 (189–402)	0.614
Procedure time, min	61.5 (43–90)	65 (40–126)	0.378
Unsuccessful reperfusion (mTICI 2a or less)	126 (23.2)	23 (39.0)	0.012
Outcomes			
Any hemorrhagic transformation	167 (30.8)	33 (55.9)	<0.001
Parenchymal hematoma	70 (13.0)	16 (27.1)	0.006
Parenchymal hematoma, type 2	38 (7.0)	7 (11.9)	0.191
mRS at 3 months	3 (1–4)	5 (4–6)	<0.001
Good functional outcome (mRS 0–2)	264 (48.7)	7 (11.9)	<0.001
Mortality at 3 months	57 (10.5)	29 (49.2)	<0.001

Values are presented as n (%), mean ± standard deviation, or median (interquartile range). TIA, transient ischemic attack; CTA, computed tomography angiography; EVT, endovascular treatment; eGFR, estimated glomerular filtration rate; NIHSS, National Institutes of Health Stroke Scale; ASPECTS, Alberta stroke program early CT score; tPA, tissue plasminogen activator; mTICI, modified Thrombolysis in Cerebral Infarction; mRS, modified Rankin Scale. * p-value for trend. † ASPECTS was properly measured in 492 patients (92.8% of anterior circulation occlusion).

Table 2. Multivariate analysis of factors associated with acute kidney injury.

	Odds Ratio (95% Confidence Interval)	p-Value
Age, years	0.990 (0.961–1.022)	0.541
Sex, men	0.581 (0.316–1.057)	0.077
Hypertension	1.974 (0.978–4.201)	0.066
Diabetes mellitus	2.341 (1.283–4.269)	0.005
Statin medication prior to admission	1.734 (0.654–4.211)	0.242
Baseline renal function		

Table 2. *Cont.*

	Odds Ratio (95% Confidence Interval)	*p*-Value
eGFR ≥90 mL/min/1.73 m^2	Ref	
eGFR 60–89 mL/min/1.73 m^2	0.616 (0.270–1.424)	0.249
eGFR 30–59 mL/min/1.73 m^2	0.521 (0.211–1.309)	0.160
eGFR <30 mL/min/1.73 m^2	1.434 (0.432–4.697)	0.551
CTA before EVT	2.112 (0.786–7.406)	0.181
Contrast dose, per 10 mL increase	1.107 (1.032–1.187)	0.004
NIHSS score on admission	1.041 (0.993–1.092)	0.095
Unsuccessful reperfusion	1.909 (1.019–3.520)	0.040

eGFR, estimated glomerular filtration rate; EVT, endovascular treatment; CTA, computed tomography angiography; NIHSS, National Institutes of Health Stroke Scale.

Table 3. Multivariate analysis of factors associated with a poor functional outcome at 3 months.

	Model 1		Model 2	
	Odds Ratio (95% Confidence Interval)	*p*-Value	Odds Ratio (95% Confidence Interval)	*p*-Value
Age, years	1.047 (1.025–1.071)	<0.001	1.047 (1.025–1.071)	<0.001
Sex, men	0.755 (0.501–1.134)	0.176	0.755 (0.501–1.135)	0.177
Hypertension	1.178 (0.769–1.805)	0.450	1.187 (0.775–1.820)	0.430
Diabetes mellitus	1.465 (0.934–2.309)	0.098	1.460 (0.929–2.303)	0.102
Baseline renal function				
eGFR ≥90 mL/min/1.73 m^2	Ref		Ref	
eGFR 60–89 mL/min/1.73 m^2	1.260 (0.678–2.354)	0.465	1.245 (0.670–2.324)	0.490
eGFR 30–59 mL/min/1.73 m^2	0.914 (0.456–1.824)	0.798	0.894 (0.446–1.784)	0.750
eGFR <30 mL/min/1.73 m^2	1.145 (0.396–3.423)	0.805	1.117 (0.385–3.346)	0.840
Presence of acute kidney injury	5.145 (2.177–13.850)	<0.001		
Stage of acute kidney injury				
No acute kidney injury			Ref	
Stage 1			2.938 (0.888–11.699)	0.094
Stage 2			13.709 (2.108–280.187)	0.022
Stage 3			6.028 (1.452–42.593)	0.030
Contrast dose, per 10 mL increase	1.080 (1.013–1.155)	0.021	1.078 (1.011–1.153)	0.025
White blood cell count	1.076 (1.011–1.148)	0.024	1.076 (1.011–1.149)	0.024
NIHSS score on admission	1.129 (1.089–1.174)	<0.001	1.130 (1.089–1.174)	<0.001
Onset to puncture time, min	1.001 (1.0001–1.002)	0.034	1.001 (1.0001–1.002)	0.029
Procedure time, min	1.012 (1.006–1.018)	<0.001	1.012 (1.006–1.018)	<0.001
Unsuccessful reperfusion	2.686 (1.640–4.468)	<0.001	2.672 (1.630–4.445)	<0.001
Parenchymal hematoma, type 2	4.438 (1.792–12.877)	0.003	4.510 (1.818–13.098)	0.002

Univariate analysis of factors associated with poor functional outcome is described in the Table S2. eGFR, Estimated glomerular filtration rate; NIHSS, National Institutes of Health Stroke Scale.

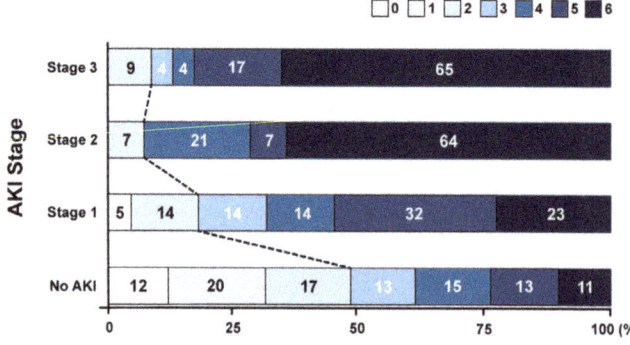

Figure 2. Modified Rankin Scale at 3 months according to acute kidney injury stage. AKI, acute kidney injury.

Table 4. Multivariate analysis of factors associated with mortality at 3 months.

	Model 1		Model 2	
	Odds Ratio (95% Confidence Interval)	*p*-Value	Odds Ratio (95% Confidence Interval)	*p*-Value
Age, years	1.006 (0.978–1.036)	0.675	1.006 (0.978–1.037)	0.667
Sex, men	1.377 (0.785–2.450)	0.269	1.300 (0.733–2.330)	0.372
Diabetes mellitus	1.212 (0.663–2.168)	0.524	1.247 (0.676–2.252)	0.471
Statin medication prior to admission	1.776 (0.624–4.809)	0.267	1.705 (0.580–4.751)	0.317
Baseline renal function				
eGFR ≥90 mL/min/1.73 m^2	Ref		Ref	
eGFR 60–89 mL/min/1.73 m^2	2.515 (0.988–6.916)	0.062	2.438 (0.936–6.868)	0.078
eGFR 30–59 mL/min/1.73 m^2	4.264 (1.598–12.361)	0.005	4.012 (1.465–11.935)	0.009
eGFR <30 mL/min/1.73 m^2	3.949 (1.048–15.280)	0.043	3.609 (0.904–14.548)	0.068
Presence of acute kidney injury	8.164 (4.046–16.709)	<0.001		
Stage of acute kidney injury				
No acute kidney injury			Ref	
Stage 1			2.355 (0.660–7.265)	0.155
Stage 2			20.845 (5.907–82.054)	<0.001
Stage 3			13.670 (4.740–41.925)	<0.001
Contrast dose, per 10 mL increase	1.039 (0.958–1.125)	0.345	1.027 (0.944–1.113)	0.530
White blood cells	0.968 (0.891–1.047)	0.433	0.969 (0.889–1.050)	0.452
Platelets	1.008 (1.004–1.013)	<0.001	1.008 (1.004–1.012)	<0.001
NIHSS score on admission	1.115 (1.063–1.172)	<0.001	1.116 (1.063–1.173)	<0.001
Procedure time, min	1.004 (0.998–1.010)	0.193	1.005 (0.999–1.011)	0.085
Unsuccessful reperfusion	2.383 (1.294–4.377)	0.005	2.475 (1.332–4.586)	0.004
Parenchymal hematoma, type 2	5.176 (2.450–10.836)	<0.001	5.212 (2.422–11.074)	<0.001

Univariate analysis of factors associated with mortality is described in the Table S3. eGFR, estimated glomerular filtration rate; NIHSS, National Institutes of Health Stroke Scale.

4. Discussion

This study assessed the frequency of AKI and the association between AKI and clinical outcomes in ischemic stroke patients who had undergone EVT. Our data showed that about 9.8% of the ischemic stroke patients developed AKI after EVT. However, renal replacement therapy was required for less than 1% of the patients who underwent EVT. The rate does not differ significantly from the 9.6% incidence rate of AKI after stroke in meta-analysis [5]. However, the incidence of AKI in our study is higher than those in CTA studies of ischemic stroke patients [19] or in studies of general ischemic stroke patients [4]. Our study included patients who underwent EVT and who had experienced a relatively severe stroke, which may have influenced the development of higher incidences of AKI. The rate in our study is also higher than in other recently reported studies using EVT patients. This is probably because the patients enrolled in this study are older, with worse ASPECTS and a lower successful reperfusion rate [12]. However, the result is lower than the 20.9% of stroke patients who were admitted to the neurology intensive care unit [6].

In this study, the presence of diabetes mellitus was independently associated with AKI after EVT in ischemic stroke patients. In a previous CTA study of ischemic stroke patients, diabetes mellitus was also associated with contrast-induced nephropathy [20]. Diabetes mellitus was also found to affect the occurrence of AKI in a previous study of patients who underwent percutaneous coronary interventions [21]. However, the precise pathophysiologic mechanisms of CA-AKI remain unclear [2]. Several studies suggested that AKI can be caused by ischemia due to the vasoconstrictive properties of the contrast media or the direct toxic effects of the contrast media on endothelial cells and renal tubules [22]. Patients with diabetes have an increased sensitivity to renal vasoconstrictors and renal ischemia, as well as decreased nitric-oxide-dependent vasodilatation [23,24]. Therefore, patients with diabetic nephropathy are more vulnerable to renal ischemia caused by a contrast medium.

The total amount of contrast medium and the final reperfusion status were also associated with AKI after EVT. Previous studies of patients undergoing coronary interventions have also identified these dose-dependent impairments of renal function [25,26]. In another study of acute myocardial infarction, the use of more than 100 mL of contrast agent increased the risk of AKI [27]. In coronary angiography, contrast medium refluxes into the aorta and renal arteries. However, contrast material administered into the intracranial arterial circulation is intravenous from the perspective of the kidneys.

For this reason, it is somewhat different from coronary angiography. However, as our findings showed the relationship between the contrast dose and AKI, practitioners should keep in mind it is best to avoid the use of excessive amounts of contrast medium during EVT if possible.

Reperfusion status is directly related to the short-term prognosis as well as the long-term outcome in stroke patients with large artery occlusion. Patients with successful reperfusion required the use of fewer EVT techniques and smaller amounts of the contrast medium. In patients with poor reperfusion, the possibility of complications such as brain edema or pneumonia increases [28,29]. Using osmotic diuretics such as mannitol or broad-spectrum antibiotics may increase the risk of AKI [30,31]. It is well known that initial stroke severity is related to the risk of AKI [32,33]. At a given severity of stroke, the risk of AKI was higher in patients without successful reperfusion than in patients with successful reperfusion. This may be related to the fact that, unlike in other studies that did not consider reperfusion, the initial NIHSS score was not significantly associated with AKI risk in our study.

The performance of CTA before EVT was not independently associated with AKI after EVT. In previous CTA or CTP studies, intravenous contrast agents did not increase AKI risk in patients with acute stroke [34–36]. In a study of 12,508 propensity-score-matched patients, intravenous contrast material used for computed tomography did not increase AKI risk [37]. In a reperfusion study examining intravenous tissue plasminogen activator in acute ischemic stroke patients, CTA also did not affect renal function [38]. It is substantially higher following catheter-based procedures with intra-arterial contrast agent administration than it is following imaging procedures with intravenous contrast agent administration [1,39,40]. Although there is a tendency for this to raise the risk of AKI, the implementation of CTA is considered relatively safe in ischemic stroke patients, regardless of whether they undergo EVT.

Our study also showed that the presence of AKI and the severity of AKI were associated with poor functional outcomes and mortality at 3 months. It is well known that AKI affects mortality and functional outcomes in acute ischemic stroke patients [4,5]. CA-AKI also increases mortality, lengthens hospitalization, and increases the cost burden [41]. Therefore, interventions to prevent AKI may improve outcomes after stroke, especially in patients with diabetes mellitus or severe renal impairment [22].

There were several limitations to this study. First, it was a retrospective analysis of a prospectively enrolled registry, which may have led to bias. Second, as with other studies examining CA-AKI that occur after EVT, there is no control; therefore, it is not known whether AKI was caused by other factors. Third, about 14% of patients were excluded due to lack of a follow-up renal function test. These individuals had better baseline renal function prior to the EVT and showed better clinical outcomes. They probably had relatively good renal function in the admission period, which indicates AKI was likely overestimated. Fourth, we could not obtain an accurate amount of the contrast agent that is related to risk of AKI. Further study is needed to overcome these shortcomings and to confirm our results. However, our study is meaningful in that it investigated the factors related to the risk of AKI and the characteristics of patients with AKI after EVT. Moreover, the number of included patients was larger than that in previous studies.

5. Conclusions

In conclusion, the incidence of AKI after EVT was approximately 9.8%. Diabetes mellitus, the total amount of contrast medium, and unsuccessful reperfusion were independently associated with the development of AKI in patients who underwent EVT. AKI may also affect the outcomes of ischemic stroke patients undergoing EVT. When implementing EVT, practitioners should be aware of these risk factors.

Supplementary Materials: The following are available online at http://www.mdpi.com/2077-0383/9/5/1471/s1, Table S1: Characteristics of included and excluded patient, Table S2: Factors associated with functional outcome at 3 months, Table S3: Factors associated with mortality at 3 months.

Author Contributions: Conceptualization: J.Y., S.-I.S.; methodology: J.Y., S.-I.S.; formal analysis: J.Y.; investigation: J.Y., J.-H.H., S.-J.L., Y.-W.K., J.M.H., C.-H.K., J.W.C., D.-H.K., Y.-S.K., Y.-H.H., J.S.L., S.-I.S.; writing–original draft preparation: J.Y., S.-I.S.; writing–review and editing: J.Y., J.-H.H., S.-J.L., Y.-W.K., J.M.H., C.-H.K., J.W.C., D.-H.K., Y.-S.K., Y.-H.H., J.S.L., S.-I.S.; supervision: S.-I.S.; funding acquisition: J.Y., S.-I.S. All authors have read and agreed to the published version of the manuscript.

Funding: This study was supported by a grant from the National Research Foundation of Korea Grant, which is funded by the Korean Government and the Korea Health Technology R&D Project through the Korea Health Industry Development Institute by the Korean Government (NRF-2017R1C1B5076990 and MSIP: No.2014R1A5A2010008), and a faculty research grant of National Health Insurance Service Ilsan Hospital (NHIMC2020CR040).

Conflicts of Interest: The authors declare no conflicts of interest.

References

1. Wichmann, J.L.; Katzberg, R.W.; Litwin, S.E.; Zwerner, P.L.; De Cecco, C.N.; Vogl, T.J.; Costello, P.; Schoepf, U.J. Contrast-Induced Nephropathy. *Circulation* **2015**, *132*, 1931–1936. [CrossRef]
2. Mehran, R.; Dangas, G.D.; Weisbord, S.D. Contrast-Associated Acute Kidney Injury. *N. Engl. J. Med.* **2019**, *380*, 2146–2155. [CrossRef]
3. Gadalean, F.; Simu, M.; Parv, F.; Vorovenci, R.; Tudor, R.; Schiller, A.; Timar, R.; Petrica, L.; Velciov, S.; Gluhovschi, C.; et al. The impact of acute kidney injury on in-hospital mortality in acute ischemic stroke patients undergoing intravenous thrombolysis. *PLoS ONE* **2017**, *12*, e0185589. [CrossRef]
4. Saeed, F.; Adil, M.M.; Khursheed, F.; Daimee, U.A.; Branch, L.A., Jr.; Vidal, G.A.; Qureshi, A.I. Acute renal failure is associated with higher death and disability in patients with acute ischemic stroke: Analysis of nationwide inpatient sample. *Stroke* **2014**, *45*, 1478–1480. [CrossRef]
5. Arnold, J.; Ng, K.P.; Sims, D.; Gill, P.; Cockwell, P.; Ferro, C. Incidence and impact on outcomes of acute kidney injury after a stroke: A systematic review and meta-analysis. *BMC Nephrol.* **2018**, *19*, 283. [CrossRef]
6. Wang, D.; Guo, Y.; Zhang, Y.; Li, Z.; Li, A.; Luo, Y. Epidemiology of acute kidney injury in patients with stroke: A retrospective analysis from the neurology ICU. *Intern Emerg. Med.* **2018**, *13*, 17–25. [CrossRef]
7. Goyal, M.; Menon, B.K.; van Zwam, W.H.; Dippel, D.W.; Mitchell, P.J.; Demchuk, A.M.; Davalos, A.; Majoie, C.B.; van der Lugt, A.; de Miquel, M.A.; et al. Endovascular thrombectomy after large-vessel ischaemic stroke: A meta-analysis of individual patient data from five randomised trials. *Lancet* **2016**, *387*, 1723–1731. [CrossRef]
8. Powers, W.J.; Rabinstein, A.A.; Ackerson, T.; Adeoye, O.M.; Bambakidis, N.C.; Becker, K.; Biller, J.; Brown, M.; Demaerschalk, B.M.; Hoh, B.; et al. Guidelines for the Early Management of Patients With Acute Ischemic Stroke: 2019 Update to the 2018 Guidelines for the Early Management of Acute Ischemic Stroke: A Guideline for Healthcare Professionals from the American Heart Association/American Stroke Association. *Stroke* **2019**, *50*, e344–e418. [CrossRef]
9. Kim, Y.D.; Heo, J.H.; Yoo, J.; Park, H.; Kim, B.M.; Bang, O.Y.; Kim, H.C.; Han, E.; Kim, D.J.; Heo, J.; et al. Improving the Clinical Outcome in Stroke Patients Receiving Thrombolytic or Endovascular Treatment in Korea: From the SECRET Study. *J. Clin. Med.* **2020**, *9*, 717. [CrossRef]
10. Loh, Y.; McArthur, D.L.; Vespa, P.; Shi, Z.S.; Liebeskind, D.S.; Jahan, R.; Gonzalez, N.R.; Starkman, S.; Saver, J.L.; Tateshima, S.; et al. The risk of acute radiocontrast-mediated kidney injury following endovascular therapy for acute ischemic stroke is low. *AJNR Am. J. Neuroradiol.* **2010**, *31*, 1584–1587. [CrossRef]
11. Sharma, J.; Nanda, A.; Jung, R.S.; Mehta, S.; Pooria, J.; Hsu, D.P. Risk of contrast-induced nephropathy in patients undergoing endovascular treatment of acute ischemic stroke. *J. Neurointerv. Surg.* **2013**, *5*, 543–545. [CrossRef]
12. Diprose, W.K.; Sutherland, L.J.; Wang, M.T.M.; Barber, P.A. Contrast-Associated Acute Kidney Injury in Endovascular Thrombectomy Patients With and Without Baseline Renal Impairment. *Stroke* **2019**, *50*, 3527–3531. [CrossRef]
13. Lee, J.S.; Lee, S.J.; Yoo, J.S.; Hong, J.H.; Kim, C.H.; Kim, Y.W.; Kang, D.H.; Kim, Y.S.; Hong, J.M.; Choi, J.W.; et al. Prognosis of Acute Intracranial Atherosclerosis-Related Occlusion after Endovascular Treatment. *J. Stroke* **2018**, *20*, 394–403. [CrossRef]

14. Lee, S.J.; Hong, J.M.; Choi, J.W.; Park, J.H.; Park, B.; Kang, D.H.; Kim, Y.W.; Kim, Y.S.; Hong, J.H.; Yoo, J.; et al. Predicting Endovascular Treatment Outcomes in Acute Vertebrobasilar Artery Occlusion: A Model to Aid Patient Selection from the ASIAN KR Registry. *Radiology* **2020**, *294*, 628–637. [CrossRef]
15. Kidney Disease: Improving Global Outcomes (KDIGO) Acute Kidney Injury Work Group. KDIGO clinical practice guideline for acute kidney injury. *Kidney Int. Suppl.* **2012**, *2*, 19–36. [CrossRef]
16. Thomas, M.E.; Blaine, C.; Dawnay, A.; Devonald, M.A.; Ftouh, S.; Laing, C.; Latchem, S.; Lewington, A.; Milford, D.V.; Ostermann, M. The definition of acute kidney injury and its use in practice. *Kidney Int.* **2015**, *87*, 62–73. [CrossRef]
17. Tomsick, T.; Broderick, J.; Carrozzella, J.; Khatri, P.; Hill, M.; Palesch, Y.; Khoury, J. Revascularization results in the Interventional Management of Stroke II trial. *AJNR Am. J. Neuroradiol.* **2008**, *29*, 582–587. [CrossRef]
18. Fiorelli, M.; Bastianello, S.; von Kummer, R.; del Zoppo, G.J.; Larrue, V.; Lesaffre, E.; Ringleb, A.P.; Lorenzano, S.; Manelfe, C.; Bozzao, L. Hemorrhagic transformation within 36 hours of a cerebral infarct: Relationships with early clinical deterioration and 3-month outcome in the European Cooperative Acute Stroke Study I (ECASS I) cohort. *Stroke* **1999**, *30*, 2280–2284. [CrossRef]
19. Ehrlich, M.E.; Turner, H.L.; Currie, L.J.; Wintermark, M.; Worrall, B.B.; Southerland, A.M. Safety of Computed Tomographic Angiography in the Evaluation of Patients With Acute Stroke: A Single-Center Experience. *Stroke* **2016**, *47*, 2045–2050. [CrossRef]
20. Rowe, A.S.; Hawkins, B.; Hamilton, L.A.; Ferrell, A.; Henry, J.; Wiseman, B.F.; Skovran, S.A.; Mosadegh, M.S.; Hare, M.E.; Kocak, M.; et al. Contrast-Induced Nephropathy in Ischemic Stroke Patients Undergoing Computed Tomography Angiography: CINISter Study. *J. Stroke Cerebrovasc. Dis.* **2019**, *28*, 649–654. [CrossRef]
21. Fan, P.C.; Chen, T.H.; Lee, C.C.; Tsai, T.Y.; Chen, Y.C.; Chang, C.H. ADVANCIS Score Predicts Acute Kidney Injury After Percutaneous Coronary Intervention for Acute Coronary Syndrome. *Int. J. Med. Sci.* **2018**, *15*, 528–535. [CrossRef]
22. Calvin, A.D.; Misra, S.; Pflueger, A. Contrast-induced acute kidney injury and diabetic nephropathy. *Nat. Rev. Nephrol.* **2010**, *6*, 679–688. [CrossRef]
23. Frauchiger, B.; Nussbaumer, P.; Hugentobler, M.; Staub, D. Duplex sonographic registration of age and diabetes-related loss of renal vasodilatory response to nitroglycerine. *Nephrol. Dial. Transplant.* **2000**, *15*, 827–832. [CrossRef]
24. Epstein, F.H.; Veves, A.; Prasad, P.V. Effect of diabetes on renal medullary oxygenation during water diuresis. *Diabetes Care* **2002**, *25*, 575–578. [CrossRef]
25. Laskey, W.K.; Jenkins, C.; Selzer, F.; Marroquin, O.C.; Wilensky, R.L.; Glaser, R.; Cohen, H.A.; Holmes, D.R., Jr. Volume-to-creatinine clearance ratio: A pharmacokinetically based risk factor for prediction of early creatinine increase after percutaneous coronary intervention. *J. Am. Coll. Cardiol.* **2007**, *50*, 584–590. [CrossRef]
26. Marenzi, G.; Assanelli, E.; Campodonico, J.; Lauri, G.; Marana, I.; De Metrio, M.; Moltrasio, M.; Grazi, M.; Rubino, M.; Veglia, F.; et al. Contrast volume during primary percutaneous coronary intervention and subsequent contrast-induced nephropathy and mortality. *Ann. Intern. Med.* **2009**, *150*, 170–177. [CrossRef]
27. McCullough, P.A.; Wolyn, R.; Rocher, L.L.; Levin, R.N.; O'Neill, W.W. Acute renal failure after coronary intervention: Incidence, risk factors, and relationship to mortality. *Am. J. Med.* **1997**, *103*, 368–375. [CrossRef]
28. Finlayson, O.; Kapral, M.; Hall, R.; Asllani, E.; Selchen, D.; Saposnik, G. Risk factors, inpatient care, and outcomes of pneumonia after ischemic stroke. *Neurology* **2011**, *77*, 1338–1345. [CrossRef]
29. Hassan, A.E.; Chaudhry, S.A.; Zacharatos, H.; Khatri, R.; Akbar, U.; Suri, M.F.; Qureshi, A.I. Increased rate of aspiration pneumonia and poor discharge outcome among acute ischemic stroke patients following intubation for endovascular treatment. *Neurocrit. Care* **2012**, *16*, 246–250. [CrossRef]
30. Jensen, J.U.; Hein, L.; Lundgren, B.; Bestle, M.H.; Mohr, T.; Andersen, M.H.; Thornberg, K.J.; Loken, J.; Steensen, M.; Fox, Z.; et al. Kidney failure related to broad-spectrum antibiotics in critically ill patients: Secondary end point results from a 1200 patient randomised trial. *BMJ Open* **2012**, *2*, e000635. [CrossRef]
31. Lin, S.Y.; Tang, S.C.; Tsai, L.K.; Yeh, S.J.; Shen, L.J.; Wu, F.L.; Jeng, J.S. Incidence and Risk Factors for Acute Kidney Injury Following Mannitol Infusion in Patients With Acute Stroke: A Retrospective Cohort Study. *Medicine (Baltimore)* **2015**, *94*, e2032. [CrossRef]
32. Tsagalis, G.; Akrivos, T.; Alevizaki, M.; Manios, E.; Theodorakis, M.; Laggouranis, A.; Vemmos, K.N. Long-term prognosis of acute kidney injury after first acute stroke. *Clin. J. Am. Soc. Nephrol.* **2009**, *4*, 616–622. [CrossRef]

33. Khatri, M.; Himmelfarb, J.; Adams, D.; Becker, K.; Longstreth, W.T.; Tirschwell, D.L. Acute kidney injury is associated with increased hospital mortality after stroke. *J. Stroke Cerebrovasc. Dis.* **2014**, *23*, 25–30. [CrossRef]
34. Krol, A.L.; Dzialowski, I.; Roy, J.; Puetz, V.; Subramaniam, S.; Coutts, S.B.; Demchuk, A.M. Incidence of radiocontrast nephropathy in patients undergoing acute stroke computed tomography angiography. *Stroke* **2007**, *38*, 2364–2366. [CrossRef]
35. Brinjikji, W.; Demchuk, A.M.; Murad, M.H.; Rabinstein, A.A.; McDonald, R.J.; McDonald, J.S.; Kallmes, D.F. Neurons Over Nephrons: Systematic Review and Meta-Analysis of Contrast-Induced Nephropathy in Patients with Acute Stroke. *Stroke* **2017**, *48*, 1862–1868. [CrossRef]
36. Demel, S.L.; Grossman, A.W.; Khoury, J.C.; Moomaw, C.J.; Alwell, K.; Kissela, B.M.; Woo, D.; Flaherty, M.L.; Ferioli, S.; Mackey, J.; et al. Association Between Acute Kidney Disease and Intravenous Dye Administration in Patients with Acute Stroke: A Population-Based Study. *Stroke* **2017**, *48*, 835–839. [CrossRef]
37. McDonald, J.S.; McDonald, R.J.; Carter, R.E.; Katzberg, R.W.; Kallmes, D.F.; Williamson, E.E. Risk of intravenous contrast material-mediated acute kidney injury: A propensity score-matched study stratified by baseline-estimated glomerular filtration rate. *Radiology* **2014**, *271*, 65–73. [CrossRef]
38. Aulicky, P.; Mikulik, R.; Goldemund, D.; Reif, M.; Dufek, M.; Kubelka, T. Safety of performing CT angiography in stroke patients treated with intravenous thrombolysis. *J. Neurol. Neurosurg. Psychiatry* **2010**, *81*, 783–787. [CrossRef]
39. Karlsberg, R.P.; Dohad, S.Y.; Sheng, R. Contrast medium-induced acute kidney injury: Comparison of intravenous and intraarterial administration of iodinated contrast medium. *J. Vasc. Interv. Radiol.* **2011**, *22*, 1159–1165. [CrossRef]
40. Dong, M.; Jiao, Z.; Liu, T.; Guo, F.; Li, G. Effect of administration route on the renal safety of contrast agents: A meta-analysis of randomized controlled trials. *J. Nephrol.* **2012**, *25*, 290–301. [CrossRef]
41. Aubry, P.; Brillet, G.; Catella, L.; Schmidt, A.; Benard, S. Outcomes, risk factors and health burden of contrast-induced acute kidney injury: An observational study of one million hospitalizations with image-guided cardiovascular procedures. *BMC Nephrol.* **2016**, *17*, 167. [CrossRef] [PubMed]

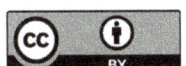

© 2020 by the authors. Licensee MDPI, Basel, Switzerland. This article is an open access article distributed under the terms and conditions of the Creative Commons Attribution (CC BY) license (http://creativecommons.org/licenses/by/4.0/).

MDPI
St. Alban-Anlage 66
4052 Basel
Switzerland
Tel. +41 61 683 77 34
Fax +41 61 302 89 18
www.mdpi.com

Journal of Clinical Medicine Editorial Office
E-mail: jcm@mdpi.com
www.mdpi.com/journal/jcm

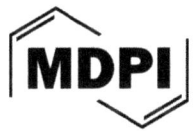